Health Care Management

Donald J. Lombardi and John R. Schermerhorn, Jr.
with *Brian Kramer*

Ohio University

Credits

Publisher
Anne Smith

Associate Editor
Beth Tripmacher

Marketing Manager
Jennifer Slomack

Senior Editorial Assistant
Tiara Kelly

Production Manager
Kelly Tavares

Production Assistant
Courtney Leshko

Creative Director
Harry Nolan

Cover Designer
Hope Miller

This book was set in Times New Roman, printed and bound by R. R. Donnelley.

The cover was printed by Phoenix Color.

To order books or for customer service please, call 1-800-CALL WILEY (225-5945).

ISBN-13 978-0-471-79078-8

ISBN-10 0-471-79078-8

Printed in the United States of America

10 9 8 7 6 5 4 3 2 1

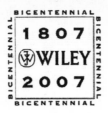

THE WILEY BICENTENNIAL—KNOWLEDGE FOR GENERATIONS

*E*ach generation has its unique needs and aspirations. When Charles Wiley first opened his small printing shop in lower Manhattan in 1807, it was a generation of boundless potential searching for an identity. And we were there, helping to define a new American literary tradition. Over half a century later, in the midst of the Second Industrial Revolution, it was a generation focused on building the future. Once again, we were there, supplying the critical scientific, technical, and engineering knowledge that helped frame the world. Throughout the 20th Century, and into the new millennium, nations began to reach out beyond their own borders and a new international community was born. Wiley was there, expanding its operations around the world to enable a global exchange of ideas, opinions, and know-how.

For 200 years, Wiley has been an integral part of each generation's journey, enabling the flow of information and understanding necessary to meet their needs and fulfill their aspirations. Today, bold new technologies are changing the way we live and learn. Wiley will be there, providing you the must-have knowledge you need to imagine new worlds, new possibilities, and new opportunities.

Generations come and go, but you can always count on Wiley to provide you the knowledge you need, when and where you need it!

William J. Pesce

PRESIDENT AND CHIEF EXECUTIVE OFFICER

Peter Booth Wiley

CHAIRMAN OF THE BOARD

PREFACE

College classrooms bring together learners from many backgrounds with a variety of aspirations. Although the students are in the same course, they are not necessarily on the same path. This diversity, coupled with the reality that these learners often have jobs, families, and other commitments, requires a flexibility that our nation's higher education system is addressing. Distance learning, shorter course terms, new disciplines, evening courses, and certification programs are some of the approaches that colleges employ to reach as many students as possible and help them clarify and achieve their goals.

Wiley Pathways books, a new line of texts from John Wiley & Sons, Inc., are designed to help you address this diversity and the need for flexibility. These books focus on the fundamentals, identify core competencies and skills, and promote independent learning. The focus on the fundamentals helps students grasp the subject, bringing them all to the same basic understanding. These books use clear, everyday language, presented in an uncluttered format, making the reading experience more pleasurable. The core competencies and skills help students succeed in the classroom and beyond, whether in another course or in a professional setting. A variety of built-in learning resources promote independent learning and help instructors and students gauge students' understanding of the content. These resources enable students to think critically about their new knowledge, and apply their skills in any situation.

Our goal with *Wiley Pathways* books—with its brief, inviting format, clear language, and core competencies and skills focus—is to celebrate the many students in your courses, respect their needs, and help you guide them on their way.

CASE Learning System

To meet the needs of working college students, *Health Care Management* uses a four-step process: The CASE Learning System. Based on Bloom's Taxonomy of Learning, CASE presents key healthcare management topics in easy-to-follow chapters. The text then prompts analysis, synthesis, and evaluation with a variety of learning aids and assessment tools. Students move efficiently from reviewing what they have learned, to acquiring new information and skills, to applying their new knowledge and skills to real-life scenarios:

▲ Content
▲ Analysis
▲ Synthesis
▲ Evaluation

Using the CASE Learning System, students not only achieve academic mastery of healthcare management *topics*, but they master real-world healthcare management *skills*. The CASE Learning System also helps students become independent learners, giving them a distinct advantage whether they are starting out or seek to advance in their careers.

Organization, Depth and Breadth of the Text

▲ **Modular format.** Research on college students shows that they access information from textbooks in a non-linear way. Instructors also often wish to reorder textbook content to suit the needs of a particular class. Therefore, although *Health Care Management* proceeds logically from the basics to increasingly more challenging material, chapters are further organized into sections that are self-contained for maximum teaching and learning flexibility.

▲ **Numeric system of headings.** *Health Care Management* uses a numeric system for headings (for example, 2.3.4 identifies the fourth sub-section of section 3 of chapter 2). With this system, students and teachers can quickly and easily pinpoint topics in the table of contents and the text, keeping class time and study sessions focused.

▲ **Core content.** Topics in the text are organized into twelve chapters and four parts

Part I: Stepping Into Management

Chapter 1, Meeting the Challenge, is designed to help students understand the healthcare supervisor's job, roles, functions, and authority. Among the topics presented are descriptions of today's healthcare work environment; what patients, staff, and managers expect of a healthcare manager; the typical levels of management, and the functions, skills, and responsibilities associated with each; and the difference between professional and managerial work. Industry trends and changes, communication channels, and the most commonly used tools and techniques of healthcare managers are also described.

Chapter 2, Doing the Right Thing, outlines social responsibilities and what constitutes ethical behavior in today's healthcare workplace. Common types of ethical dilemmas and ways to respond to them are discussed, as are common rationalizations for unethical behavior. Influences on a person's ethics, ways to encourage high ethical standards, and socially responsible responses to difficult situations are presented. A seven-step process for ethical decision making rounds out the chapter.

Part II: Organizing

Chapter 3, Organizing the Workplace, explores the fundamentals of organizational structures by reviewing traditional patterns of organizing healthcare services, as well as the trend toward increasing productivity with newer functions, divisions, and matrix structures. Organizational tools such as committees, teams, and task forces, are also described.

Chapter 4, Managing Teams, aims to help students lead and develop work teams that are efficient, focused, and flexible. The chapter opens with the basics: the characteristics of strong teams, principles of team orientation, phases of team development, and key ways that teams develop. It goes on to describe methods that team leaders can use to enhance individual members and overall team orientation. The pros and cons of team decision making are also highlighted.

Chapter 5, Managing Resources, addresses how to get the most from today's workforce by examining the legal and labor issues that impact human resource management. Employee recruitment, hiring, orientation, and training tools are outlined, followed by descriptions of performance appraisals for individuals and teams. Methods of keeping, developing, and terminating employees are also presented, along with techniques for dealing with office politics and interdepartmental conflict.

Part III: Planning and Controlling

Chapter 6, Managerial and Supervisory Planning, prepares students for the road ahead by explaining the benefits of planning, the common types of plans, and the five steps of the planning process. Students then learn the relative merits of widely used planning tools and techniques, including the SWOT analysis; the critical factors that distinguish them; and how organizations can benefit from using them. How to adapt plans to account for uncertainty and change, and how to evaluate their effectiveness round out the discussion.

Chapter 7, Keeping Things in Check, outlines the four steps of the control process, identifies the characteristics of effective controls, and explains how controls are used to assess performance, improve processes, and boost quality. The three main types of controls are described, along with specific control techniques for discipline, information, and finances. Operational control strategies, including schedules, budgets, inventory, and quality, are also reviewed. Ways to successfully manage by objectives and the traits of internal control and self-management conclude the chapter.

Chapter 8, Making Major Choices, explains the two responsibilities of strategic management, describes the levels of organizational strategy, and highlights essential values for making decisions. The Portfolio Planning Approach to decision making, along with tools for preparing to make decisions, strategies for analyzing situations, and models for implementing decisions are presented. Ways to communicate strategic decisions and measure their effectiveness are also addressed.

Part IV: Leading and Influencing

Chapter 9, Leading Others, underscores the relationship between vision and leadership, and how to call people to action. The characteristics of strong leadership are described, along with the relative effectiveness of various leadership models, types, and styles. Three types of position power and two types of personal power are reviewed, along with a variety of ways to empower others while continuing to develop as a leader. The role of gender, morals, and ethics in leadership rounds out the chapter.

Chapter 10, Motivating Others, encourages students to strive for great results and outstanding contributions. The chapter opens by explaining the relationship between needs and motivation, and presents three theories of needs-based motivation, including Maslow's Hierarchy. Discussions of process-based motivation, strategies for successful goal setting, and ways to reinforce behaviors follow. The chapter concludes with a discussion of non-traditional work arrangements.

Chapter 11, Change Leadership in the Workplace, offers advice on guiding others through challenging times. The reasons for change in the workplace and the characteristics of positive change leadership are reviewed. Common change goals are examined, followed by an explanation of the phases of planned change. The chapter then presents commonly used change strategies and explores reasons why people and groups resist change, culminating in a discussion of stress management techniques.

Chapter 12, Communicating, presents strategies for developing out-standing interpersonal skills. Key elements of the communication process, typical sources of messaging, and common communication barriers are explained, along with perceptions that affect communication, and strate-gies for improving communication. Conflict management techniques, and steps and pitfalls in the negotiation process conclude the text.

Pre-Reading Learning Aids

Each chapter of *Health Care Management* features the following learn-ing and study aids to activate students' prior knowledge of the topics and orient them to the material.

▲ **Pre-test.** This pre-reading assessment tool in multiple-choice format not only introduces chapter material, but it also helps students anticipate the chapter's learning outcomes. By focus-ing students' attention on what they do not know, the self-test provides students with a benchmark against which they can measure their own progress. The pre-test is available online at www.wiley.com/college/Lombardi.

▲ **What You'll Learn in This Chapter and After Studying This Chapter.** These bulleted lists tell students what they will be learning in the chapter and why it is significant for their careers. They also explain why the chapter is important and how it relates to other chapters in the text. "What You'll Learn..." lists focus on the *subject matter* that will be taught (e.g. what "man-agement by objectives" is). Each bullet in the list corresponds to a chapter section. "After Studying This Chapter..." lists emphasize *capabilities and skills* students will learn (e.g. how to apply management by objectives techniques).

▲ **Goals and Outcomes.** These lists identify specific student capabilities that will result from reading the chapter. They set students up to synthesize and evaluate the chapter material, and relate it to the real world.

Within-Text Learning Aids

The following learning aids are designed to encourage analysis and synthesis of the material, and to support the learning process and ensure success during the evaluation phase:

▲ **Introduction.** This section orients the student by introducing the chapter and explaining its practical value and relevance to

the book as a whole. Short summaries of chapter sections preview the topics to follow.

▲ **"For Example" boxes.** Found within each section, these
boxes tie section content to real-world organizations, scenarios,
and applications.

▲ **Figures and tables.** Line art and photos have been carefully
chosen to be truly instructional rather than filler. Tables distill
and present information in a way that is easy to identify,
access, and understand, enhancing the focus of the text on
essential ideas.

▲ **Self-Check.** Related to the "What You'll Learn" bullets and
found at the end of each section, this battery of short answer
questions emphasizes student understanding of concepts and
mastery of section content. Though the questions may either
be discussed in class or studied by students outside of class,
students should not go on before they can answer all questions correctly. Each *Self-Check* question set includes a link to
a section of the pre-test for further review and practice.

▲ **Key Terms and Glossary.** To help students develop a professional vocabulary, key terms are bolded in the introduction,
summary and when they first appear in the chapter. A complete list of key terms with brief definitions appears at the end
of each chapter and again in a glossary at the end of the book.
Knowledge of key terms is assessed by all assessment tools
(see below).

▲ **Summary.** Each chapter concludes with a summary paragraph
that reviews the major concepts in the chapter and links back
to the "What you'll learn" list.

Evaluation and Assessment Tools

The evaluation phase of the CASE Learning System consists of a
variety of within-chapter and end-of-chapter assessment tools that test
how well students have learned the material. These tools also encourage students to extend their learning into different scenarios and
higher levels of understanding and thinking. The following assessment
tools appear in every chapter of *Health Care Management:*

▲ **Summary Questions** help students summarize the chapter's
main points by asking a series of multiple choice and
true/false questions that emphasize student understanding of

concepts and mastery of chapter content. Students should be able to answer all of the *Summary Questions* correctly before moving on.

▲ **Review Questions** in short answer format review the major points in each chapter, prompting analysis while reinforcing and confirming student understanding of concepts, and encouraging mastery of chapter content. They are somewhat more difficult than the *Self-Check* and *Summary Questions,* and students should be able to answer most of them correctly before moving on.

▲ **Applying this Chapter** Questions drive home key ideas by asking students to synthesize and apply chapter concepts to new, real-life situations and scenarios.

▲ **You Try It Questions** are designed to extend students' thinking, and so are ideal for discussion or writing assignments. Using an open-ended format and sometimes based on Web sources, they encourage students to draw conclusions using chapter material applied to real-world situations, which fosters both mastery and independent learning.

▲ **Assess Your Understanding Post-test** should be taken after students have completed the chapter. It includes all of the questions in the pre-test, so that students can see how their learning has progressed and improved.

Instructor and Student Package

Health Care Management is available with the following teaching and learning supplements. All supplements are available online at the text's Book Companion Website, located at *www.wiley.com/college/Lombardi.*

▲ **Instructor's Resource Guide.** Provides the following aids and supplements for teaching an Introduction to Healthcare management course:

• *Diagnostic Evaluation of Grammar, Mechanics, and Spelling.* A useful tool that instructors may administer to the class at the beginning of the course to determine each student's basic writing skills. The Evaluation is accompanied by an Answer Key and a Marking Key. Instructors are encouraged to use the Marking key when grading students' Evaluations, and to duplicate and distribute it to students with their graded evaluations.

- *Sample syllabus.* A convenient template that instructors may use for creating their own course syllabi.
- *Teaching suggestions.* For each chapter, these include a chapter summary, learning objectives, definitions of key terms, lecture notes, answers to select text question sets, and at least 3 suggestions for classroom activities, such as ideas for speakers to invite, videos to show, and other projects.

▲ **PowerPoints.** Key information is summarized in 10 to 15 PowerPoints per chapter. Instructors may use these in class or choose to share them with students for class presentations or to provide additional study support.

▲ **Test Bank.** One test per chapter. Each includes true/false, multiple choice, and open-ended questions. Answers and page references are provided for the true/false and multiple choice questions, and page references for the open-ended questions. Available in Microsoft Word and computerized formats.

ACKNOWLEDGMENTS

Taken together, the content, pedagogy, and assessment elements of *Health Care Management* offer the career-oriented student the most important aspects of the healthcare management field as well as ways to develop the skills and capabilities that current and future employers seek in the individuals they hire and promote. Instructors will appreciate its practical focus, conciseness, and real-world emphasis. We would like to thank the following reviewers for their feedback and suggestions during the text's development. Their advice on how to shape *Health Care Management* into a solid learning tool that meets both their needs and those of their busy students is deeply appreciated.

Peter Cruise, *California State University—Chico*
Sara Grostick, *University of Alabama—Birmingham*
Deryl Gulliford, *DeVry University*
Russell Porter, *Clayton State University*

BRIEF CONTENTS

CONTENTS

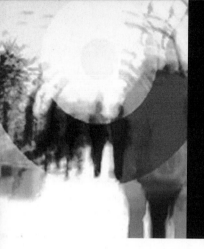

1

MEETING THE CHALLENGE
The Supervisor's Job, Roles, Functions, and Authority in Today's Health Care Workplace

Starting Point

Go to www.wiley.com/college/Lombardi to assess your knowledge of the basic job of a health care supervisor.
Determine where you need to concentrate your effort.

What You'll Learn in This Chapter

▲ The characteristics and components of today's health care work environment
▲ Patient expectations
▲ Expectations for today's health care manager
▲ Typical levels of management
▲ Four management functions
▲ Contrasts between professional and managerial work

After Studying This Chapter, You'll Be Able To

▲ Distinguish common characteristics of patients
▲ Discuss the three top expectations for health care managers
▲ Distinguish levels of management and respective responsibilities
▲ Compare the four core management functions
▲ Differentiate between professional and managerial experiences

Goals and Outcomes

▲ Master terminology related to today's health care workplace, patients, and management roles
▲ Recognize common tools and techniques of health care managers at various levels
▲ Describe trends and changes in health care management
▲ Discuss duties and expectations for health care managers
▲ Compare managerial tasks, skills, roles, and responsibilities
▲ Connect with others within and outside a health care organization
▲ Evaluate management concerns and responses

INTRODUCTION

In the new health care workplace, everyone must respond and adapt to rapid changes in society and science, as well as to the shifting needs of today's health care patient. Managers must be accountable for productivity while encouraging a high-quality, diverse work environment. Managers exist at a variety of levels in a health care organization, and each level of management has specific roles, expectations, and duties. The experience of a manager stands in contrast to the daily work of nonmanagerial professionals.

1.1 Exploring Today's Health Care Workplace

We live and work in a challenging environment, filled with both dramatic uncertainty and great opportunity. As the manager in a health care organization, your personal and organizational responsibilities require that you work in and create an environment that promotes participation, empowerment, involvement, teamwork, flexibility, self-management, and more. Along with these ideals, there are continuing calls for higher performance, greater efficiency, and lower costs. Health care organizations and the patients they serve demand nothing less than the best from every employee—and managers are no exception!

An **organization,** from a large corporation to a governmental agency to the local convenience store, is a collection of people working together to achieve a common purpose. In so doing, members of the organization are able to accomplish tasks that are far beyond the reach of anyone acting alone. In health care, organizations can take a variety of forms—small nonprofit clinics, networks of health care specialists, large for-profit research hospitals, and privately run physicians' offices, to name but a few options. When describing health care organizations, experts often speak of where the organization falls along the **continuum of care,** the complete spectrum of available health care services today.

The **purpose** of an organization is to produce goods and/or services that satisfy the needs of customers. While many of today's health care organizations focus primarily on producing services (immunizing infants, testing for diseases, treating illnesses, or providing long-term nursing care, to suggest just a few examples), all organizations exist because they contribute something useful to society.

Technologies, experts, and resources are all important components of organizations, but people are at the center of any organization. People—what they know, what they learn, and what they do with it—are the ultimate foundations of organizational performance. People are so valuable that nowadays most economists and top executives refer to an organization's employees as its **intellectual capital** of talents, knowledge, and experience. Intellectual capital is indispensable in creating long-term success.[1]

To further understand today's workplace, you can also divide the workplace into general and specific environments.

FOR EXAMPLE

U.S. Department of Health and Human Services

To get a nationwide view of the health care industry—including the most recent reports on the economic, social, legal, and technological issues surrounding health care organizations and workers today—spend some time getting to know the U.S. Department of Health and Human Services (HHS; www.hhs.gov). HHS is the principal agency for protecting the health of all Americans, managing more than 300 agencies, 67,000 employees, and a multibillion-dollar annual budget (almost a quarter of all federal spending, in fact). The agency's Web site is packed with industry-wide reports, as well as useful links to virtually every governmental agency.

1.1.1 The General Environment

Health care services are provided in a broad range of physical environments today, including hospitals, nursing care facilities, clinics, mobile medical vehicles, and within patients' own homes. However, this book focuses on the **general environment** of health care organizations, which includes all the background and external conditions for the organization. This part of the environment provides a situational context for managerial decision making.

Major external environmental issues include

- ▲ **economic conditions,** including inflation, income levels, gross national productivity, unemployment, and other related indicators of economic health;
- ▲ **social-cultural conditions,** including the prevailing social values on human rights, the natural environment, education, marriage, and family;
- ▲ **legal-political conditions,** including the philosophies and objectives of political parties running the government, as well as laws and government regulations;
- ▲ **technological conditions,** including the development and availability of the latest computers, software, research tools, drugs, medical procedures, and health care devices;
- ▲ **natural environment conditions,** including conditions of the natural or physical environment, which includes levels of public concern expressed through environmentalism.

1.1.2 The Specific Environment

The **specific environment** consists of the actual organizations, groups, and persons with whom an organization must interact in order to survive and prosper.

Figure 1-1

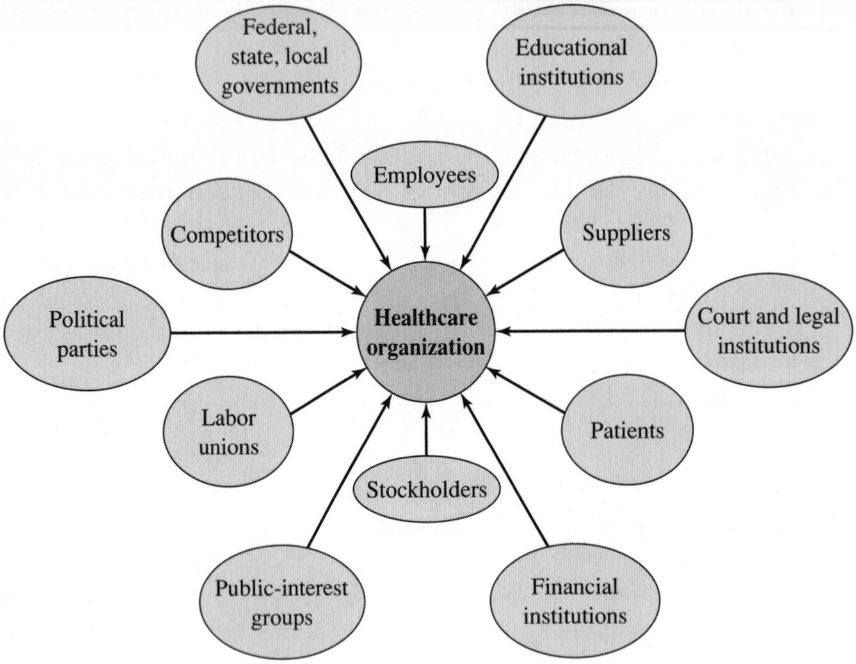

The many stakeholders in today's health care organizations.

These are environmental elements of direct consequence to the organization as it operates on a day-to-day basis.

The specific environment is often described in terms of **stakeholders**—the people, groups, and institutions who are affected in one way or another by the organization's performance. Figure 1-1 shows multiple stakeholders as they may exist in the external environment of a typical business firm.

Sometimes the specific environment and the stakeholders are distinct for each organization. They can also change over time according to the company's unique customer base, operating needs, and circumstances. Important stakeholders common to the specific environment of organizations include

▲ **patients,** who are the groups, individuals, and organizations that purchase the organization's goods and/or use its services. Section 1.2 covers the particularities of today's patients;

▲ **suppliers,** who are specific providers of the human, information, and financial resources and raw materials needed by the organization to operate;

▲ **competitors,** who are specific organizations that offer the same or similar goods and services to the same consumer-patients;

▲ **regulators,** which include specific government agencies and representatives, at the local, state, and national levels, that enforce laws and regulations affecting the organization's operations.

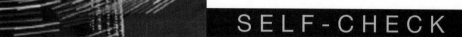

SELF-CHECK

- Identify and define **organization, purpose, environment, and stakeholders.**
- List five conditions that make up the general environment of an organization.
- Describe major stakeholders for a health care organization.

1.2 Getting to Know Today's Patient

Patient is the term used most consistently in the book to refer to the individuals who utilize the goods and services produced by health care organizations. Three critical dynamics figure prominently when considering today's patient: public scrutiny, customer expectation, and customer demand.

1.2.1 Public Scrutiny

Public scrutiny of health care organizations and institutions is at an all-time high because

- ▲ individual patients are paying a larger portion of their health care costs due to higher insurance deductibles and rising costs;
- ▲ the media, insurance companies, and government regulators are focusing more attention on cost-versus-quality issues.

Health care patients are increasingly aware of the quality of services they receive as well as certain quantity indicators, such as time and expense. Consumers pay closer attention to their local health care providers and the services they provide.

In your role as health care manager, you must be acutely aware of this scrutiny and how your organization is perceived by its paying public.

1.2.2 Customer Expectation

In the media, modern health care is often referred to as a *public trust,* and access to appropriate health care is an inalienable American right. These assertions, combined with the reality that most Americans do pay for their health care, demand that expectation and effort be at the forefront of the health care manager's thinking at all times.

Patients expect more, and when they are in the care of a health care organization, they are unquestionably the highest priority. The amount and quality of effort demonstrated by a manager and his or her staff, as perceived by the patient, is the most critical indicator of whether you are upholding your organization's charter as a public trust. This dynamic applies to any health care department or organization, in any institution, regardless of financial structure.

Health care managers recognize the importance of always maintaining a service-oriented image and realize that the patient drives the organization, not vice versa. Managers must set an example of strong commitment to each patient and establish this commitment as a criterion of service for all staff members.

1.2.3 Customer Demands

Today's health care patient also demands a broader range of newer technologies and services. As a result, health care managers must constantly determine how their departments can satisfy these new consumer expectations.

To meet patient needs and fulfill expectations and demand, health care providers are diversifying their delivery systems to include numerous nonmedical goods and services. In the 1970s, for example, it would have been unique for a community hospital to have a drug-awareness program or a rehabilitation program. Today, it would be unusual for a large community hospital not to have both.

Health care managers can contribute to this demand for organizational diversity by seeking out opportunities for your department to provide new and better services. In dynamic organizations, great ideas are generated from the

---

FOR EXAMPLE

Health Advocates

A new type of health care professional has emerged in the last few years to help guide patients through complex medical decisions. Health advocates help seriously ill patients research new treatments, cut through medical bureaucracy, coordinate treatment and expertise from various specialists, and assist with insurance-related questions. The service is available through private for-profit providers and through nonprofit groups (which usually focus on a specific disease or aspect of health care, such as insurance problems). As the complexity of health care decisions continues to increase, the use of health advocates is likely to increase. For more information about leading nonprofit health advocate services available through the University of Wisconsin Law School, visit www.law.wisc.edu/patientadvocacy.

bottom up; team leaders and lower-level managers develop and execute some of today's most important new health care programs and initiatives.

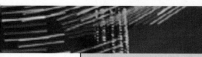

SELF-CHECK

- Identify and define **patient**.
- Discuss reasons for increases in patient scrutiny.
- Explain how patient expectations and demands affect health care organizations.

1.3 Managing in the New Workplace

This book is about managers in today's new, exciting, and highly demanding health care workplace. A **manager** is anyone in an organization who supports and is responsible for the work performance of one or more other persons. Managers can have a variety of titles (including supervisor, team leader, division head, administrator, vice president, and more), but all managers share some common traits:

▲ Managers mobilize people and resources to accomplish the work of organizations and their subunits.

▲ Managers share responsibility—with people they report to and with people who report to them—in order to accomplish high-performance results.

▲ Managers accomplish their goals through the process of organizing, planning, controlling the use of resources, leading, and influencing.

Although specific day-to-day responsibilities vary greatly, managers within health care organizations typically[2]

▲ plan meetings and work schedules;
▲ clarify goals and tasks and gather ideas for improvement;
▲ appraise productivity and team-member performance;
▲ recommend pay increases and new assignments;
▲ recruit, train, and develop team members;
▲ encourage high performance and teamwork;
▲ inform team members about goals and expectations;
▲ inform higher levels of team needs and accomplishments;
▲ coordinate with other teams and support their work efforts.

In addition to these day-to-day duties, today's health care manager deals with a few overarching concerns, specifically accountability, quality of work life, and diversity.

1.3.1 Accountability

In this context, all managers must face and master a common problem: They must create the work environments in which individuals and groups contribute to organizational productivity. Furthermore, they must do this while being held *accountable* for results achieved. Formally defined, **accountability** is the requirement of one person to answer to a higher authority and show results achieved for assigned duties.

Every manager's daily challenge is to fulfill performance accountabilities for the results achieved by a team or work unit. To do so, however, every manager depends on the accomplishments of others to make this performance possible. Truly effective managers fulfill this accountability while utilizing organizational resources in ways that result in the members of their work teams achieving both high-performance outcomes and high levels of personal satisfaction.

1.3.2 Quality of Work Life

Productivity is a measure of high-performance results; by contrast, **quality of work life (QWL)** is an indicator of the overall quality of human experiences in the workplace. The QWL concept expresses a true respect for people at work and their rights to job satisfaction—an important theme that is addressed frequently throughout this book.

Practically speaking, a high quality of work life is one that offers the individual such things as

- ▲ fair pay;
- ▲ safe working conditions;
- ▲ respect for talents;
- ▲ opportunities to learn and use new skills;
- ▲ room to grow and progress in a career;
- ▲ protection of individual rights;
- ▲ pride in the work itself and in the organization.

Part of any manager's accountability is to achieve high-performance outcomes while supporting a high quality of work life for those who actually make this performance possible. Simply put, in the new workplace, productivity and a high-quality work life can and should go hand in hand.

1.3.3 Valuing Diversity

Closely associated with the quality of work life concept is another aspect of managerial accountability—valuing diversity.[3] **Workforce diversity** describes demographic differences among employees, principally differences in age, gender, race, ethnicity, able-bodiedness, religious affiliation, and sexual orientation. Today's workforce is increasingly diverse not only in demographics, but also in cultural

---

FOR EXAMPLE

U.S. Plans for Workforce Diversity

The U.S. federal government places great value on the goals of creating, defending, and ensuring workplace diversity in every U.S. state, county, and city. In particular, the Department of the Interior Office for Equal Opportunity serves as an organizing hub for national plans, reports, and news about workplace diversity. Visit the DOI's Web page dedicated to workplace diversity (www.doi.gov/diversity/workforce_diversity.html) to review the United States's official 5-year plan for maintaining a diverse workforce, as well as the most recent annual survey of workplace demographics in U.S. businesses and organizations.

---

traditions and lifestyles. This presents both a challenge in terms of required employer support and an opportunity with respect to potential performance gains.[4]

Managers should value diversity and help everyone work to their full potential. But what does this really mean? A female vice president answered the question this way: "consciously creating an environment where everyone has an equal shot at contributing, participating, and most of all advancing."[5]

Diversity barriers in organizations can exist as prejudice involving negative, irrational attitudes of some members toward people different from themselves. It can take the form of discrimination that puts such people at a disadvantage by denying them the full benefits of organizational membership. It can also result in what some call the **glass-ceiling effect**—the existence of an invisible screen that prevents disfavored people or minorities from rising above a certain level of organizational responsibility.[6]

SELF-CHECK

- Identify and define **manager, accountability, quality of work life, workplace diversity,** and **glass-ceiling effect.**
- Cite typical traits of managers and list typical managerial responsibilities.
- Describe characteristics of a job with high quality of work life (QWL).
- Explain reasons why workforce diversity is valuable in today's health care organizations.

1.4 Management at Various Levels

Mangers exist at a variety of levels within today's health care organizations. While the trend toward less hierarchy (i.e., few middle and upper managers) is definitely in effect, most organizations continue to have managers at three main levels:

▲ A top manager (or perhaps a few top senior managers) establishes an organization's major performance objectives and ensures that the rest of the company accomplishes the goals in accordance with the organization's purpose. The CEO of Johnson & Johnson and the director of the Centers for Disease Control are examples of top, senior-level managers. Top managers are responsible for the performance of an organization as a whole or for one of its major parts. They pay special attention to the external environment, are alert to potential long-term problems and opportunities, and develop appropriate ways of dealing with them. The best top managers are future-oriented strategic thinkers who make good decisions under highly competitive and uncertain conditions. Other common job titles at this level are *chief executive officer, chief operating officer, president,* and *vice president.*

▲ Middle managers are in charge of relatively large departments or divisions consisting of several smaller work units. Examples are clinic directors in hospitals, division managers, and regional managers. Middle managers report to top managers and develop and implement action plans consistent with organizational objectives. They must be team-oriented and able to work well with peers to help coordinate activities across the organization. Middle managers must often implement complex projects that require the contributions of people from many different parts of an organization.

▲ Team leaders and supervisors are in charge of smaller groups of nonmanagerial workers. Although most people enter the workforce as technical specialists—such as accounting clerk, information system technicians, medical professionals, or customer care representatives—sooner or later, many advance to positions of initial managerial responsibility. Job titles at this level vary greatly but include *department head, group leader,* and *unit manager.* These managers ensure that their work teams or units meet performance objectives that are consistent with the plans of middle and top management.

Among the many changes affecting managerial work today, the concept of the "upside-down pyramid" is one of the most symbolic. As shown in Figure 1-2, this new way of looking at organizations puts customers and clients at the top of the pyramid, followed by operating workers who interact directly with customers. These groups are supported by managers located below them, and top

Figure 1-2

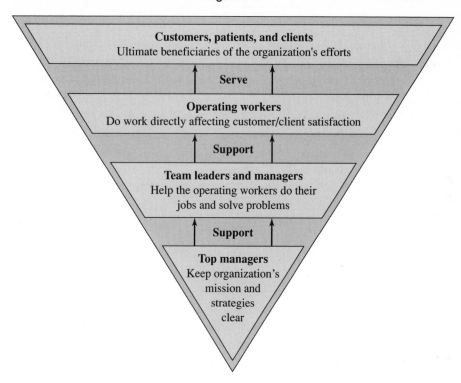

The "upside-down pyramid" view of today's organizations.

managers support everyone. In a sense, everyone in the upside-down pyramid becomes a **value-added worker**—someone who does things that create eventual value for best serving the customers.

The implications of this new perspective are dramatic for day-to-day work:

▲ Today's best managers are known more for helping and supporting, rather than directing and order-giving.

▲ Even in this age of high technology, people and their talents are critical building blocks of organizational success.

▲ Jobs in the new workplace put more emphasis on teamwork.

1.4.1 Appreciating Managerial Skills

Two ways to further define what exactly a manager is in today's health care organization is to explore the position in terms of skills and roles.

A **skill** is an ability to translate knowledge into an action that results in desired performance. Many skills are required to master the challenging nature of managerial work, and the most important ones allow managers to help others be highly productive.

One important distinction for management skills is effective versus affective. **Effective management skills** are abilities that support the effort to complete work on time and within budget. Key effective skills include estimating, scheduling, assigning work, supplying feedback, and analyzing processes. **Affective skills** are abilities managers use to manage their own emotions and their interaction with others in the workplace. Key affective skills include self-awareness, self-management, and relationship management.

Robert L. Katz classifies the essential skills of managers into three categories: technical, human, and conceptual.[7] Although all three skills are essential for managers, their relative importance tends to vary by level of managerial responsibility, as shown in Figure 1-3.

A **technical skill** is the ability to use a special proficiency or expertise to perform particular tasks. Accountants, engineers, market researchers, and computer scientists, for example, possess technical skills. These skills are initially acquired through formal education and are further developed by training and job experience. Technical skills are most important at lower levels of management.

A **human skill** is the ability to work well with other people. Trust, enthusiasm, and genuine involvement in interpersonal relationships are all examples of human skills. A manager with good human skills has a high degree of self-awareness and a capacity to understand or empathize with the emotions and feelings of others. Given the highly interpersonal nature of managerial work, human skills are critical for all managers.

A **conceptual skill** is the ability to think analytically and solve complex problems. All good managers ultimately have the ability to view situations

Figure 1-3

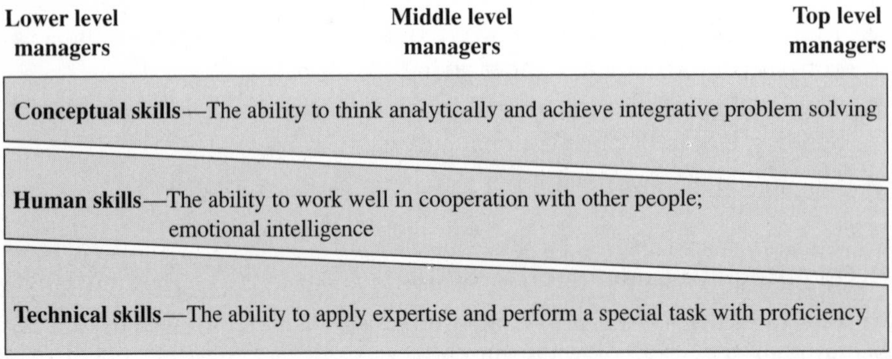

Lower level managers	Middle level managers	Top level managers

Conceptual skills—The ability to think analytically and achieve integrative problem solving

Human skills—The ability to work well in cooperation with other people; emotional intelligence

Technical skills—The ability to apply expertise and perform a special task with proficiency

Essential managerial skills.

Figure 1-4

Interpersonal roles	Informational roles	Decisional roles
How a manager interacts with other people • Figurehead • Leader • Liaison	How a manager exchanges and processes information • Monitor • Disseminator • Spokesperson	How a manager uses information in decision making • Entrepreneur • Disturbance handler • Resource allocator • Negotiator

Ten managerial roles.

broadly and find solutions to problems. Conceptual skills involve the capacity to break down problems into smaller parts, to see the relations between the parts, and to recognize the implications of any one problem for others. As managers assume ever-higher responsibilities in organizations, they must deal with more ambiguous problems that have longer-term consequences. Conceptual skills gain in relative importance for higher management levels.

1.4.2 Appreciating Managerial Roles

In trying to define the position and importance of managers in the workplace, classic managerial researcher Henry Mintzberg systematically divided and described the nature of managerial work into a set of 10 roles, which Figure 1-4 depicts graphically.

The roles managers must be prepared to perform fall into three categories:[8]

▲ A manger's **interpersonal** roles involve interactions with people inside and outside the work unit.

▲ The **informational** roles involve the giving, receiving, and analyzing of information.

▲ The **decisional** roles involve using information to make decisions, to solve problems, or to address opportunities.

1.4.3 Responding to Change

The nature of managerial work is always evolving as organizations change and develop with time. A *Wall Street Journal* article described the transition this way: "Not so long ago, [managers] may have supervised 10 people sitting outside their offices. Today they must win the support of scores more—employees of different backgrounds, job titles, and even cultures . . . these new managers are expected to be skilled at organizing complex subjects, solving problems, communicating ideas, and making swift decisions."[9]

We live in times of dramatic and continuous change. Values, cultures, and societies are changing along with today's health care organizations. In many ways, change is only constant in today's workplace, especially within the dynamic health care industry. Prominent trends include[10]

▲ **preeminence of technology:** New opportunities appear with each new development in computer and information technology. Technology continually changes the way organizations operate and how people work; all workers need to be open to incorporating new technology into their work processes;

▲ **emphasis on knowledge:** Knowledge and *knowledge workers* (employees who primarily know how things work and share this understanding with other employees or patients) are increasingly driving organizations. Because knowledge constantly makes itself obsolete, the pressure is on everyone to learn and continually apply new knowledge to problems and opportunities;

▲ **demise of command-and-control:** Traditional hierarchical structures with "do as I say" bosses are proving too slow, conservative, and costly to do well in today's competitive environments. While most health care organizations still have upper, middle, and lower management, fewer layers of power now exist between workers and top management. As a result, every manager and worker must take greater responsibility for the success of their career, department, and organization;

▲ **focus on speed:** Everything moves fast today. The health care organization that provides a needed service first will always have an advantage in the vast array of health care options available to patients;

▲ **embrace of networking:** Like traditional corporate entities, health care organizations are increasingly communicating and coordinating with external partners, contractors, suppliers, and customers to provide a greater array of services to patients in more efficient and effective manners;

▲ **belief in empowerment:** Today's workplaces demand highly involved workers who utilize their knowledge, experience, and commitment on a daily basis to solve problems and provide solutions to patients. The days of relying on upper management to "fix" situations or make all the tough decisions are ending. Today's health care managers are increasingly expected to figure things out on their own, working with the resources available to them;

▲ **reexamination of ethics:** Prompted by recent business and governmental scandals, the public has increased its demand for ethical behavior and socially responsible actions within health care organizations. Managers must do the "right" things, not just the convenient things, or else potentially lose customer-clients to organizations that are viewed as ethical and socially responsible. Monitoring organizations, such as the Joint Commission on Accreditation of Healthcare Organizations (www.jcaho.org), evaluate thousands of hospitals, clinics, and health care providers each year to determine whether these organizations are fulfilling both their medical and ethical responsibilities;

▲ **emphasis on teamwork:** Today's health care organizations are increasingly driven by teams that combine individuals with different expertise into one, high-functioning unit. For example, it's not uncommon to find "treatment teams" consisting of a physician, several nurses, a social worker, a therapist, an office manager, and several specialized medical assistants all working closely together on a daily basis to serve the needs of patients;

▲ **concern about work-life balance:** As society increases in complexity, workers are forcing organizations to pay more attention to balance in the often-conflicting demands of work and personal affairs. Demands for flexible scheduling, job sharing, part-time employment, and telecommuting are prompting managers in health organizations to come up with ever more creative ways to get work done.

1.4.4 Meeting the Challenges Ahead

Those who want to succeed in the twenty-first-century workplace must be self-starters and leaders who find continuing ways to add value to employers even as the environment continues to change. They must be willing to "do the right things" every day and continuously learn from experience to remain as capable in the future as they are in the present.

FOR EXAMPLE

Mayo Clinic Responds to Change

More than a century ago, brothers and physicians Charlie and Will Mayo realized that medical professionals needed to be organized differently in order to respond to the rapidly changing health care needs of patients in early twentieth-century America. The brothers created the first group practice, a health care system in which multiple physicians with various expertise can work together to provide the best care for patients. Today, Mayo Clinic continues to respond to the rapidly changing needs of patients with state-of-the-art research, complementary treatment programs, and experimental medicine. Find out more about Mayo's history—and its future plans—at www.mayoclinic.org/about/index.html.

In this context, new managers must be well educated, and they must continue their educations throughout their careers. Success in turbulent times comes only through continuous learning.

SELF-CHECK

- Define the three levels of management and give examples of responsibilities and duties at each level.
- Define **skill** and discuss the three types of managerial skills.
- Compare Mintzberg's three categories of managerial roles.
- Discuss the most prominent changes in health care today.

1.5 Tackling Managerial Duties

The ultimate "bottom line" in every manager's job is to succeed in helping an organization achieve high performance while utilizing all of its human and material resources. For many organizations, high productivity (in the form of high levels of performance effectiveness and efficiency) is a measure of organizational success. Managers are largely responsible for ensuring its achievement.

The job descriptions of most health care managers are extensive yet also open-ended. Managers monitor and endeavor to improve the daily operations of their departments or teams. They also need to think strategically about the future—how to improve the efficiency and productivity of their staffs and departments, and how to grow their own careers.

The duties and responsibilities outlined in this section cover many of the most common managerial duties.

1.5.1 The Management Process

On a daily basis, health care managers must recognize performance problems and opportunities, make good decisions, and take appropriate action. Managers do this through the process of **management**—organizing, planning, controlling the use of resources, and leading to accomplish performance goals. These functions of management and their interrelationships are shown in Figure 1-5.

All managers, regardless of title, level, type, and organizational setting, are responsible for the following four functions:[11]

▲ **Organizing** is the process of assigning tasks, allocating resources, and arranging and coordinating the activities of individuals and groups to implement plans. Through organizing, managers seek to understand and

Figure 1-5

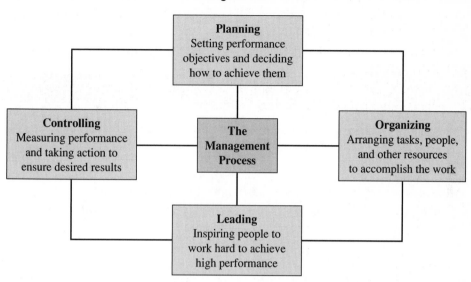

Functions of management.

give shape to the complex nature of the workplace. Defining jobs, assigning personnel, and supporting staff with formal plans, specific technology, and other resources are all organizing tasks. Chapters 3 and 4 focus on organizing.

▲ **Planning** is the process of setting performance objectives and determining what actions should be taken to accomplish them. Through planning, a manager identifies desired work results, makes decisions, and lays the path for others to achieve the results. Chapters 6 and 8 focus on planning.

▲ **Controlling** is the process of measuring work performance, comparing results to objectives, and taking corrective action as needed. Through controlling, managers maintain active contact with people in the course of their work, gather and interpret reports on performance, and use this information to plan constructive action and change. Chapter 7 covers controlling.

▲ **Leading** is the process of arousing people's enthusiasm to work hard to fulfill plans and accomplish objectives. Through leading, managers build commitments, encourage activities that support goals, and influence others to do their best work on the organization's behalf. Chapters 9, 10, and 11 address leading.

While all managers are responsible for these functions, managers do not often accomplish these functions in a linear step-by-step fashion. In the real world, managers quickly move from task to task, utilizing multiple, sometimes overlapping, functions.

1.5.2 Time Management

Successful managers must learn, early on, to manage their time—in terms of how much time they spend working and how they allot the time spent.

Without a set shift or nine-to-five routine, a manager's time is never really his or her own. The amount of time a manager spends on the job largely is dictated by the needs of the organization and the manager's department. Some new managers overact to the time demands, assuming that the only way to meet their new objectives is to spend 18 hours a day at work while virtually forgoing a personal life. This quickly results in burnout and failure in the management role.

Not only is the number of hours different between managers and nonmanagers, but also the way this time is allotted is usually quite different. Nonmanagerial health care professionals spend about 80% of their time in professional activities—conducting laboratory work, treating patients, filling prescriptions, or repairing equipment. Health care managers tend to divide their time quite differently, as shown in Figure 1-6.[12]

As Figure 1-6 shows, almost two-thirds of managerial time involves *people-management activities* (motivating employees, setting work objectives, dealing with employee performance problems, assisting employees in accomplishing their work goals). This category also includes handling patient requests and complaints, working with peers, and engaging in other people-intensive activities.

Figure 1-6

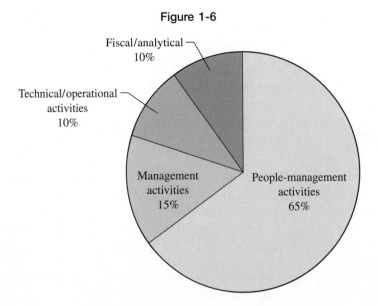

Typical management responsibilities.

Additionally, 15% of managerial time is dedicated to *management activities*. Meetings, which consume a big part of this managerial time, are necessary as the business itself changes and new objectives are established. Other management activities include training employees, participating on councils and committees, and collaborating with colleagues and upper managers.

The remaining 20% of the chart in Figure 1-5 is divided equally between fiscal-analytical responsibilities and technical-operational responsibilities.

▲ **Fiscal-analytical responsibilities** include budgeting, financial paperwork, and cost-benefit analyses. In some management roles, this 10% quotation can easily be replaced or supplemented with administrivia, a popular term that relates to the paperwork (for example, compliance reports and organizational inventories) in many organizations.

▲ **Technical-operational** activities include participating in conferences related to your department's specific area of technical expertise or participating in educational activities aimed at improving your technical proficiency.

1.5.3 Agenda-Setting

Successful health care managers develop action priorities for their jobs by setting **agendas,** plans that include specific long- and short-term goals. Agendas are usually incomplete and loosely connected in the beginning but become more specific as the manager utilizes information that is continually gleaned from many different sources.

Forward-thinking managers keep their agendas in mind and are ready to share details whenever opportunities arise, such as when the general manger unexpectedly visits or team members express concerns about the appropriateness of a manager's decision.

Good managers implement their agendas by working with a variety of people inside and outside the organization.

1.5.4 Connecting with Other Departments

The old expression says that "no man is an island," and by extension, the same can be said of health care managers. Savvy managers understand how their department or team relates to other departments or teams in the broader organization.

For example, as the personnel manager in a large metropolitan hospital, your departments would connect with a large employee population—nursing, support services, and operations, for example. Or if you managed a drug-rehabilitation team, all other rehabilitation-related departments (such as physical therapy, occupational rehabilitation, and social work) are closely related to your day-to-day work.

To determine which departments are closely related to yours, consider the following four questions:

▲ Which department(s) seem to have a natural similarity to the department I manage?
▲ Which department(s) do I communicate with the most frequently?
▲ Which department(s) do I find myself spending the most time in?
▲ Which areas have similar personnel and mission objectives and work with the same type of patient as my department?

Wise health care managers learn as much as possible about these closely related departments. Open communication and a spirit of freely shared information can lead to greater action and better productivity for all departments.

1.5.5 Networking

Networking is the process of building and maintaining positive relationships with people (typically outside of your current organization or business) whose help you may need to someday implement your work agendas. Networks are indispensable to managerial success in today's complex health care environments, and the best managers devote time and effort to developing their network.

Entire books are written on the process of networking, but the following techniques are some of the most effective means for developing these important connections:

▲ **Collect business cards.** Whenever you meet a management counterpart in the course of your personal or professional activities, exchange business cards. Counterpoints may be professionals at other hospitals, clinics, health care suppliers, governmental agencies, or nonprofit organizations. Even if another professional's job tasks seem far removed from your duties, keep the person's card; contacts are all potential sources of information.

▲ **Join a professional organization.** Membership in a strong national or regional professional organization can help you develop in your area of expertise. The organization may be related to a specific technical area, or it could be a general health care management development organization. Professional associations offer tremendous educational and networking opportunities, as well as a range of publications that can help developing management skills.

▲ **Become involved in community activities.** One of the unique qualities of health care is its standing within a community and its people-orientation. Try to participate in a range of community activities to build your base of contacts while providing you with information about how your organization

FOR EXAMPLE

American College of Healthcare Executives

The American College of Healthcare Executives (ACHE; www.ache.org) is a leading professional organization for health care managers in the United States and abroad. The society's membership includes more than 30,000 professionals, representing a wide range of health care managers working in hospitals, health care systems, nonprofit health care initiatives, and other organizations. ACHE's Congress on Healthcare Management is a popular national event, drawing more than 4,000 participants annually. ACHE publishes the *Journal of Healthcare Management* and *Healthcare Executive,* in addition to dozens of research, career development, and public policy papers every year. A significant portion of ACHE's content is also available free and online.

is perceived throughout the community. Community-based contacts may include religious organizations, schools, social service agencies, and more.

▲ **Ask questions.** When you meet a new contact, ask as many questions as you can without becoming impolite or intrusive. Ask about the person's background, areas of interest, and knowledge. Furthermore, ask about other individuals he or she may know who might help you gain specific knowledge in key areas. Most individuals are flattered by such questions and will be more than happy to provide you with critical information.

▲ **Read critically.** Take full advantage of journals, newsletters, abstracts, and other professional literature. Even the daily newspaper in your area, given health care's prominence on the public scene, is also a great source of useful information.

SELF-CHECK

- Identify and define **management, productivity, agenda, and networking.**
- Define and describe the four functions of management: organizing, planning, controlling, and leading.
- Discuss the four typical, daily management activities.
- Explain the purpose of agendas and agenda-setting.
- Suggest ways to effectively network with outside departments and individuals.

1.6 Differentiating between Professional and Managerial Experiences

Whatever your career history and goals, working as a team member (as a specialist, technician, assistant, or some other title) and working as a manager—even within the same health care organization—are two distinct experiences.

The following sections identify four of the biggest contrasts between health care professional and health care manager.[13]

1.6.1 Self-Direction versus Selfless Service

As a health care professional, you are in a position that is more **self-directed.** Your job description reflects a range of activities that you pretty much control and that require mastery of some technical discipline. (Here, *technical discipline* includes specific medical skills, as well as expertise in accounting, information technology, customer care, and a host of other specific skills.) In your daily work, you make technical judgments without undue reliance on others, and external and internal organizational dynamics have little impact on your daily activities. In essence, professionals are responsible first and foremost for their own performance: you are the key factor in determining the level of success you experience and what contribution you make to your organization.

As a health care manager, by contrast, you are in an area of selfless service. Rather than focusing on self-performance, health care managers supervise the activities of others. You have a great degree of control over and responsibility for others' activities. Your time is governed by the work activities and needs of your reporting staff, as well as the needs of your organization. Your work is constantly interrupted by people problems, organizational mandates, and change in work direction generated by upper management. Furthermore, your first responsibility is to the individuals you supervise, not to yourself. This means that your priorities and interests often take a backseat.

1.6.2 Autonomy versus Circumstantial Control

As a health care professional, you have *autonomous control* over your work responsibilities. In many cases, your work activity is primarily governed by a job description, and you perform your tasks based on deadlines, processes, and procedures. Unless an emergency arises, you can work at your own pace and accomplish the goals you desire, based on your own performance and motivation.

As a manager, circumstances and situations control your action flow. The organizational contribution your department makes is the main factor in determining your workflow and your daily responsibilities. As emergencies arise, you must mobilize your entire department and determine who will work to attain specific objectives. Flexibility is a key factor in your success; you must be positively reactive, adaptable, and versatile in undertaking your management responsibilities.

1.6.3 Quantitative versus Qualitative Outcomes

The roles of most health care professionals usually lead to a variety of **quantitative outcomes.** In general, your performance as a professional is assessed based on meeting quantitative outcomes on a regular basis. For example:

▲ A lab technician conducts analysis and assays, which produces numerical (quantitative) outcomes.

▲ A staff pharmacist is responsible for filling a set amount of prescriptions on a daily basis.

▲ A staff nurse has a certain number of procedures and activities that, if successfully undertaken, dictates whether you had a good day.

As a manager, you deal largely in **qualitative outcomes,** which means measuring your success is more difficult. You deal with personalities and perceptions rather than measurable results. Even the most important indicator of successful health care management performance—patient satisfaction—is very difficult to measure numerically and is definitely qualitative in scope.

1.6.4 Focusing on Definitive Criteria versus Focusing on Overall, Comprehensive Goals

Health care professionals deal with definite outcomes. For example, you either complete a lab analysis or not; fill a prescription correctly or fail to note contraindications. Having clear-cut criteria provides a degree of satisfaction: You can recognize clearly the contribution you make toward providing stellar health care. Furthermore, this clarity of outcome provides a building-block-like sequence, whereby you can improve your performance each day and compare it with a previous goal.

Health care management offers few black-and-white performance criteria. Given all the dynamics of change and expectations mentioned earlier in this

---

FOR EXAMPLE

Healthcare.Monster.com

Over the last decade, Monster.com has transformed the way people search, prepare, apply, and interview for jobs. To assist both new and experienced health care professionals to successfully find and transition to new jobs, Monster created a free health care-specific information hub (http://healthcare. monster.com). In addition to listing thousands of open positions nationwide, the site's lively discussion forum offers a place for individuals searching for new work or transitioning to new responsibilities to ask questions and share insights.

chapter, it is very difficult to measure performance, clearly identify key performance criteria, and establish reliable goals for optimum performance. As a result, you must adapt your thinking to look at the breadth of activity, as opposed to the depth of activity. This means looking at the big picture as it relates to all your department's activities, establishing overall, comprehensive goals, and closely monitoring performance with an open mind—all without ever losing sight of the objective of providing excellent health care.

SELF-CHECK

- Identify and define the four biggest contrasts between professional and managerial work.
- Contrast self-direction with selfless service.
- Discuss forces that control professional and managerial work experiences.
- Define **quantitative** and **qualitative** outcomes.
- Compare definitive criteria and comprehensive goals.

SUMMARY

Careers in health care offer both fantastic opportunities and considerable challenges. Today's health care organizations must respond to many dynamic changes, while today's patient has new demands and expectations. As in any workplace, health care managers must be accountable, create a quality of work life, and value diversity. Although managerial levels, roles, and responsibilities vary within organizations, all managers must respond effectively to change. Every day managers must organize, plan, control, and lead in order to achieve the goals of their health care organizations.

KEY TERMS

Accountability	The requirement of one person to answer to higher authority and show results achieved for assigned duties.
Affective skills	Abilities managers use to manage their own emotions and their interaction with others in the workplace.
Agendas	Action plans set by managers that include specific long- and short-term goals.

Continuum of care	The complete spectrum of available health care services.
Controlling	The managerial process of measuring work performance, comparing results to objectives, and taking corrective action as needed.
Effective skills	Managerial abilities that support the effort to complete work on time and within budget.
General environment	The background and external conditions for an organization.
Glass-ceiling effect	The existence of an invisible screen that prevents disfavored people or minorities from rising above a certain level of organizational responsibility.
Human skill	the ability to work well with other people
Intellectual capital	An organization's employees, including their talents, knowledge, and experience.
Leading	The managerial process of arousing people's enthusiasm to work hard to fulfill plans and accomplish objectives.
Management	The process of organizing, planning, controlling the use of resources, and leading to accomplish performance goals.
Manager	Anyone in an organization who supports and is responsible for the work performance of one or more other persons.
Networking	The process of building and maintaining positive relationships with people, typically outside of your current organization or business.
Organization	A collection of people working together to achieve a common purpose.
Organizing	The managerial process of assigning tasks, allocating resources, and arranging and coordinating the activities of individuals and groups to implement plans.
Patient	Individual who utilizes the goods and services produced by health care organizations.
Planning	The managerial process of setting performance objectives and determining what actions should be taken to accomplish them.
Productivity	Performance effectiveness and efficiency within the organization.

Purpose	Why an organization exists; organizations exist to produce goods and/or services that satisfy the needs of customers.
Qualitative outcome	A nonmeasurable result, usually involving personalities and perceptions rather than specific figures.
Quality of work life (QWL)	An indicator of the overall quality of human experiences in the workplace.
Quantitative outcome	A measurable result.
Skill	An ability to translate knowledge into action that results in desired performance.
Specific environment	The actual organizations, groups, and persons with whom an organization must interact in order to survive and prosper.
Stakeholders	The people, groups, and institutions who are affected in one way or another by the organization's performance.
Technical skill	The ability to use a special proficiency or expertise to perform particular tasks.
Value-added worker	Someone who does things that create eventual value for best serving customers.
Workforce diversity	Demographic differences among employees, principally differences in age, gender, race, ethnicity, able-bodiedness, religious affiliation, and sexual orientation.

ASSESS YOUR UNDERSTANDING

Go to www.wiley.com/college/Lombardi to evaluate your knowledge of the basic job of a health care supervisor.
Measure your learning by comparing pretest and post-test results.

Summary Questions

1. Prevailing social values on the environment, human rights, education, and family are part of an organization's
   (a) economic conditions.
   (b) legal-political conditions.
   (c) technological conditions.
   (d) social-cultural conditions.

2. The only stakeholder that matters for today's health care organization is the patient. True or false?

3. The amount and quality of effort demonstrated by the staff of a health care organization, as perceived by the patient, is the most critical indicator of whether the organization is upholding its charter as a public trust. True or false?

4. Regardless of the industry, business, or organization, managers do all of the following, except
   (a) alleviate uncertainty.
   (b) share responsibility.
   (c) mobilize people and resources.
   (d) accomplish goals through organizing and planning.

5. A high quality of work life offers employees
   (a) room to grow and progress in a career.
   (b) safe working conditions.
   (c) fair pay.
   (d) all of the above.

6. Managers who ensure that their teams or units meet performance objectives that are consistent with plans can be described as
   (a) middle managers.
   (b) team leaders or supervisors.
   (c) top managers.
   (d) technical specialists.

7. In the "upside-down pyramid" model, top management is at the top of the pyramid and their plans and recommendations flow down to

middle management, team leaders, and, finally, customer-patients. True or false?

8. Change is the only constant in today's health care workplace. All of the following are change-related trends in health care, except

   (a) the revision of traditional, hierarchical reporting structures.

   (b) worker demands for flexible scheduling, telecommuting, and other benefits.

   (c) decreased reliance on diagnostic testing.

   (d) reexamination of ethics and socially responsible behaviors.

9. The managerial functions of organizing, planning, controlling, and leading are interconnected and do not flow in a linear fashion. True or false?

10. The majority of managerial time—typically more than 60% of any given day—is spent on

    (a) people-management activities.

    (b) management activities.

    (c) fiscal-analytical activities.

    (d) technical-operational activities.

11. An effective technique for networking is

    (a) posting your resume online.

    (b) joining a professional organization.

    (c) consulting with a career counselor.

    (d) donating money to a community organization.

12. As a manager, you have autonomous control of your work, setting your own pace and accomplishing goals based on your desires. True or false?

13. An example of a qualitative outcome is

    (a) the number of blood tests conducted daily.

    (b) the cost savings from terminating an ineffective lab technician.

    (c) the number of postsurgical patients a physical therapist can see in a day.

    (d) the satisfaction of a pharmacy customer when offered generic drugs.

Review Questions

1. Health care organizations are only as strong as their intellectual capital. What is intellectual capital, and what are some specific types of capital?

2. What are the actual organizations, groups, and people with whom an organization interacts collectively referred to?

3. What are some reasons that public scrutiny of health care is at an all-time high?

4. An employee is prevented from rising above a certain level in an organization based on his or her gender. What might the employee be experiencing?

5. Workplace diversity encourages, maintains, and defends (when necessary) demographic differences among employees. What are the key demographic factors of workplace diversity?

6. The floor nurse at a university hospital is known for being able to almost instantly connect with patients, sensing how they really feel about a situation. What category of managerial skill is the nurse exemplifying?

7. Managers must have a variety of skills to do their jobs effectively. The ability to think analytically and solve complex problems is what type of skill?

8. How does the upside-down pyramid model change the basic responsibilities and duties of managers?

9. Today's health care workplaces must embrace networking to a greater degree than ever before. With whom might today's health care manager be likely to network?

10. Which function of the management process are you exemplifying when you ask staff to tally and log the exact number of syringes they use each day?

11. About 15% of a typical manager's day is spent doing management activities. What sorts of things are considered "management activities"?

12. Every time you meet a new co-worker or contact, you add their name and pertinent contact information to your electronic organizer. Which networking activities are you essentially doing?

13. As a manager, you must respond with great flexibility to emergencies as they arise, mobilizing your staff and resources to attain specific objectives. How could you describe the controls involved here?

14. In what ways is managerial work "selfless service"?

Applying This Chapter

1. In a speech to investors, the CEO of a medical research firm complains about the current environment as being "bad for business," due to new governmental regulations, high unemployment, and public demands for limited tests on animal subjects. What environment is the CEO referring to? What are some conditions the CEO is referring to?

2. Today's health care patient has new expectations and demands. What are some of these expectations and what are some of the demands? How do these expectations and demands compare and contrast?

3. The manager of a radiology department sets up an interdepartmental exchange program in which her radiological technicians can spend one afternoon a month shadowing an MRI technician. In exchange, MRI technicians get to spend similar time each month in radiology learning about the department and its procedures. Which aspect of the quality of work life is the manager trying to address?

4. A large suburban hospital has several levels of management—lower level, middle level, and top level. If you were the director of Human Resources, how would you compare the relative levels of technical, human, and conceptual skills required at each level within your organization?

5. As the manager of a small-town health clinic, you want to introduce a diabetes-screening program for your patients and the community at large. What would be at least one task/duty to be addressed for each of the four functions of the management process?

6. A busy four-physician medical office has a small front office staff, including a front-desk receptionist and a general office manager. Although these two individuals work in the same office, how might their work experiences differ based on the characteristics described in section 1.6?

You and Your Environment

Take a moment and think of yourself as a company or organization. Just like any successful health care organization, you personally need to be aware of your general environment if you want to make yourself the most successful job candidate or employee. In your general environment, what are the economic, social-cultural, legal-political, technological, and environmental conditions that affect your ability to find and prosper in a health care job?

The Patients' Bill of Rights

Based on a mandate from President Bill Clinton, the Advisory Commission on Consumer Protection and Quality in the Health Care Industry presented a seven-part "Patients' Bill of Rights" in 1998. Since then, many health care organizations have adopted the document as a way to treat patients. Review the seven parts of the Patients' Bill of Rights at www.consumer.gov/qualityhealth/rights.htm and determine which portions protect the "customer" and the "patient" portions of today's patient approach to delivering health care.

Daily Managerial Duties

Take another look at the list of typical day-to-day responsibilities of health care managers in section 1.3. Go through the list and consider what percentage of an average day you anticipate you'll spend doing each of the nine general tasks on the list. After you make sure your percentage estimates total 100, ask at least two health care managers how they spend their time on an average day. Compare your findings with your estimates. Which differences surprised you the most?

Your Managerial Skills

Evaluate your resume in terms of the three categories of skills that are expected of managers in today's health care workplace. (If you haven't begun creating a resume that chronicles your health care-related experiences, begin doing so immediately. Even if you don't plan to enter the workforce for several years, a detailed resume helps you figure out what skills and experiences you have and still require.) Does your resume include specific examples of technical, human, and conceptual skills? If you don't have health care-specific examples of human and conceptual skills, brainstorm instances in which you helped someone else do or learn something new (human skills). Also list any event or major project that you planned or led (conceptual skills). Consider incorporating the best examples of human and/or conceptual skills on your resume.

Network Now

The health care organization you currently work for represents your biggest bank of career advancement contacts—even if you don't plan to move into a management position within your current employer. Many managers within your health care organization have expertise in areas that interest you and already have their own networks established. Make a list of health care practitioners you respect and feel comfortable talking with. (You can start building your health care contacts, even if you're not currently working at a health care facility, simply by listing physicians, therapists, nurses, social workers, and others who you and your family and friends have had positive health care experiences.) Ask each person on your list, "Do you know someone who...?" This approach not only solidifies the person you're asking as part of your network, but it also yields valuable answers and information that can further enhance your own network.

Professional versus Manager

Consider the four major contrasts of professional versus managerial work outlined in section 1.6. As you review the four dynamics, consider when in your work, school, and personal life you experienced each side of the dynamic. Do you prefer working in a self-directed manner, or do you prefer selfless serving of others or an organization? How do you feel about controls in your workday— do you like to be in control or can you work with circumstantial control? Are you more comfortable achieving quantitative or qualitative outcomes? Do you enjoy working toward definite outcomes, or do you prefer working toward a general goal? Your thoughts, experiences, and feelings toward each of these dynamics can play a significant role in your ability to acquire and enjoy management work in today's health care environment.

31

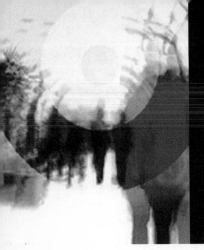

2

DOING THE RIGHT THING
Ethical Behavior and Social Responsibilities in Today's Health Care Workplace

Starting Point

Go to www.wiley.com/college/Lombardi to assess your knowledge of the basics of ethics in health care.
Determine where you need to concentrate your effort.

What You'll Learn in This Chapter

▲ Common types of ethical dilemmas
▲ Four ways to respond to ethical dilemmas
▲ Common rationalizations for unethical behavior
▲ Three influences on a person's ethics
▲ Three ways to encourage high ethical standards
▲ Socially responsible responses to difficult situations

After Studying This Chapter, You'll Be Able To

▲ Demonstrate ethics and socially responsible behavior
▲ Analyze typical ethical dilemmas
▲ Practice health care-specific ethical considerations
▲ Use the seven-step process for ethical decision making
▲ Compare the three common influences on an individual's ethics
▲ Distinguish between ethics and social responsibility
▲ Examine ways to incorporate social responsibility into today's workplace

Goals and Outcomes

▲ Master the terminology related to ethical and socially responsible behavior
▲ Recognize common ethical dilemmas and responses
▲ Compare the four views on ethical behavior
▲ Analyze the reasons behind an ethical choice
▲ Formulate ethical responses
▲ Propose ways to encourage high ethical standards and behavior
▲ Evaluate ethical dilemmas and possible responses

INTRODUCTION

Often ambiguous and unexpected, ethical dilemmas are part of the challenge of working in today's health care organization. While individuals approach ethical questions differently and generate their own unique responses, a basic framework for ethical decision making does exist and can be a useful tool for health care managers. Throughout the decision-making process, managers need to be aware of what influences their ethics. Proactive managers can establish and encourage high ethical standards. Socially responsible behavior extends beyond ethics, encouraging health care managers to make a difference in patients' lives and the world at large.

2.1 Acting Ethically

Ethics are a collection of moral principles that set standards of good or bad, or right or wrong, in one's conduct and thereby guide the behavior of a person or group within an organization.[1] Ethics help people make choices among alternative courses of action. **Ethical behavior** is what is accepted to be "good" and "right" as opposed to "bad" or "wrong" in the context of the governing moral code. For example, is it ethical to

- ▲ take longer than necessary to do a job?
- ▲ make personal telephone calls on company time?
- ▲ call in sick and then take the day off for leisure activities?
- ▲ fail to report rule violations by a co-worker?

None of these acts is strictly illegal, but many people consider one or more of them to be unethical. Indeed, most ethical problems arise when people are asked to do something that violates their personal conscience.

For some people, if an act is legal, they proceed with confidence. For others, however, their ethical tests go beyond legality, extending to a question of **personal values** (or morals)—the underlying beliefs and attitudes that help determine individual behavior. Because values vary among people, different people interpret situations differently and may consider the same behavior ethical or unethical.

2.1.1 Identifying Ethical Dilemmas

An **ethical dilemma** is a situation that requires you to make a choice or take action that, although offering the potential for personal or organizational benefit, may be considered unethical. In ethical dilemmas, action often must be taken, but there isn't a clear consensus on what is right and wrong. In these murky situations, you bear the burden of making good choices. One manager, speaking from experience, sums up ethical dilemmas this way: "I define an unethical situation as one in which I have to do something I don't feel good about."[2]

Many managerial decisions have ethical overtones. Some areas where managers can feel caught in ethical dilemmas (and even cross the line into questions of legality) include[3]

▲ **discrimination:** For example, a manager denies promotion or appointment to a job candidate because of the candidate's race, religion, gender, age, or other non-job-related criterion;

▲ **sexual harassment:** A manager makes a co-worker feel uncomfortable with inappropriate comments or actions regarding sexuality;

▲ **conflicts of interest:** A manager takes a bribe—perhaps money or an extraordinary gift—in return for making a decision favorable to the gift giver;

▲ **organizational resources:** A manager uses company stationery or an e-mail account to communicate personal opinions or requests to community organizations.

Additionally, the health care field has its own set of ethical considerations that other managers and workers in other businesses or professions may not encounter. While each health care organization has unique organizational values (refer to your organization's mission statement or other literature for specifics), most health care organizations affirm the following as part of their organizational ethic:

▲ **Care:** Whether you're processing insurance claims or preparing a patient for knee surgery, care means providing health services to patients with an added human touch element. All health care staff should demonstrate care when dealing with each consumer.

FOR EXAMPLE

Most Common Ethical Dilemmas

In a survey of Harvard Business Review (http://harvardbusinessonline.hbsp. harvard.edu) subscribers (which included both business and health care leaders), many of the ethical dilemmas reported by managers involved conflicts with superiors, customers, and subordinates.[4] The most frequent issues involved dishonesty in communications with top management, clients, and government agencies. Problems in dealing with special gifts, entertainment, and kickbacks were also reported. Significantly, the managers' bosses were singled out as sometimes pressuring their subordinates to engage in such unethical activities as supporting incorrect viewpoints, signing false documents, overlooking the boss's wrongdoings, and doing business with the boss's friends.

▲ **Concern:** The staff should show concern not only to patients and their physical, emotional, and mental well-being, but also to each other. Staff should be concerned about the wellness and development of fellow employees, helping each other through crises as well as sharing in the joy of daily victories.

▲ **Compassion:** Compassion is a cornerstone of successful health care organizations and should be present at all levels—including in interactions with patient-consumers and co-workers.

▲ **Community:** A sense that "we're all in this together" is helpful in bettering the health of patients—and it comes in quite handy when working with others on a team or department.

▲ **Confidentiality:** While federal and state laws—as well as organizational guidelines—spell out in detail who is allowed to know personal, health care-related information, there are appropriate times to share information, as well as to protect others' privacy.

2.1.2 Approaching Ethical Choices Differently

Figure 2-1 shows four alternative views of how people make ethical decisions and how they behaved in an ethical manner.[5] None of these four viewpoints on ethics is necessarily better; the differences simply reflect how complex the question of ethical behavior is and how different people may evaluate the same situation and end up with different ethical responses.

▲ **Utilitarian view:** the **utilitarian view** of ethical behavior focuses on delivering the greatest good to the greatest number of people. Also known as

Figure 2-1

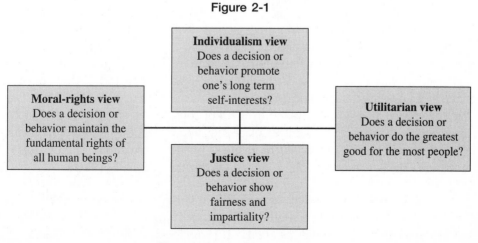

Four views of ethical behavior.

results-oriented point of view, this ethical standpoint tries to assess the moral implications of a decision in terms of its consequences.

Decision makers in business—including top management in today's health care organizations—often use profits, efficiency, and some other performance criteria to judge what is best for the most people in the organization. For example, the manager of a 24-hour pharmacy may make the utilitarian decision to eliminate one full-time pharmacist from her staff in order to keep her pharmacy profitable and save jobs for the remaining staff of 20 pharmacists, technicians, and customer service representatives.

▲ **Individualism view:** The **individualism view** of ethical behavior is based on the belief that your primary commitment is to the advancement of your long-term self-interests. If self-interests are pursued from a long-term view, the argument goes, such things as lying and cheating for short-term gain should not be tolerated.

For example, a call center manager may set up a training plan that is based primarily on his workers' decision to improve their customer-service skills. The manager asserts that anyone who truly wants to do a good job as a phone rep needs to take the personal responsibility to improve themselves.

While the individualism view is supposed to promote honesty and integrity, it can backfire in today's demanding health care economy. Individualism can result in an environment where individuals stretch the limits of laws, disregard rules that aren't agreeable or easy, or aggressively compete with one another for supremacy.[6]

▲ **Moral-rights view:** the **moral-rights view** of ethical behavior respects and protects the fundamental rights of people. Decisions are made in response to an ideal or moral, not based on personal or individual circumstances.

In the United States, for example, the rights of all citizens to life, liberty, and fair treatment under the law are considered inviolate. All laws in the United States must mesh with these ideals. In health care organizations today, this concept extends to ensuring that employee rights—such as the right to privacy, due process, free speech, free consent, safety, and freedom of conscience—are always protected. For example, a manager can put in place regulations about when employees are allowed to converse about nonwork matters, but the regulations cannot violate employee's rights to free speech, as guaranteed in the U.S. Bill of Rights.

▲ **Justice view:** The **justice view** of ethical behavior is based on the belief that all ethical decisions should treat people impartially and fairly, according to guiding rules and standards. This approach evaluates the ethical aspects of any decision on the basis of whether it is "equitable" for everyone affected.

Several principles follow this line of ethical thinking, including

▲ **all policies and rules are to be fairly administered.** For example, a sexual harassment charge against a senior executive should receive the same full hearing as one made against a shift supervisor;

▲ **people should be treated the same regardless of individual characteristics** based on ethnicity, race, gender, age, or other particular criteria. For example, a woman with the same qualifications and experience as a man should receive the same consideration for a promotion;

▲ **others should be treated with dignity and respect.** For example, a supervisor should take the time to fully explain to a team member why he or she was not selected for a special training program.[7]

2.1.3 Rationalizing Unethical Behavior

Why might otherwise reasonable people act unethically? Take a look at some of the ethical scenarios described in the preceding sections and think about examples from your experiences. Consider the possibility of being offered money to alter a patient's medical records. Perhaps the patient is requesting the change so he can be considered for an experimental treatment, or perhaps the patient wants to receive a larger reimbursement from his health insurance provider. Whatever the case, falsifying medical records is a violation of federal law, as well as contradictory to many people's moral codes. And yet, unethical behavior happens all the time in today's workplace.

At least part of the answer for why people behave unethically at times can be found in the way people rationalize their unethical choices. At least four justifications are commonly asserted to rationalize behavior:[8]

▲ **"My behavior is not really illegal."** This rationalization expresses a mistaken belief that one's behavior is acceptable, especially in ambiguous conditions. When dealing with "shady" or "borderline" situations in which you are having a hard time precisely defining right from wrong, the advice is quite simple: When in doubt about a decision to be made or an action to be taken, don't do it.

▲ **"My behavior is really in everyone's best interests."** This response involves the mistaken belief that because someone can be found to benefit from the behavior, the behavior is also in the individual's or the organization's best interests. Overcoming this rationalization depends in part on the ability to look beyond short-term results to address longer-term implications. It also requires looking beyond results in general to the ways in which they are obtained.

▲ **"Nobody will ever find out what I've done."** Sometimes rationalizers mistakenly believe that a questionable behavior is really "safe" and will never be found out or made public. Unless it is discovered, the argument implies, no wrong was really committed. Lack of accountability, unrealistic pressures to perform, and a boss who prefers "not to know" can all reinforce such thinking. In this case, the best deterrent is to make sure that everyone knows that wrongdoing will be punished whenever it is discovered.

▲ **"My company/boss/organization will protect me."** This rationalization is misperceived loyalty. You believe that the organization's best interests stand above all others. In return, you believe that top managers will condone your behavior and protect you from harm. Again, the advice is straightforward: Loyalty to the organization is not an acceptable excuse for misconduct.

2.1.4 Making Ethical Decisions

Numerous guidelines for making ethical decisions exist, but the following seven-step process offers a convenient, concise method for confronting ethical dilemmas. For more information on the process of making decisions, see section 8.1.

In particular, the following process serves as a reminder that good decision making typically involves double checking before taking action. For example, the key issue in the checklist may well be Step 6, which requires you (and the organization you're making decisions for) to essentially "look in the mirror" and evaluate the risk of public disclosure of your action and your willingness to bear it.[9]

Step 1: Recognize the ethical dilemma.

Step 2: Get the facts.

Step 3: Identify your options.

Step 4: Test each option: Is it legal? Is it right? Is it beneficial?

Step 5: Decide which option to follow.

Step 6: Double-check your decision by asking two questions:

> *"How would I feel if my family found out about my decision?"*

> *"How would I feel about this if my decision were printed in the local newspaper?"*

Step 7: Take action.

Be sure to turn to Chapter 8 for more information on the process of making decisions within a health care organization.

SELF-CHECK

- Identify and define **ethical behavior, ethical dilemma, ethics,** and **personal values.**
- List common ethical dilemmas.
- Discuss health care-specific ethical responses.
- Distinguish among the four most common ethical views: utilitarian, individualism, moral rights, and justice.
- Describe common rationalizations for unethical behavior.
- Explain a seven-step process for making ethical decisions.

2.2 Identifying Ethical Influences

Confronting ethical dilemmas from the safety of a textbook or a college classroom is almost too easy. In the real world, you are often challenged to choose ethical courses of action in situations that arise unexpectedly. The pressures to respond or act may be contradictory and great.

As shown in Figure 2-2, three main influences affect your ability to make ethical choices.

2.2.1 Personal Influences

Family influences; religious values; personal standards; and personal needs, financial and otherwise, all help determine your ethical conduct in any given circumstance.

Figure 2-2

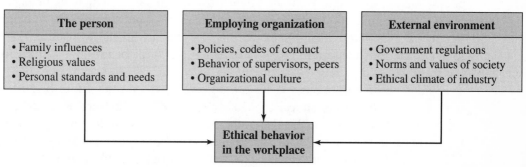

Factors influencing ethical behavior at work.

Managers who lack a strong and consistent set of personal ethics find that their decisions vary from situation to situation as they strive to maximize self-interests or please an ever-changing roster of supervisors and co-workers. Those who operate with strong ethical frameworks, positive personal rules or morals, or strategies for ethical decision making are more consistent and confident because their choices are made against a stable set of ethical standards.

2.2.2 Organizational Influences

The organization itself is another source of important influences on your ethical choices at work. Your supervisors can affect your behavior significantly. For example, what exactly a supervisor requests and the ways in which certain actions are rewarded or punished in an organization affect your decisions and actions. For example, if no one has ever been promoted to floor nurse in your organization without dumping difficult patients on newer staff members, you are more likely to burden lesser-experienced staff with tough cases in an effort to prove you'd be a good candidate for floor nurse.

Similarly, the expectations and reinforcements provided by your peers and group norms are likely to affect your behavior, and ultimately your ethics. For example, if asking for help when you become overwhelmed with end-of-the-month invoices is considered a sign of weakness in the medical billing office you work in, you're much less likely to assist an overwhelmed co-worker or to ask for an hour or two of assistance for yourself.

Formal policy statements and written rules, although they cannot guarantee results, are also very important in establishing an ethical climate for the organization as a whole. They support and reinforce the organizational culture, which can have a strong influence on your ethical behavior.

Ethics training—structured programs to help participants understand the ethical aspects of decision making—can help people incorporate high ethical standards into their daily behaviors.

However, the purpose of ethics training must be kept in perspective. Most ethics training programs focus on dramatized dilemmas in which participants brainstorm and discuss possible responses. The focus of most training is on helping people deal with ethical issues while under time or financial pressure—and to avoid the four common rationalizations for unethical behavior discussed in the section 2.1.3.

Senior health care managers have the power to shape the entire organization's policies and set its ethical tone. They can and should serve as models of appropriate ethical behavior for the entire organization. Not only must their day-to-day behavior be examples of high ethical conduct, but top managers must also regularly communicate similar expectations throughout the organization.

However, the responsibility to "lead by example" in regards to high ethical standards is not only top management's responsibility. All managers at all levels in all organizations are in positions to influence the ethical behavior of the people who work for and with them. Every manager is an ethical role model and must always bear this in mind when making decisions and interacting with others.

Codes of ethics are official written guidelines on how to behave in situations where ethical dilemmas are likely to occur. The codes of ethics for many health care organizations mirror the code of ethics of the medical professions. Within medical professions, ethical codes try to ensure that individual behavior is consistent with the historical and shared norms of the professional group.

Items frequently addressed in codes of ethics include

▲ workforce diversity;

▲ bribes and kickbacks;

▲ political contributions and activities;

▲ the honesty of records and patient information;

▲ appropriate employee relationships with patients;

▲ confidentiality of patient information;

▲ confidentiality of organizational information.

Although interest in codes of ethical conduct is growing, codes cannot cover all situations, and they cannot guarantee universal ethical conduct. The value of any formal code of ethics still rests on the underlying human resource foundations of the organization—its managers and other employees.

There is no replacement for effective hiring practices that staff an organization with honest and moral people. And there is no replacement for the leadership of committed managers who are willing to set the examples and act as ethical role models to ensure desired results.

FOR EXAMPLE

Answering Ongoing Ethical Questions at Beth Israel

Beth Israel Deaconess Medical Center (www.bidmc.harvard.edu) in Boston has responded to the ethical concerns of its patients, families, and staff by establishing the BIDMC Ethics Support Service. Medical personnel can contact a toll-free number 24 hours a day, 7 days a week and discuss ethics questions in a supportive manner. Following formal consultation, the service notes its assessment and recommendations in a patient's medical records, but any final decisions are the responsibility of the attending physician and patient. Additionally, the team also holds regular "ethics rounds" in which staff gathers to discuss recent ethical questions at Beth Israel and other health care organizations worldwide.

2.2.3 Environmental Influences

As section 1.1 discusses, all organizations operate in external environments, which include competitors, government laws and regulations, and social norms and values, among other influences. Laws interpret social values to define appropriate behaviors for organizations and their members; regulations help governments monitor these behaviors and keep them within acceptable standards.

The climate of competition in an industry also sets a standard of behavior for those who hope to prosper within it. Sometimes the pressures of competition contribute further to the ethical dilemmas of managers. Outside groups and stakeholder organizations can also influence the ethical environment.

SELF-CHECK

- Identify and define **ethics training** and **code of ethics.**
- Compare the three types of ethical influences: personal, organizational, and environmental.
- Describe three ways organizations attempt to influence and encourage ethical behavior.
- List topics that are frequently covered by formal codes of ethics.

2.3 Taking Social Responsibility

Concerns for ethical behavior must extend beyond the behaviors of individual workers and managers. Ethical concerns must also apply to the organization as a whole. Chapter 1 describes the environment of a health care organization as a network of other organizations and institutions with which it must interact.

Social responsibility is defined by health care organizations and other businesses in a variety of ways, including concerns for ecology and environmental quality, patient care and protection, and ongoing aid in community education. Many health care organizations also include direct service to community needs, positive employment practices, positive diversity practices, progressive labor relations, employee assistance, and general corporate philanthropy, as part of their social responsibility.

Regardless of the activities an organization considers as part of its social responsibility, social responsibility in the broadest sense is an obligation of the organization to act in ways that serve both

▲ its own interests and
▲ the interests of individuals and groups affected by the behavior of an organization.

2.3.1 Making the Case for Social Responsibility

Organizations choose to be socially responsible for various reasons, including some or all the following:

- ▲ People do their best in healthy work environments that permit job involvement, respect for contributions, and a good balance of work and family life.
- ▲ Organizations function best over the long run when located in healthy communities with high qualities of life.
- ▲ Organizations realize performance gains and efficiencies when they treat the natural environment with respect.
- ▲ The reputation of an organization must be protected to ensure consumer and stakeholder support.

The public at large now expects health care organizations to act with genuine social responsibility and to integrate social responsibility into their core values and daily activities. And on the business side of health care organizations, the argument that social responsibly efforts negatively affect the organization's bottom line is hard to defend. Increasing evidence shows that socially responsible organizations also exhibit strong financial performance (and, at worst, socially responsible organizations experience no adverse financial impact). Businesses can serve the public good as well as a broad pool of stakeholders (including financial shareholders).

2.3.2 Putting Social Responsibility into Action

Some health care organizations perform a **social audit** to report on and systematically assess an organization's commitments and accomplishments in the areas of social responsibility. Often conducted at regular intervals—annually, every other year, or every 5 years are common intervals—social audits give organizations a sense of how well they're meeting their socially responsible goals and how their contributions compare to other similar organizations.

Social audits typically cover four areas of organizational responsibility (as you move down the list, the types of responsibilities become increasingly socially responsible):

- ▲ **Economic responsibility:** A for-profit organization meets its economic responsibility when it earns a profit by selling a certain amount of goods and services, thus satisfying investors' expectations. A not-for-profit organization meets its economic responsibility when it earns enough money to fully pay for its programs, employees, and long-term endowment investments.
- ▲ **Legal responsibility:** When an organization operates within the law (including federal, state, and local regulations), its meets its legal responsibility.

FOR EXAMPLE

Global Alliance for Vaccines and Immunization

The Global Alliance for Vaccines and Immunization (GAVI) began in 2000 as a coalition of private, public, and governmental groups united by an overarching mission to "save children's lives and protect people's health through the widespread use of vaccines." To meet a complex array of economic, legal, ethical, and discretionary responsibilities, GAVI relies on an executive board to set policies of its numerous working groups worldwide. Five renewable members (WHO, UNICEF, the World Bank, the Bill & Melinda Gates Foundation, and the Vaccine Fund), along with 12 rotating members with medical, financial, and/or philanthropic expertise, regularly meet and discuss how to balance GAVI's inspiring global vision with its demanding financial needs. The board's decisions are frequently published online at www.vaccinealliance.org.

▲ **Ethical responsibility:** An organization meets its ethical responsibility when its actions *voluntarily* conform not only to legal expectations but also to the broader values and moral expectations of society.

▲ **Discretionary responsibility:** The highest level of social performance comes through the satisfaction of an organization's discretionary responsibility. Here, the organization *voluntarily* provides leadership in advancing the well-being of individuals, communities, and society as a whole.[10]

2.3.3 Obeying the Law

Governments often pass laws and establish regulatory agencies to ensure that organizations act responsibly. You probably know these agencies best by their acronyms: FAA (Federal Aviation Administration), EPA (Environmental Protection Agency), OSHA (Occupational Safety and Health Administration), and FDA (Food and Drug Administration), among many others.

Executives within the business community and the health care industry sometimes complain that laws and regulatory agencies are overly burdensome. Many express concerns that regulations raise costs by increasing the paperwork and staff necessary to comply with regulations. Many executives feel that regulation diverts their attention from important productivity, profit, or patient-consumer concerns.

In reality, the legal environment is both complex and constantly changing. Many themes discussed as being key areas of social responsibility in this chapter are backed by major federal, state, and local laws. Managers must stay informed about new and pending laws, as well as existing ones.

As a reminder of the positive side of legislation, consider a few examples of how the U.S. government takes an active role in regulating businesses, including health care organizations.

▲ **Occupational safety and health:** The Occupational Safety and Health Act of 1970 firmly established that the federal government was concerned about worker health and safety on the job.

▲ **Fair labor practices:** The Equal Employment Opportunity Act of 1972 and many following regulations are designed to eliminate discrimination in labor practices based on race, gender, age, national origin, and marital status.

▲ **Consumer protection:** The Consumer Product Safety Act of 1972 gives government authority to examine and force a business to withdraw from selling any product that it feels is hazardous to the consumer.

▲ **Environmental protection:** The Air Pollution Control Act of 1962 was the first in a series designed to eliminate careless pollution of the air, water, and land.

2.3.4 Making the Difference—One Manager at a Time

As public demands grow for organizations to be accountable for ethical and social performance, the manager stands in the middle. A manager's decisions affect quality-of-life outcomes in the critical boundaries between people and organizations and between organizations and their environments. Everyone must be more than willing to increase the weight given to ethical and social responsibility considerations when making decisions.

Figure 2-3 presents the manager's or team leader's challenge this way: to fulfill accountabilities for achieving performance objectives, while always doing so

Figure 2-3

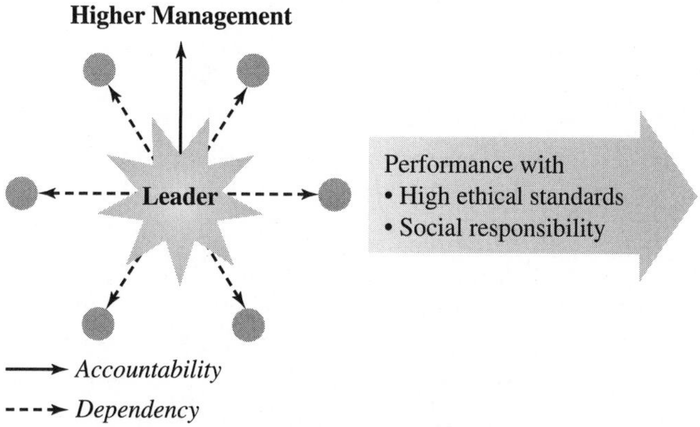

Central nature of ethics and social responsibility
in leadership and the managerial role.

in an ethical and socially responsible manner. The full weight of this responsibility holds in every organizational setting—small to large, private or public, for-profit or not-for-profit. There is no escaping the ultimate reality: being a manager is a very socially responsible job!

Today's health care workplace expects and demands managers who fully accept the responsibilities of ethical leadership, which is moral leadership that meets the test of being "good" rather than "bad," and "right" rather than "wrong." Trends in the evolution of social values point to ever-increasing demands from governments and other stakeholders that managerial decisions reflect ethical as well as high-performance goals. Today's workers and managers, as well as tomorrow's, must accept personal responsibility for doing the "right" things. Broad social and moral criteria must be used to examine the interests of multiple stakeholders in this dynamic and complex environment.

SELF-CHECK

- Identify and define **social responsibility** and **social audit**.
- List reasons for organizations to act in a socially responsible manner.
- Describe the four areas typically covered in a social audit.
- Identify major laws and governmental organizations that impact an organization's social responsibility.

SUMMARY

Not only must today's health care managers strive to manage people and processes for maximum productivity, these individuals must also be ethical leaders for their staffs and organizations. Ethical dilemmas abound in today's workplace, but managers can still respond to situations ethically, based on various ethical viewpoints and standardized decision-making processes. While a person's ethics and morals are affected by his or her personal background and overarching environmental influences, organizations can also influence ethical behavior through ethics training, ethical leadership, and codes of ethics. Social responsibility takes ethics a step further, requiring organizations to act in ways that are legally appropriate and encourage the well-being of individuals, communities, and society as a whole.

KEY TERMS

Codes of ethics	Official written guidelines on how to behave in situations where ethical dilemmas are likely to occur.
Ethical behavior	What is accepted to be "good" and "right" as opposed to "bad" or "wrong" in the context of the governing code.
Ethical dilemma	A situation that requires you to make a choice or take action that, although offering the potential for personal or organizational benefit, may be considered unethical.
Ethics	Collection of moral principles within a group or organization that set standards of good or bad, or right or wrong, for one's conduct.
Ethics training	Structured programs to help participants understand the ethical aspects of decision making.
Individualism view	Based on the belief that your primary commitment is to the advancement of your long-term self-interests.
Justice view	Based on the belief that all ethical decisions should treat people impartially and fairly, according to guiding rules and standards
Moral-rights view	Respects and protects the fundamental rights of people. Decisions are made in response to an ideal or moral, not based on personal or individual circumstances.
Personal values	Morals, or the underlying beliefs and attitudes that help determine individual behavior.
Social audit	A systematic assessment of an organization's commitments and accomplishments in the areas of social responsibility.
Social responsibility	Having concern for issues beyond business-related issues, including ecology and environmental quality, patient care and protection, and community involvement.
Utilitarian view	Also known as **results-oriented point of view**, this ethical standpoint tries to assess the moral implications of a decision in terms of its consequences.

ASSESS YOUR UNDERSTANDING

Go to www.wiley.com/college/Lombardi to evaluate your knowledge of the basics of ethics in health care.
Measure your learning by comparing pretest and post-test results.

Summary Questions

1. The only purpose of ethics is to help people determine whether an action is legal and illegal. True or false?

2. Ethical dilemmas frequently involve questions regarding
   (a) conflicts of interest.
   (b) use of company resources.
   (c) preferential treatment.
   (d) all of the above.

3. Many health care organizations have an organizational ethic that relates to how patients are treated. This ethic relates to
   (a) confidentiality.
   (b) care.
   (c) concern.
   (d) community.

4. An individualism view of ethics can promote honesty and integrity in the workplace, but it can also lead to disregard for rules that aren't agreeable with the individual. True or false?

5. Laws and regulations are what type of ethical influence?
   (a) Personal
   (b) Organizational
   (c) Environmental
   (d) Legal

6. Personal influences on ethical choices can include all of the following except
   (a) financial needs.
   (b) employee handbook.
   (c) family influences.
   (d) religious beliefs.

7. "Leading by example" is largely the responsibility of upper management in a health care organization. True or false?

8. Each organization defines *social responsibility* for itself, often including concerns, employment equality, labor relations, and corporate philanthropy. True or false?

9. One reason organizations should choose to be socially responsible is that
   (a) organizations function best over the long run when located in healthy communities.
   (b) organizations are held accountable by the EPA for environmental damage.
   (c) organizations owe their employees the best possible work environment.
   (d) organizations grow more quickly when they are profitable.
10. Social audits compare an organization's code of ethics with other similar organizations, attempting to determine the best possible plan for going forward. True or false?
11. Previous governmental legislation has encouraged organizations to act in a socially responsible manner in which of the following areas?
   (a) Environmental protection
   (b) Fair labor practices
   (c) Occupational health and safety
   (d) All of the above

Review Questions

1. A health care worker shares patient information with a pharmaceutical representative to assist the rep in putting together a survey that could potentially help the patient gain access to a new drug. What sort of ethical dilemma is the worker engaged in?
2. Using greater profits and efficiency to justify a difficult decision is typical of what ethical viewpoint?
3. You routinely take paper towels for personal use from your department's supply room because you know that no one really monitors the inventory for paper products. What rationalization are you engaging in?
4. What are three questions that you can use to test your options in ethical decision making?
5. In addition to laws and regulations, what are some environmental influences on ethical behavior?
6. Where might an employee turn for help dealing with questions of whether he or she can make a contribution to a political party?
7. What are some appropriate topics for an organization's formal code of ethics to address?
8. In the broadest sense, social responsibility is an obligation of an organization to serve the interests of what two groups?
9. What four areas of social responsibility do social audits usually pay attention to?

10. In what ways is discretionary responsibility the highest level of social responsibility?

11. Which governmental agencies help ensure that organizations act in a socially responsible manner?

Applying This Chapter

1. A drug-treatment program's mission statement says that "every human being has the right to live free from addictions and chemical vices." Consider the ethics that support this mission statement. Which ethical viewpoint does this mission statement align with?

2. A medical assistant at an in-house corporate health center frequently helps workers pass annual drug screenings by altering urine samples. The assistant feels that drug-screening is unnecessary because no employees operate heavy machinery or do anything that risks the lives of themselves or others. Besides, the assistant reasons that what workers do on their own time is their personal business. What type of rationalization for unethical behavior is the assistant using?

3. When the CEO of an insurance company states in an interview that her company will not share customer information with a direct marketing firm, even though the relationship could be profitable for the insurance company, how is the CEO helping maintain high ethical standards?

4. A nursing home's annual report to patients and their families notes that the facility has operated debt and litigation-free for the last 16 years, although many of its competitors have accrued significant financial liability and entered into expensive lawsuits. What two levels of organizational responsibility is the facility highlighting?

5. You manage a team of customer service representatives at an insurance call center. Several on your team have been complaining about new federal restrictions on privacy and the additional paperwork they must process for each claim. How might you respond to these team members, letting them know the importance and necessity of complying with the new laws?

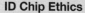

ID Chip Ethics

For years, people with life-threatening allergies or diseases have worn metal identification necklaces or bracelets to alert emergency caregivers to special medical conditions. Several technology firms recently began offering embeddable microchips that do the same job as wearable ID While potentially lifesaving, embeddable chips can also give hospitals instant access to much more patient information, including personal and financial data. An organization of emergency physicans formally supported the ID chips, taking a utilitarian view and saying that the benefits of ID chips to provide life-saving emergency medical care outweigh the potential risk of abuse. What would be a positive response based on individualism to the ID chips? What would be a response based on moral rights or justice?

Evaluate a Plan's Ethics

As the manager of a student health clinic on a small college campus, you meet daily with students to discuss and screen for sexually transmitted diseases. In the last month, you and your staff have noted a dramatic increase in chlamydia cases for students residing in one co-education dorm facility. You and your staff decide to post flyers about the symptoms and risks of chlamydia in the dorm bathrooms and lead a short educational session during the next all-dorm meeting. Is your plan legal, right, and beneficial? Run through the seven-step process for ethical decision making, paying particular attention to Steps 4 and 6.

Your Ethical Influences

Recall an ethical decision you made in the last year. Perhaps you had to make a difficult choice related to your education, career, employment, or personal life. What were some of the pros and cons of going with the decision you made? What specifically influenced your decision? Were these influences personal, organizational, or environmental? Was there a combination of influences?

Responding with Social Responsibility

One technique to encourage socially responsible behavior is to utilize a *stress-positive approach* to dealing with news reports. Television, magazines, newspapers, and online information sources today seem to be filled with potentially alarming information about the state of health care, our government, and the world in general. Rather than letting yourself feel overwhelmed by the information, ask yourself how these news items might affect your studies, your career goals, or how you do your job. The next time you encounter a potentially alarming news story, remind yourself that news reports are simply information; you can respond with negative stress (worrying about your job prospects or even distressing about the future of the world), or you can use the information to educate yourself and help focus your studies or work behaviors to act in a more socially responsible manner.

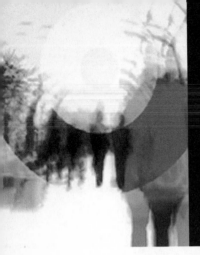

3

ORGANIZING THE WORKPLACE
Exploring the Fundamentals of Organizing Structures

Starting Point

Go to www.wiley.com/college/Lombardi to assess your knowledge of the basics of workplace organization.
Determine where you need to concentrate your effort.

What You'll Learn in This Chapter

▲ Traditional and more recently developed organizational structures
▲ Functional, divisional, and matrix structures
▲ The importance of teams and teamwork in today's health care workplace
▲ Trends and changes in organizing the health care workplace
▲ Organizational tools such as divisions, committees, teams, and task forces

After Studying This Chapter, You'll Be Able To

▲ Compare formal and informal organizational structures
▲ Employ common team structures
▲ Analyze ways in which health care organizations are adapting to workplace trends
▲ Compare organizational design options

Goals and Outcomes

▲ Master the terminology and tools related to organizational structures
▲ Choose the best organizational structures—including functional, divisional, and matrix structures for various situations
▲ Compare the purposes of teams, committees, divisions, and departments as organizational structures
▲ Respond effectively to organizational trends and changes
▲ Use delegation techniques
▲ Establish subsystems within organizations
▲ Design effective, efficient organizations
▲ Evaluate the effectiveness of organizational structures

INTRODUCTION

Health care organizations are trying a variety of new forms and structures in the quest for greater productivity, improved patient care, and competitive advantage. Some organizations follow traditional patterns based on functional, divisional, and matrix structures, while others experiment with nontraditional directions—emphasizing teams, networks, and even "boundaryless" organizations. Today's health care organizations must effectively and creatively respond to trends in the modern workplace changes, including shorter chains of command, increased delegation, and decentralization. Subsystems, work process evaluation, and teams are useful adaptations to include when designing an organization.

3.1 Understanding Common Organizational Structures

Formally defined, **organizing** is the process of arranging people and other resources to work together to accomplish a goal. Organizing involves both dividing up the tasks to be performed and coordinating results to achieve a common purpose.

Figure 3-1 shows the central role organizing plays in the management process. As the figure shows, managers are responsible for carrying out plans. Planning activities often precede organizing tasks, but the sequence varies based on the needs and culture of each health care organization. (Chapter 6 covers the planning process in detail.) Many beginning health care managers must first follow long-standing plans and procedures that upper managers or former managers created before creating new plans of their own. Whatever the specifics of your situation, organizing and planning tasks often happen in close conjunction; be flexible and adjust your management duties to suit the situation.

Figure 3-1

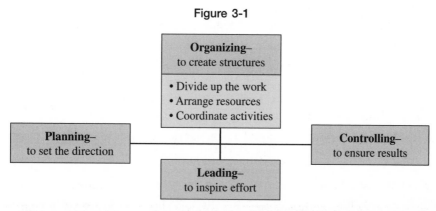

Organizing, as it relates with other management functions.

At the most basic level, organizing includes

▲ implementing a clear mission, core values, objectives, and strategy;
▲ identifying who is to do what, who is in charge of whom, and how different people and parts of the organization relate to one another.

The challenge of organizing effectively is to choose the best form or structure to fit the demands of a given situation.[1]

The **organization structure** is the system of tasks, workflow, reporting relationships, and communication channels that link the diverse parts of an organization. The specific structures vary greatly between health care organizations, but generally, any structure must both allocate or assign tasks and provide for the coordination of performance results.

Unfortunately, talking about good structures is easier than actually creating them. This is why you often read and hear about **restructuring,** the process of changing an organization's structure in an attempt to improve performance.

Organization structures can be described and classified in several ways based on formality, function, divisions, and more.

3.1.1 Formal and Informal Structures

You may know the concept of structure best in the form of an organization chart. A typical **organization chart** identifies, by diagram, key positions and job titles within an organization. It shows the lines of authority and communication between them.[2]

An organizational chart shows the **formal structure,** the intended or official structure. The diagram depicts the way the organization is intended to function. Organizational charts can tell much about an organization, including

▲ **the division of work:** Positions and titles show how work responsibilities are assigned;
▲ **supervisory relationships:** Lines among positions show who reports to whom;
▲ **communication channels:** Lines among positions show formal communication channels;
▲ **major subunits:** Positions reporting to a common manager are identified as a group;
▲ **levels of management:** Layers of management from top to bottom are shown.

Figure 3-2 shows the formal organizational chart for a midsize teaching hospital.

However, behind every formal structure typically lies an **informal structure.** This is a "shadow" organization made up of the unofficial, but often critical,

Figure 3-2

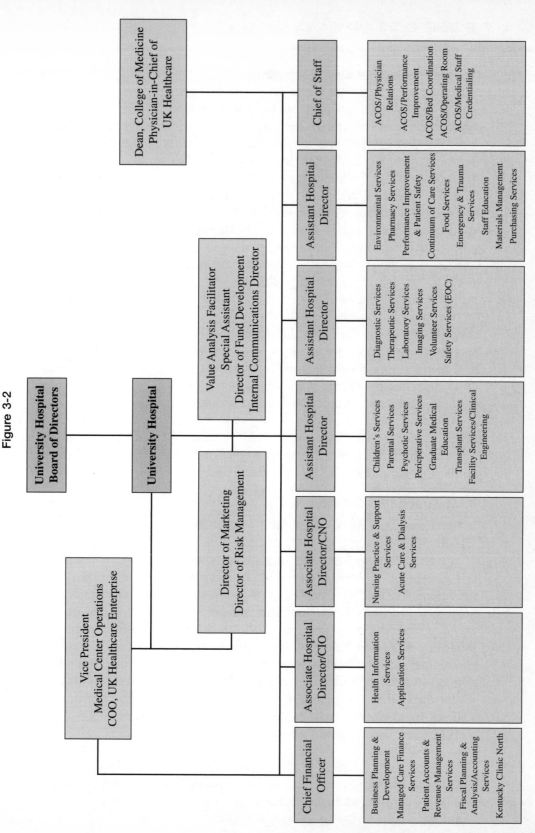

Formal organizational chart for a midsize teaching hospital.

working relationships among organizational members. If you drew an organization's informal structure, it would show who talks to and interacts regularly with whom, regardless of their formal titles and relationships. Informal structures include people meeting for coffee, exercise groups, friendship cliques, and many other possibilities. The lines of informal structures often cut across levels and move from side to side, rather than solely up and down.

Because of the complex nature of organizations and constantly shifting performance demands, informal structures can be very helpful in accomplishing large and small tasks. Through the emergent and spontaneous relationships of informal structures, people gain access to interpersonal networks of emotional support and friendship that satisfy important social needs. They also benefit from contacts with others who can help them better perform their jobs and tasks. Valuable learning and knowledge sharing takes place as people interact informally throughout the workday and in a variety of unstructured situations.

Savvy organizations identify and capitalize on their informal structures. For example, a study by the Center for Workforce Development found that the cafeteria can be a "hotbed for informal learning," as workers at a variety of levels tend to share ideas, problems, and solutions with one another over snacks and meals. Dynamic health care managers can mobilize these types of informal learning opportunities as resources for organizational improvement.[3]

Of course, informal structures also have potential disadvantages. They can be susceptible to rumor, carry inaccurate information, breed resistance to change, and even divert work efforts from important objectives. People who feel left out of informal groupings may become dissatisfied.[4]

3.1.2 Functional Structures

In **functional structures,** people with similar skills and performing similar tasks are grouped together.

Figure 3-3 shows functional organizations on a large and small scale. In the first example, a health care organization is organized by the functions of marketing/public relations, finance, patient services, and human resources. In this functional structure, patient problems are the responsibility of the patient vice president, marketing problems are the province of the marketing and PR vice president, and so on. In the second chart, a midsize medical clinic is run by a clinic supervisor and four function-specific managers of nursing, office administration, accounting, and laboratory services. Members of each function work within their areas of expertise. In both diagrams, if each function does its job well, the expectation is that the businesses will operate successfully.

The major advantages of a functional structure include

▲ efficient use of resources within and between functional areas;

▲ consistent and appropriate task assignments based on expertise and training within each functional area;

▲ high-quality technical problem-solving;

Figure 3-3

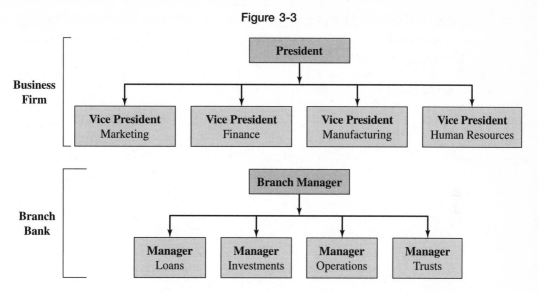

Functional structures for a health care organization and a medical clinic.

▲ in-depth training and skill development within functions;

▲ clear career paths within functions.

However, focusing strongly on functions, functional expertise, and functional careers can sometimes create problems within organizations:

▲ **Functional chimneys:** When members of a specific functional group develop self-centered and narrow viewpoints, become uncooperative with other groups, and lose the ability to focus on the larger picture, a **functional chimney** develops. Each function ends up communicating, coordinating, and problem-solving up and down its chain of command (like a chimney) without extending sideways to other function groups.

▲ **Reliance on upper management:** When problems occur between function groups, they are too often referred up to higher levels for resolution rather than being addressed directly at the level of action. Running problems up the managerial flagpole slows decision making and problem-solving—and over time can result in a loss of competitive advantage.

▲ **Confusion and responsibility-shifting:** Focusing too heavily on function groups can create responsibility confusion for issues that actually every group (and indeed, person) in the organization should be accountable for. For example, cost containment, timeliness, patient care, and ongoing responses to legal and business changes are duties that everyone in an organization—both the newly hired payroll clerk and the experienced director of pediatric medicine—need to consider, discuss within their functional groups, and share ideas between functional groups.

3.1.3 Divisional Structures

Another traditional way to discuss organizations is to focus on divisional structure. **Divisional structures** group together people who

▲ provide the same services;

▲ work within the same processes;

▲ serve similar patients;

▲ are located in the same area or geographical region.

As illustrated in Figure 3-4, divisional structures are common in complex organizations that have multiple and differentiated products and services, pursue diversified strategies, and/or operate in several competitive environments.[5]

The potential advantages of divisional structures include the following:

▲ More flexibility in responding to environmental changes.

▲ Improved coordination across functional departments.

Figure 3-4

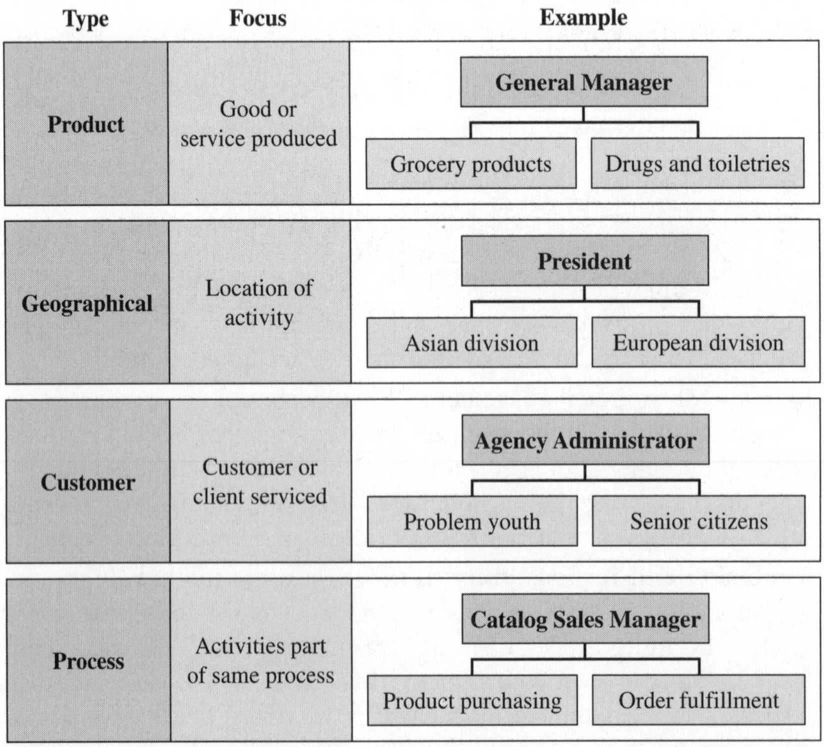

Type	Focus	Example
Product	Good or service produced	**General Manager** → Grocery products | Drugs and toiletries
Geographical	Location of activity	**President** → Asian division | European division
Customer	Customer or client serviced	**Agency Administrator** → Problem youth | Senior citizens
Process	Activities part of same process	**Catalog Sales Manager** → Product purchasing | Order fulfillment

Divisional structures based on service, geography, patient, and process.

▲ Clearer points of responsibility for delivery of services or products.

▲ Expertise focused on specific patients or customers, products, and regions.

▲ Greater ease in changing size by adding or deleting divisions.

Of course, divisional structures also have potential disadvantages as well:

▲ **Redundancy:** Divisional structures can reduce efficiencies and increase costs by duplicating resources and efforts across divisions. A divisional structure based on geographic region, for example, may require a full-time lab technician at all 20 clinic locations spread throughout a state, rather than having a central lab facility with 12 full-time technicians.

▲ **Internal competition:** Unhealthy rivalries can emerge as divisions compete for resources and attention or focus heavily on the performance of their division compared to similar divisions within the organization. Rewarding individual divisions for outstanding performance can encourage increased productivity and improve workplace attitudes, but it can also lead divisions to forget the larger goals and mission of the entire health care organization.

▲ **Tunnel vision:** Divisional structures can encourage a division to focus on its needs and goals rather than the best interests of the organization as a whole. (Of course, this "tunnel vision" can happen with functional structures, too.)

3.1.4 Matrix Structures

A **matrix structure** combines elements of both the functional and divisional structures. The goal is to combine the advantages of each, while minimizing disadvantages. As shown in Figure 3-5, a matrix structure uses permanent **cross-functional teams** to integrate functional expertise with a divisional focus. Workers in a matrix structure belong to at least two formal groups at the same time—a functional group and a product, program, or project team. They also report to two bosses—one within the function and the other within the team. The cross-functional team members work closely together to share functional expertise and information to solve problems in a timely manner.

The potential advantages of matrix structures include

▲ more interfunctional cooperation in operations;

▲ increased flexibility in meeting changing demands;

▲ better customer service championed by individual project managers;

▲ better performance accountability through the project managers;

Figure 3-5

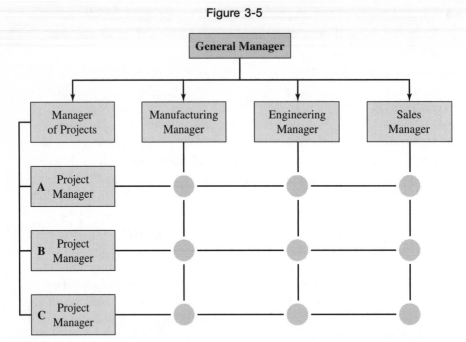

Functional personnel assigned to both projects and their respective functional departments

Matrix structure for a small public health organization.

▲ improved problem-solving at the team level, where the best information is available;

▲ improved strategic management, as top managers can focus on broader strategic issues (PR, patient care, and communications in Figure 3-5) rather than day-to-day specific tasks.

Predictably, the matrix structure also has potential disadvantages:

▲ **Power struggles:** The two-boss system is susceptible to confusion and conflict, especially when functional supervisors and team leaders vie with one another as to who has the ultimate authority for the project.

▲ **Priority confusion:** Members of the matrix may have difficulty determining which tasks to do first or where to focus their energies, especially when team members receive orders from more than one boss or manager.

▲ **Tunnel vision:** Like other structures this section discusses, matrix teams may develop "groupitis" or strong loyalties that focus attention more on the team than on larger organizational goals.

▲ **Expense:** The use of formal team leaders in a matrix structure can result in increased personnel costs.

FOR EXAMPLE

The Center for Collaborative Organizations

Begun as a student-run organization within the psychology department at the University of North Texas in 1990, the Center for Collaborative Organizations (www.workteams.unt.edu) is now a dynamic institution with eight full-time staff members and a nationally noted reputation for examining the ways in which companies are organized. With a mission of helping all organizations "design and implement work systems to maximize collaboration for organizational effectiveness," the Center hosts conferences and public workshops, as well as publishes original research, papers, and a free bimonthly newsletter on organizational structures in today's workplace. More than 20 free papers on organizational trends are available at www.workteams.unt.edu/literature/free.html; sign up for a free bimonthly newsletter and read previously published newsletters at www.workteams.unt.edu/newsletter.html.

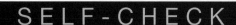

S E L F - C H E C K

- Identify and define **organizing, organizing structure,** and **restructuring.**
- Explain the role of organizing within the four functions of management.
- Compare formal structure and informal structure within an organization.
- Discuss advantages and disadvantages of organizing by functional structure, divisional structure, and matrix structure.

3.2 Exploring Recent Developments in Organization Structures

The global economy and the demands of hypercompetition have health care managers everywhere searching for organizational structures that better meet today's ever-changing environmental challenges.

Throughout the health care industry, traditional **vertical structures** are being dismantled in favor of more horizontal ones. In general, **horizontal structures** emphasize integration and cross-functional teamwork, often while gaining the advantages of networking through information technology.

The following sections discuss several of the most significant changes in organization structures in recent years.

3.2.1 The Team Approach

Teams are the building blocks of today's new and more-horizontal organizational forms. Team structures formally designate and use permanent and temporary teams extensively to accomplish tasks.[6]

As Figure 3-6 illustrates, a nursing care facility organized into teams can solve problems and explore opportunities in a more flexible manner. **Cross-functional teams** composed of members from different functional areas can work together on a part-time or full-time basis, depending on the needs of the organization.

The intention of a team-based approach is to break down functional chimneys (see section 3.1.2), increase information sharing, and create more effective lateral relations that improve problem-solving and performance. At a community health clinic, for example, staff may be assigned to one or more projects (community outreach, infant immunization, and disease education and prevention, to name just a few possibilities). With each project under the direction of a team leader, traditional hierarchy takes a backseat to the focus on team activities and project accomplishments.

The potential advantages of team structures are numerous and include

▲ better communication across functions;

▲ shared responsibility by all team members for meeting performance targets;

▲ fewer barriers between departments;

▲ improved morale, as people from different parts of an organization get to better know one another;

▲ improved speed and quality because the teams focus shared knowledge and expertise on specific problems.

Of course, teams and teamwork create many challenges as well. These include conflicting loyalties among members to both team and functional assignments,

Figure 3-6

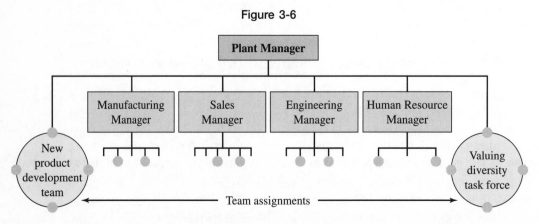

Team structure utilizing cross-functional teams for improved lateral relations.

> ## FOR EXAMPLE
>
> ### Attaching Goals and Timelines to Organizational Structures
>
> The Veterans Administration (VA) medical system in Hawaii (www.va.gov/hawaii) consists of four separate facilities on four islands. To effectively communicate its unique organizational structures as well as its ongoing goals, VA of Hawaii reviews its organizational chart annually and attaches goals and timelines to each relationship in its organizational chart. VA of Hawaii then publishes the organizational chart along with organizational performance and goals with its employees, physicians, and volunteers in its annual report. VA of Hawaii finds this method beneficial in getting goal commitment and understanding of reporting structures from all members in its four facilities.

issues of time management, and difficulties with interpersonal relations and group process. Sections 4.1 and 4.2 discuss ways to effectively manage and participate on teams.

3.2.2 Information and Technology Networks

Increasingly, today's health care organizations utilize advanced information technology to better link groups within the organization and with groups outside the organization.

A good example of this type of structure is the ongoing trend of groups of different medical services joining into a **health care network.** Thus, the offices of several pediatricians, an ears/nose/throat specialist, and an allergist might combine into a comprehensive children's health care network, sharing the services of one business office and laboratory. The group may even decide to work with outside contractors for some essential services (a child psychologist, for instance).

Network organizations such as this must use the latest computer and information technologies to support a shifting mix of strategic alliances and business contracts. With a technological edge, organizations can operate with fewer full-time employees and less complex internal systems. They can more easily develop and maintain partnerships, often across great distances. Networks can also help organizations stay cost competitive through reduced overhead and increased operating efficiency.

The potential disadvantages of network structures trace largely to the demands of coordinating the complex system of business relationships. If one part of the network breaks down or fails to deliver, the entire system suffers the consequences.

As information technology continues to develop, network structures are growing in number and complexity.[7] Networks can be useful for smaller organizations, including entrepreneurial ones. They are also appropriate components in larger organizations, enabling an organization to outsource specialized business functions or services rather than maintain full-time staff to do them.

3.2.3 Boundaryless Organizations

Although increasingly more common in the business world, the **boundaryless organization** combines the team and network structures described previously, with the addition of temporariness. Entrepreneurial, start-up, and dot-com businesses are often boundaryless organizations. The ability of these businesses to respond quickly to changes in their environments and create new solutions to complex problems makes boundaryless organizations an important organizational structure for health care managers to be aware of in the coming years.

▲ **Within boundaryless organizations,** context, teamwork, and communication replace formal lines of authority. Team members must react spontaneously to intense situation demands. Barriers that traditionally and structurally separate organizational members from one another are removed.

▲ **Outside boundaryless organizations,** organizational needs are met by a shifting mix of outsourcing contracts and operating alliances that form and disband with changing circumstances. The organization's configuration of external relationships today will look different from one taken tomorrow, as the form naturally adjusts to new pressures and circumstances.

Although few health organizations today are considered boundaryless organizations, many characteristics of boundaryless organizations are becoming part of the everyday structure of the modern health care workplace, specifically including the absence of hierarchy, empowerment of team members, technology utilization, and acceptance of impermanence. Work is accomplished by empowered people who come together voluntarily and temporally to apply their expertise to a task, gather additional expertise from whatever sources may be required to perform it successfully, and stay together only as long as the task is a work in process. The focus in the boundaryless form is on talent for task. The assumption is that empowered people working together without bureaucratic restrictions can accomplish great things. Such a work setting is supposed to encourage creativity, quality, timeliness, and flexibility, while reducing inefficiencies and increasing speed.

Knowledge sharing is an essential component of the boundaryless organization. People with talent work together as needed to get a job done. Meetings and spontaneous sharing can happen continuously, perhaps involving thousands of people working together in hundreds of teams that form and disband as needed. Again, the evolving opportunities of information technology help make this type of collaboration possible.

- Identify and define **team, cross-functional team, health care network,** and **boundaryless organization.**
- List characteristics and advantages of work-based teams.
- Compare teams, networks, and boundaryless organizations as tools for organizing a workplace.
- Describe challenges and solutions for health care networks and boundaryless organizations.

3.3 Responding to Recent Organizational Trends and Changes

As section 1.4 discusses, the concept of the **upside-down pyramid** is a powerful example of the new mindset evolving in health care management today. By putting patients on top, served by workers in the middle, who are in turn supported by managers at the bottom, the upside-down pyramid tries to refocus attention on the marketplace and patient needs.

Although the upside-down pyramid is more of a concept than a depiction of a formal organization structure, such thinking is representative of forces behind new trends in organizing the modern workplace. Among these trends is a common theme: managers (and indeed all workers) must make the necessary adjustments to streamline for cost efficiency and to allow increased worker involvement in all aspects of operations.

The following sections cover the most significant changes resulting from recent shifts in perspective.

3.3.1 Shorter Chains of Command

A typical organization chart shows a **chain of command,** or line of authority that vertically links all positions with successively higher levels of management. When organizations grow in size, they tend to get taller (or grow "vertically") as more levels of management are added to the chain of command. More layers of management increase overhead costs, add distance in communication, limit access between top and bottom levels, and can slow decision making. These are all reasons why "tall" organizations with many levels of management are often criticized for inefficiencies and poor productivity.

In the business world generally and the health care industry specifically, the current trend is to streamline organizations by cutting unnecessary levels of management. Flatter structures are viewed as a potential source of competitive advantage because they can respond more quickly and efficiently to situations.

Figure 3-7

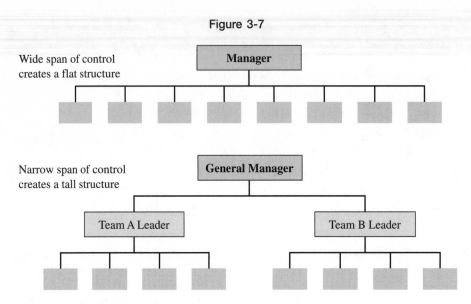

How span of control creates "flat" versus "tall" structures.

For the manager, shorter chains of command often mean broader responsibilities, greater empowerment, and people or processes to manage.

3.3.2 Wider Spans of Control

The **span of control** is the number of persons reporting directly to a manager. When span of control is narrow, only a few people are directly supervised; a wide span of control indicates that a manager supervises many people. Figure 3-7 shows the relationship between span of control and the number of management levels. Organizations with wider spans of control tend to be flat and have few levels of management. Those with narrow spans of control tend to be tall and have many levels of management.

Tall organizations are more costly and may be less efficient, less flexible, and less customer (or patient) sensitive than flatter ones. The current trend is toward wider spans of control that shorten chains of command and increase worker empowerment.

For the manager, wider spans of control often mean managing a more diverse staff, including many individuals with extensive technical skills outside the manager's training and experience.

3.3.3 Less Unity of Command

Traditional management theory emphasizes the **unity-of-command principle**— each person in an organization should report to one and only one supervisor.

This one person/one boss notion is intended to avoid the confusion created when a person gets work directions from more than one source.

The "two-boss" system of matrix structure violates unity of command. It does so on purpose and in an attempt to improve lateral relations and project teamwork. Unity of command is also less predominant in structures that use cross-functional teams or task forces. The current trend is for less, not more, unity of command in organizations.

For the manager, less unity of command often means additional effort coordinating, brainstorming, and even negotiating responsibilities and assignments for staff with other managers in the organization.

3.3.4 More Delegation and Empowerment

Managers and team leaders must decide what work they should do themselves and what should be left for others. At issue here is **delegation**—the process of distributing and entrusting work to other people.

Unfortunately, a common management mistake is failure to delegate. By not delegating, managers easily become overloaded with work that could and should be done by others. And failure to delegate denies others the opportunity to fully utilize their talents on the job. When done well, by contrast, delegation leads to empowerment. It gives people the freedom to contribute ideas and do their jobs in the best possible ways.

For today's health care manager, effectively delegating responsibilities and empowering team members to make strong, good decisions is critical for success of the work team and the entire organization. Sections 3.5 and 9.4.3 deal with the process of delegating.

3.3.5 Decentralization with Centralization

A question frequently asked by managers is, "Should most decisions be made at the top levels of an organization, or should they be dispersed by extensive delegation throughout all levels of management?"

Top-down decision making is sometimes referred to as **centralization;** dispersed decision making is called **decentralization**. Centralization/decentralization doesn't have to be an either/or choice. Today's health care organizations can operate with greater decentralization without losing centralized control. By using computer networks and advanced information systems, organizations allow higher-level managers to more easily stay informed about a wide range of day-to-day performance matters. Because the top has information on results readily available, it can allow more decentralization.[8] If something goes wrong, presumably the information system helps sound an alarm in time for corrective action to be taken quickly.

The current trend is toward more decentralization in organizations, while utilizing advances in information systems to retain centralized control. For the manager, this trend means greater reliance on technology to keep track of and quickly report productivity.

3.3.6 Reduced Use of Staff

Health care organizations often have large, diverse staffs to help provide expert advice, skills, guidance, and services. Unfortunately, a staff can grow to the point that it costs more in administrative overhead than it is worth. For this reason, staff cutbacks are a common first choice in downsizing and other cost-saving efforts.

What is best for any organization is a cost-effective, sensibly sized staff that satisfies, but doesn't overreact to, needs for specialized technical services and skills.

The current trend is for organizations to minimize the use of staff components in the quest for increased operating efficiency. Specialized services or skills are often hired on a contract basis, rather than paid for as a full-time staff position. For the manager, reduced use of staff means thinking creatively about how to meet specific technical demands in the workplace, without hiring too many full-time workers.

FOR EXAMPLE

Regional Reorganization for Catholic Healthcare West

In an effort to reduce management layers and increase local decision making at its 47 locations, Catholic Healthcare West (www.chwhealth.org) decided to undergo dramatic reorganization. The new structure streamlined reporting relationships, eliminated duplicate services in the main hospital and regional offices, and placed the hospital's CEO closer to day-to-day operations. Prior to 2001, the hospital's organizational structure consisted of 10 distinct regions in California, Nevada, and Arizona, each managed by a president/chief executive officer. After the restructuring, these 10 regions were replaced by four divisions, each managed by a division president. Although the number of hospitals remained constant, the restructuring eliminated approximately 350 corporate and administrative jobs, saving the organization more than $100 million annually. In the years following the reorganization, each division of Catholic Healthcare West has been able to respond more quickly to divisional needs, developing specialized programs and targeting specific communities.

SELF-CHECK

- Identify and define **upside-down pyramid organization, chain of command, span of control, unity of command principle, delegation, centralization,** and **decentralization.**
- Discuss how formal organizational structures are changing in terms of chains of command and spans of control.
- Describe trends in unity of control and delegation in today's workplace.
- Compare decentralization and centralization as decision-making strategies.

3.4 Designing Effective Organizations

Organizational design is the process of aligning organizational structures and cultures to best serve the organization's mission, strategy, and objectives.[9] Key directions today involve a basic shift in attention away from traditional, vertical, authority-driven organizations and toward those that are more horizontal and task-driven.

3.4.1 Bureaucratic versus Adaptive Designs

A **bureaucracy** is a form of organization based on logic, order, and the legitimate use of formal authority. Originally described by theorist Max Weber as "ideal" organizational forms, bureaucracies are supposed to be fair and highly efficient.[10] They operate with a clear-cut division of labor, a strict hierarchy of authority, formal rules and procedures, and career advancement based on competency. Today, most organizations recognize that there are limits to bureaucracy.[11] Organizations that rely too much on rules and procedures can become unwieldy, rigid, and slow in responding to changing environments.

However, a bureaucratic form can sometimes be appropriate for an organization. In a classic research study conducted in England during the early 1960s, Tom Burns and George Stalker concluded that different organizational forms could be successful, depending on the nature of an organization's external environment.[12] Specifically, more bureaucratic or "mechanistic" forms of organization work best in stable environments, while less bureaucratic and more "organic" forms perform best in changing and uncertain environments.

The left-hand portion of Figure 3-8 lists additional characteristics of bureaucratic organizations, including centralized authority, many rules and procedures, a precise division of labor, narrow spans of control, and formal means of coordination.

Figure 3-8

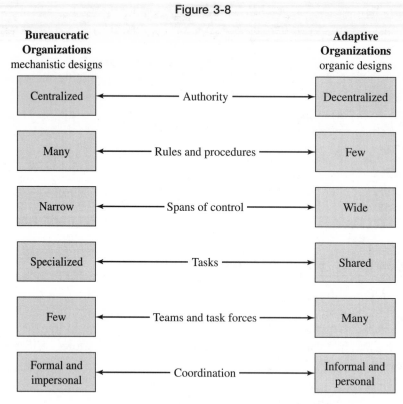

A continuum of organizational alternatives, from bureaucratic to adaptive organizations.

In today's modern workplace—including the rapidly changing health care industry—the ability to respond quickly to shifting challenges in rapidly changing environments often distinguishes successful organizations from less successful ones.[13] High performance in these circumstances is achieved by **adaptive organizations** with a minimum of bureaucratic features and with cultures that encourage worker empowerment and participation.

The right-hand portion of Figure 3-8 contrasts the characters of adaptive organizations with bureaucratic organizations. In general, adaptive organizations operate with more decentralized authority, fewer rules and procedures, less precise division of labor, wider spans of control, and more personal means of coordination. Adaptive organizations are flatter systems in which a lot of work gets done through informal structures and networks of interpersonal contacts.

The horizontal design features value teamwork and legitimate cross-functional linkages. They try to give otherwise capable employees the freedom to do what they can do best—get the job done. Above all, adaptive organizations are built upon eliminating restrictive centralized controls and trusting that people will do the right things on their own initiative.

3.4.2 Making Design Decisions

Good organizational design decisions satisfy situational demands and allow all resources to be used to best advantage.

The notion that "structure follows strategy" is an important premise of organizational design.[14]

▲ **When your strategy is stability oriented,** the premise is that little significant change will be occurring in the external environment. The supporting organization's structure should be well defined and predictable, as found in bureaucratic organizations using more mechanistic design alternatives.

▲ **When your strategy is growth oriented,** operating objectives are likely to include the need for innovation and flexible responses to changing competition in the environment. The most supportive structure is likely to be one that is more decentralized and empowered, as found in adaptive organizations using more organic design alternatives.

Size is another factor that plays a role in organizational design. Although research indicates that larger organizations tend to have more mechanistic structures than smaller ones, it is clear that this is not always best for them. In fact, a perplexing managerial concern is that organizations tend to become more bureaucratic as they grow in size and consequently have difficulty adapting to changing environments.

Good managers constantly search for unique ways to overcome the disadvantages of large size. They are creative in forming teams and smaller units, and allowing them to operate with considerable autonomy within the larger organizational framework. Such simultaneous structures combine mechanistic and organic designs to meet the need for both production efficiency and continued innovation.

Managers who want to design organizations and work processes that make good sense for their teams or departments, as well as the broader organization, can run through the following five critical questions, or checks, whenever they change, add to, or eliminate something from the design of an organization:

Check 1: Does the design fit well with the major problems and opportunities of the external environment?

Check 2: Does the design support the implementation of strategies and the accomplishment of key operating objectives?

Check 3: Does the design support core technologies and allow them to be used to best advantage?

Check 4: Can the design handle changes in organizational size and different stages in the organizational life cycle?

Check 5: Does the design support and empower workers and allow their talents to be used to best advantage?

FOR EXAMPLE

Facilitating Change at the Food and Drug Administration

The Office of Regulatory Affairs in the U.S. Food and Drug Administration (www.fda.gov/ora) established a special organizational development (OD) team to assist field offices throughout the United States in creating and implementing organizational changes. The OD team includes managerial and staff-level employees (two full-time OD specialists plus 10 to 12 others who spend a portion of their weekly time on organizational development tasks). The OD team is trained together on organizational topics and meets by video conference to share information. The Office of Regulatory Affairs regional and divisional managers can request the OD team's help to plan changes, assess departmental readiness for change, clarify vision, and implement change strategies.

3.4.3 Incorporating Subsystems

Small departments, work units, or teams headed by managers are **subsystems** that perform specialized tasks within organizations. Ideally, the work of each subsystem is efficient and well integrated to meet the needs of the larger organization.

Research in subsystems design by Paul Lawrence and Jay Lorsch of Harvard University[15] found that not only did successful firms match their overall organizational designs to their respective environmental challenges, but they also matched their subsystem designs to the challenges of their respective subenvironments. So, as an example, a successful inner-city hospital might include divisions targeting the needs of its community (emergency care, chemical dependency, pediatric medicine, and so on) as well as having special programs within a division further targeting the needs of the community (subsidized early childhood vaccines within pediatric medicine, for instance).

Additionally, Lawrence and Lorsch's research found that subsystems within successful organizations

▲ **included different structures** to better accommodate the special problems and opportunities of their unique operating situations. This illustrates **differentiation,** or the degree of difference that exists between the internal components of the organization;

▲ **worked well with one another,** even though they had very different structures. This illustrates **integration,** the level of coordination achieved among an organization's internal components.

Figure 3-9 shows how research, patient-care, and community relations divisions in a single hospital can operate differently in response to unique needs, yet still provide outstanding medical services to all its constitutes.

Figure 3-9

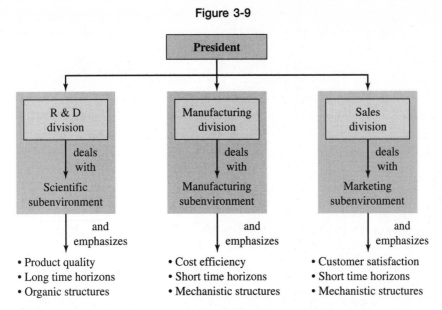

Differentiation among research, patient-care, and community relations divisions.

As Figure 3-9 shows, four common sources of differentiation exist among these and other subsystems:

▲ **Differences in time orientation become characteristic of work units themselves.** This occurs as the planning and action horizons of managers vary from short term to long term. In the hospital described in Figure 3-9, for example, the patient-care subsystem may have a shorter-term outlook than does the research group. These differences can make it difficult for personnel from the two units to work well together.

▲ **Different tasks assigned to work units may result in differences in objectives.** For example, a cost- and efficiency-conscious shift manager and a volume-conscious public relations manager may have difficulty agreeing on solutions to common problems.

▲ **Differences in interpersonal orientation can affect subsystem relations.** To the extent that patterns of communication, decision making, and social interaction vary, it may be harder for personnel from different subsystems to work together.

▲ **Differences in formal structure can also affect subsystem behaviors.** Someone who is used to flexible problem-solving in an organic setting may find it very frustrating to work with representatives from a mechanistic setting that operates with very strict rules.

As described by the Lawrence and Lorsch study, successful organizations operate with both differentiated structures and appropriate integrating mechanisms. A basic paradox, however, makes this a particularly challenging task in organizational design: Increased differentiation among organizational subsystems creates the need for greater integration, but integration becomes harder to achieve as differentiation increases.

Bottom line: Subsystems need to be different, but integrating subsystems is a challenge. Keep the following tips in mind when attempting to improve subsystem integration:[16]

▲ Clearly specify required activities (such as rules and procedures everyone must follow).

▲ Refer problems between divisions upward, to a common boss if possible.

▲ Plan and set clear targets and goals so everyone is heading in the same direction.

▲ Assign formal coordinators to act as liaisons and link subunits.

▲ Form temporary task forces to coordinate activities and solve specific problems.

▲ Form permanent teams with the authority to coordinate and solve problems as they occur over time.

▲ Create a matrix structure to improve coordination among multiple and diverse projects.

3.4.4 Evaluating Work Processes

Researcher Michael Hammer defines a **work process** as "a related group of tasks that together create a result of value for the customer."[17] Four aspects of Hammer's definition are particularly worth noting:

▲ **Group of tasks:** Tasks are viewed as part of a group rather than in isolation.

▲ **Together:** Everyone must share a common goal.

▲ **Result:** The focus is on what is accomplished, not merely on activities.

▲ **Customer:** Processes serve customers (or patients in the case of health care organizations), and the patients' perspectives are the ones that really count.

Today's health care managers are frequently asked to reorganize the way their departments, teams, and staffs work and interact. **Process reengineering** is the systematic and complete analysis of work processes and the design of new and better ones.[18] The goal of process reengineering is to focus attention on the future, on patients, and on improving ways of doing things. It tries to break people and mind-sets away from habits, preoccupation with past accomplishments, and tendencies to continue implementing old and outmoded ways of doing things. Simply put, reengineering is a radical and disciplined approach to changing the way work is carried out in organizations.

Through **process value analysis,** managers identify and carefully evaluate each step in a workflow. In rigorous process value analysis, managers must find each step important, useful, and adding value to the overall purpose of the organization. If not, the step is eliminated. Process value analysis typically involves the following steps.[19]

1. Identify the core processes.
2. Map the core processes in respect to workflows.
3. Evaluate all tasks for the core processes.
4. Search for ways to eliminate unnecessary tasks or work.
5. Search for ways to eliminate delays, errors, and misunderstandings.
6. Search for efficiencies in how work is shared and transferred among people and departments.

Patients, teamwork, and efficiency are all central to process reengineering. The goal is to redesign core processes to center control for them with an identifiable group of people and to focus the entire system on best meeting patient needs and expectations.

Process reengineering tries to eliminate duplications of work and systems bottlenecks. In so doing, it tries to reduce costs and streamline operations efficiency.

SELF-CHECK

- Identify and define **organizational design, bureaucracy, adaptive organizations, subsystems, differentiation, integration, process *reengineering,*** and **process value analysis.**
- List characteristics of bureaucratic and adaptive organizational designs.
- Describe strategies for the process of organizing a department.
- Discuss five checks to consider prior to any organizational change.
- Explain four reasons for including subsystems in an organization.
- Sequence the six steps of process value analysis.

3.5 Dividing Work among Teams

Formally defined, a *team* is a small group of people with complementary skills, who work together to achieve a shared purpose and who hold themselves mutually accountable for its accomplishment.[20]

Teamwork is the process of people working together to accomplish these goals. The ability to lead through teamwork requires a special understanding of how teams operate and the commitment to use that understanding to help them achieve high levels of task performance and membership satisfaction. One of the biggest benefits of teamwork is **synergy**—the creation of a whole that is greater than the sum of its parts. Synergy occurs when teams use their resources to the fullest and achieve, through collective performance, far more than is otherwise possible.

An important part of a manager's job is knowing when a team is the best organizing choice for a task. The second is to know how to work with and lead the team to best accomplish that task. The following section discusses the first task, using teams as an organizing tool for dividing work responsibilities. (Managing and leading teams is covered in Chapter 4.)

3.5.1 The Benefits of Teams

While synergy is an important advantage, teams are useful in other ways. Being part of a team can have a strong influence on individual attitudes and behaviors. Working in and being part of a team can satisfy important individual needs and can also improve performance. Teams, simply put, can be very good for both organizations and their members. The usefulness of teams includes[21]

▲ increasing resources for problem-solving;
▲ fostering creativity and innovation;
▲ improving the quality of decision making;
▲ enhancing members' commitments to tasks;
▲ raising motivation through collective action;
▲ helping control and discipline members;
▲ satisfying individual needs as organizations grow in size.

Of course, organizing based on a team approach is never a guaranteed success. Who hasn't been part of a team that includes members who slack off because responsibility is diffused among several people and the rest of team will take care of the work?[22] And who hasn't heard people complain about having to attend what they consider to be another "time-wasting" teaming?[23]

Fortunately, things don't have to be this way. In fact, they must not be if teams are to make their best contributions to organizations. The following sections explore some of the most common types of teams in today's workplace and recommends when each type of team is most appropriate.

FOR EXAMPLE

Attitude Surveys and Team Effectiveness

Over the last 10 years, a variety of attitude surveys have been used to gauge the effectiveness of health care teams. One survey worth noting is the **Change Readiness Index** (CRI). This scorecard system asks team members to rate their health care organization and specific teams or groups in the categories of patient service, organizational reaction and readiness to change, and overall organizational dynamics such as communication and morale. The VA Medical Center in Phoenix, Arizona, used the CRI to assess the right strategy and approach for not only the commencement of a new leadership team, but also for strategy formulation in every new venture undertaken during their growth over the past decade.

3.5.2 Committees and Task Forces

Committees and **task forces** typically bring people together outside of their daily job assignments to work in small teams for a specific purpose. They are typically led by a designated head or chairperson who, in turn, is held accountable for committee or task-force results. While committees and task forces share many similarities, a few notable differences are as follows:

▲ **Committees** usually operate with a continuing purpose, while its membership may change over time.

▲ **Task forces** are more temporary, and their official tasks are very specific and time defined. Once its stated purpose has been accomplished, a task force typically disbands.

Committees and task forces are increasingly used to bring together people from various parts of an organization to work on common problems. But to achieve the desired results, these teams must be carefully established and well run, specifically:

▲ **Select appropriate members** who will be challenged by the assignment, who have the right skills, and who seem able to work well together.

▲ **Clearly define the purpose** of the task force or committee to ensure that members and important outsiders know what is expected, why, and on what timetable.

▲ **Carefully select a leader** who has good interpersonal skills, can respect the ideas of others, and is willing to do what needs to be done.

▲ **Periodically review progress** to ensure that all task-force or committee members feel collectively accountable for results and that they receive performance feedback.

3.5.3 Cross-Functional Teams

Organizational design today emphasizes horizontal integration, problem-solving, and information sharing. It also tries to eliminate the tendency of workers to remain within their functions and restrict communication with other parts of an organization. The members of a cross-functional team come together from different functional units to work on a specific problem or task, and to do so with the needs of the whole organization in mind.

Cross-functional teams are a particularly appropriate organizing choice when the goal is sharing information, exploring new ideas, and seeking creative solutions. Team members need to be encouraged to look beyond purely functional concerns and demands, and collectively and individually to think and act in the best interests of the total system.

3.5.4 Employee Involvement Teams

Many organizations now utilize functional or cross-functional **employee involvement teams.** These are groups of workers who meet on a regular basis outside of their formal assignments, with the goal of applying their expertise and attention to continuous improvement.

Using a problem-solving framework, teams often try to bring the benefits of employee participation to bear on a wide variety of performance issues and concerns. A popular form of employee involvement team is the **quality circle,** a group of workers that meets regularly to discuss and plan specific ways to improve work quality.[24] Usually, quality circles consist of six to twelve members from a work area. After receiving special training in problem-solving, team processes, and quality issues, members of the quality circle try to come up with suggestions that the entire organization can implement to raise productivity and improve processes.

3.5.5 Virtual Teams

The Internet, intranets, and computer software have all helped give rise to the phenomenon of **virtual teams.** Members of these teams work together and solve problems through largely computer-mediated rather than face-to-face interactions.[25]

Potential advantages of virtual teams make them increasingly important. Team members from widely dispersed locations can deal collectively with issues in a time-efficient fashion and without some of the interpersonal difficulties that may otherwise occur—especially when the issues are controversial.

Electronic team meetings can cause problems, however, particularly when members' working relationships are depersonalized and some of the advantages of face-to-face interaction are lost.[26]

Virtual teams are most effective for projects that are well outlined (a detailed agenda, distributed prior to the video or phone conference makes meetings clear, efficient, and focused) or that have an extremely focused nature (the team exists solely for the purpose of drafting the department's new safety plan, for example).

3.5.6 Self-Managing Work Teams

In a growing number of organizations, the functional team consisting of a first-level supervisor and his or her immediate subordinates is disappearing. It is being replaced with **self-managing work teams.** These are teams of workers whose jobs have been redesigned to create a high degree of task interdependence and who have been given authority to make many decisions about how they go about doing the required work.[27] The expected advantages include better performance, decreased costs, and higher morale.

Self-managing teams operate with participative decision making, shared tasks, and responsibility for many of the managerial tasks performed by supervisors in more traditional settings. "Self-management" responsibilities include planning and scheduling work, training members in various tasks, sharing tasks, meeting performance goals, ensuring high quality, and solving day-to-day operating problems. In some settings, the team's authority may even extend to "hiring" and "firing" its members when necessary.

A key feature of self-managing teams is multitasking, in which team members each have the skills to perform several different jobs. The implications of self-managing teams are depicted in Figure 3-10. Members of a self-managing team report to higher management through a team leader rather than to a formal supervisor, making the traditional role of first-line supervisor unnecessary. This is an important change in organizational structure because each self-managing team handles the supervisory duties on its own. Furthermore, within a self-managing team, the emphasis is always on participation.

The leader and members of a self-managed work team are expected to work together—not only to do the required work but also to make the decisions that determine how it gets done. A true self-managing team operates with these characteristics:

▲ Members are held collectively accountable for performance results.
▲ Members have discretion in distributing tasks within the team.
▲ Members have discretion in scheduling work within the team.
▲ Members are able to perform more than one job on the team.
▲ Members train one another to develop multiple job skills.
▲ Members evaluate one another's performance contributions.
▲ Members are responsible for the total quality of team products.

Self-managed teams are an appropriate organizing choice when extreme flexibility is required by the environment or when you want to develop a new

Figure 3-10

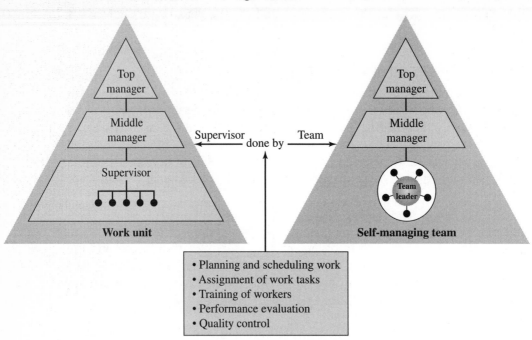

Organizational and management implications of self-managing work teams.

product, service, or way of working together. Successful self-managed teams are typically comprised of well-trained team members with training in planning, self-directing, project management, communication, and conflict resolution.

SELF-CHECK

- Identify and define **team, teamwork, synergy, committee, task force, employee involvement team, quality circle, virtual team,** and **self-managing work team.**
- Discuss the major benefits of using a team structure to organize a department.
- Compare characteristics of a task force and a committee.
- List strategies for designing and managing effective task forces and committees.
- Explain recent innovations in teaming, including the employee involvement team, quality circle, and virtual team.
- Describe characteristics of a self-managing team.

SUMMARY

The ways in which health care workplaces are structured or organized has evolved with changes in economic pressures and patient needs. Organizations rely on both formal and informal structures to arrange workers, assign responsibilities, and establish work processes. In recent years, organizing structures have developed to include teams, networks, and even boundaryless organizations. Whatever the specific organizational structures, today's health care managers must design organizations with shorter chains of command, wider spans of control, and decentralized power, among other things. Effectively designed organizations incorporate subsystems, allow for differences in work processes, and encourage integration. Team-based organizational designs are especially prevalent and effective in today's workplace; savvy managers utilize teaming in all its various forms—encouraging the ideal of self-managing teams to achieve the highest level of group productivity.

KEY TERMS

Adaptive organizations	Organizations with a minimum of bureaucratic features and with cultures that encourage worker empowerment and participation.
Boundaryless organization	An increasingly common structure in the business world, which combines teams and network structures for temporary purposes.
Bureaucracy	A form of organization based on logic, order, and the legitimate use of formal authority.
Centralization	Traditional, top-down decision.
Chain of command	Line of authority that vertically links all positions with successively higher levels of management.
Change Readiness Index (CRI)	Scorecard system asks team members to rate their health care organization and specific teams or groups in the categories such as patient service, organizational reaction and readiness to change.
Committee	Organizational group that usually operates with a continuing purpose while its membership may change over time.
Cross-functional teams	Within a matrix structure, workers belong to at least two formal groups at the same time—a functional group and a product, program, or project team.
Decentralization	Dispersed decision making.
Delegation	The process of distributing and entrusting work to other people.

Differentiation	The degree of difference that exists between the internal components of the organization.
Divisional structures	Organizational strategy in which you group together people who provide the same services, work within the same processes, serve similar audiences, or are located in the same area or geographical region.
Employee involvement team	Group of workers who meet on a regular basis outside of their formal assignments, with the goal of applying their expertise and attention to continuous improvement.
Formal structure	The intended or official structure of an organization.
Functional chimneys	Negative effect of formal structures, in which members of a specific functional group develop self-centered and narrow viewpoints, become uncooperative with other groups, and lose the ability to focus on the larger picture.
Functional structure	Organizational strategy in which people with similar skills and performing similar tasks are grouped together.
Health care network	Different medical services joining together to provide comprehensive health care, often sharing the services of one business office and laboratory.
Horizontal structures	New organizational models, which emphasize integration and cross-functional teamwork, often while gaining the advantages of networking through information technology.
Informal structure	The unofficial but often critical working relationships among organizational members, regardless of formal titles and relationships.
Integration	The level of coordination achieved among an organization's internal components.
Matrix structure	Organizational strategy that combines elements of both the functional and divisional structures.
Organizational design	The process of aligning organizational structures and cultures to best serve the organization's mission, strategy, and objectives.

Organization chart	Diagram that identifies key positions, job titles, lines of authority, and communication within an organization.
Organization structure	The system of tasks, workflow, reporting relationships, and communication channels that link the diverse parts of an organization.
Organizing	The process of arranging people and other resources to work together to accomplish a goal.
Process reengineering	The systematic and complete analysis of work processes and the design of new and better ones with the goal of focusing attention on the future, on patients, and on improving ways of doing things.
Process value analysis	Managers identify and carefully evaluate each step in a workflow. Each step must be important, useful, and add value to the overall purpose of the organization; if not, the step is eliminated.
Quality circle	A popular form of employee involvement team in which a group of workers meets regularly to discuss and plan specific ways to improve work quality.
Restructuring	The process of changing an organization's structure in an attempt to improve performance.
Self-managing work team	Workers whose jobs have been redesigned to create a high degree of task interdependence and who have been given authority to make many decisions about how they go about doing the required work.
Span of control	The number of people reporting directly to a manager within an organizational structure.
Subsystems	Small departments, work units, or teams headed by managers who perform specialized tasks within organizations.
Synergy	The creation of a whole that is greater than the sum of its parts; one of the benefits of teamwork.
Task force	Organizational group that is more temporary with official tasks that are very specific and time defined. Once its stated purpose has been accomplished, a task force typically disbands.

Team	Group of workers organized to accomplish tasks; the building blocks of today's new and more horizontal organizational forms.
Teamwork	The process of people working together to accomplish goals.
Unity-of-command principle	Each person in an organization should report to one and only one supervisor.
Upside-down pyramid	Organizational mind-set that refocuses attention on the marketplace and patient needs by putting patients on top, served by workers in the middle, who are in turn supported by managers at the bottom.
Vertical structures	Traditional top-down organizational models.
Virtual teams	Teams that work together and solve problems through largely computer-mediated rather than face-to-face interactions.
Work process	A related group of tasks that together create a result of value for the customer or patient.

ASSESS YOUR UNDERSTANDING

Go to www.wiley.com/college/Lombardi to evaluate your knowledge of the basics of workplace organization.
Measure your learning by comparing pretest and post-test results.

Summary Questions

1. Of the four major functions of management, organizing often happens in close conjunction with
   (a) leading.
   (b) planning.
   (c) controlling.
   (d) facilitating.

2. Formal structures within an organization include
   (a) recommended communication channels.
   (b) division of labor.
   (c) levels of management.
   (d) all the above.

3. Organizations that rely on functional structures can offer employees clear career paths within functions but sometimes become over-reliant on upper management to solve cross-functional disputes. True or false?

4. A potential advantage of a matrix structure is
   (a) improved problem-solving at the team level.
   (b) improved problem-solving at the technical level.
   (c) consistent and appropriate task assignments based on expertise.
   (d) efficient and effective task assignments based on training.

5. Throughout health care today, traditional horizontal work structures are being dismantled and replaced by more flexible vertical structures. True or false?

6. Organizing by teams offers numerous benefits to an organization. Benefits include all of the following except
   (a) shared responsibility by all team members for meeting performance targets.
   (b) improved morale as people in different areas better get to know one another.
   (c) streamlined interpersonal and interdepartmental relationships.
   (d) fewer barriers between departments.

7. Boundaryless organizations have qualities of teams and network structures, but they are also temporary in nature. True or false?

8. Managers in "flat" organizations tend to have wider spans of control, broader responsibilities, and shorter chains of command. True or false?

9. Decentralization in today's health care organizations is made possible by
   (a) decreased emphasis on cross-functional training.
   (b) increased reliance on degreed employees.
   (c) decreased spending on benefits.
   (d) increased use of information-share technology.

10. Bureaucratic structures have no place in today's health care workplace. True or false?

11. When you're considering new organizational structures, you should run your ideas through several of checks, including
    (a) does the design support and empower workers?
    (b) does the design support core technologies?
    (c) does the design fit with the major problems and opportunities of the external environment?
    (d) all of these.

12. Subsystems within successful health care organizations allow for both
    (a) specialization and exclusion.
    (b) communication and consistency.
    (c) differentiation and integration.
    (d) none of these.

13. One of the biggest benefits of organizing by teams is
    (a) synergy.
    (b) cost-savings.
    (c) training.
    (d) efficiency.

14. A committee usually has specific tasks and exists for a limited time frame, while a task force usually operates with continuing purpose as its membership changes over time. True or false?

15. Which of the following is NOT a characteristic of a self-managing work team?
    (a) The team shares responsibility for managerial tasks performed by supervisors in more traditional settings.
    (b) The team divides up daily tasks and solves day-to-day operation problems.
    (c) Team members follow established procedures given to them by upper management.
    (d) Team members are multitaskers, performing several different jobs.

Review Questions

1. The nurses at a large research hospital are members of a nursing team for their departments as well as disease-specific teams focusing innovative treatments for specific conditions (such as cancer, AIDS/HIV, diabetes). What sort of organization structure is this?

2. A district manager and a team leader have children who play on the same basketball team. What sort of organization are these two utilizing when they casually discuss possible solutions to a productivity problem during a game?

3. Why would a department choose to organize based on divisional structures?

4. A student health center organized by matrix structures has difficulty determining which students to see first and where to invest its limited budget. What disadvantage of matrix structure is the center experiencing?

5. Network organizations are fairly expensive to establish, requiring quality computer and information technology to link various locations. What are some benefits of network organizations?

6. In what ways might an organization be described as "boundaryless" within the organization and outside the organization?

7. The notion of one employee/one boss is being replaced in today's workplace by the two or more boss matrix structure. What does less unity of command mean for managers?

8. Hiring out specialized services on a contract basis is one common managerial response to which major organizational trend?

9. A large public health advocacy group recently eliminated all middle managers. Now several dozen project managers report to three top-level managers who focus on specific health topics. What workplace trends does this change represent?

10. How does an adaptive organization contrast with a bureaucratic organization in terms of authority and the use of teams?

11. As the manager of a small medical records team, you decide to assign responsibility for each case to a specific team member, rather than having staff work on whatever case is most pressing. Although you like the potential for increased customer service, you're concerned that this manner of working may not be effective if your hospital becomes part of a large regional health care network. What "check" for creating organizational structures are you considering?

12. In process value analysis, managers must find each step of a process important, useful, and adding value to the overall purpose of the organization. If any of these criteria are not met, what should the manager do?

13. Would a committee or a task force be a more appropriate organizational choice to deal with a significant increase in medical charting errors in the last months?

14. Virtual teams are becoming a common organizing structure in today's workplace. What two types of projects are virtual teams a particularly appropriate choice?

15. Self-managing teams are becoming an ideal in today's workplace. Why is multitasking so important to effective self-managing teams?

Applying This Chapter

1. At a community-based HIV/AIDS clinic, patients are assigned to treatment teams that focus on serving specific "clusters" patients (drug users, teens, or gay/lesbian, for example). What might be some of the advantages to this team-based approach for delivering health care services?

2. Emergency and disaster preparedness are topics of increasing importance to all health care organizations. A midsize hospital along Florida's Atlantic coast wants to establish a comprehensive plan for responding to natural disasters and other major emergencies within its organization, as well as within surrounding communities, the state of Florida, and the Atlantic coast. What sorts of team structures should the hospital put in place to achieve this goal?

3. Currently, every purchasing decision for your team must be presented to the director of purchasing in a written report and approved. The process is time-consuming and disempowering. What organizational restructuring can you as manager suggest to help save time and empower group managers to make some purchasing decisions on behalf of their teams?

4. The manager of the weekday staff at a hospice-care facility wants to redesign staff responsibilities in order to save the organization money in the next fiscal year. Specifically, the manager plans to staff each shift with one nurse practitioner rather than two RNs. (The manager also hopes that scheduling a nurse practitioner will lessen demand on doctors, thus saving the organization even more money.) To maintain head count, an additional certified nursing aide will be hired for each shift. Experienced aides and LPNs will take on additional responsibilities, as directed by the nurse practitioner. How does this plan hold up when run through the five checks described in section 3.4.2?

Following the Flow of an Organizational Chart

Take a look at the formal organizational chart for the hospital or health care organization you work for (or are interested in working for someday). You can also review the organizational chart for your school or check out the formal organizational chart for the Arkansas Regional Organ Recovery Agency (www.arora.org/about/orgchart.html). How do you describe the formal structures in place? Specifically, who reports to whom? What are the informal structures? How do decisions really get made? How long is the chain of command? How wide is the span of control?

Making Connections in Boundaryless Organizations

Although few health care workplaces today can be considered true boundaryless organizations (see section 3.2.3), workplace trends within and outside health care are requiring employees to connect with an ever-widening array of co-workers, consultants, off-site employees, and other resources. Whatever form a boundaryless organization takes, sharing knowledge is critical to the organization's success. Consider ways in which you currently share knowledge—with fellow students and professors, with family and friends, and with co-workers. What techniques have been most effective for sharing information and ideas? What techniques were ineffective? How might these techniques be applied or modified in a health care work environment?

Shorter and Wider

Current organizational trends suggest that in an effort to keep costs in check, health care organizations will continue to streamline layers of management (especially middle management) and expand the control of all remaining managers. Carefully consider the organizational chart at your current health care or non-health-care employer (or refer to the organizational chart for Penobscot Valley Hospital at www.pvhhealthcare.org/welcome/orgchart.asp). Consider the implications to you and your department if one of the departments or layers of management above you were eliminated for cost-saving reasons. What additional responsibilities might you or your department need to assume? What responsibilities would need to be assumed by other managers or departments? What additional resources or staffing would your department require to meet the new responsibilities?

Stability and Growth

Over its lifetime, an organization will most likely pursue organizational designs that are stability and growth oriented. Review the characteristics of a stability orientation and a growth orientation (section 3.4.2) and then consider the evolution of your department or employer over a period of at least 5 years. (If you don't have an employer or if you don't know enough about the strategic history of your employer, take a look at the history of Fulton State Hospital at www.dmh.missouri.gov/fulton/history.htm.) What changes and organizational designs reflect a growth orientation? What changes and organizational designs reflect a stability orientation? In your opinion, has the organization had more a growth or stability orientation during its history?

Steps Toward Self-management

Consider your next group assignment or project as an opportunity to try working as a self-managing team. Rather than selecting a leader for the project, use participative decision-making strategies (see section 4.5 for specific tools and ideas) to create a group in which all members are collectively accountable for performance results. As a group, discuss and decide on who will do which tasks. Consider how the role of multitasking will affect your group—for example, how can group members perform more than one job on the team and still complete the assignment on time and effectively? In what way could the group members evaluate one another's performance or contributions?

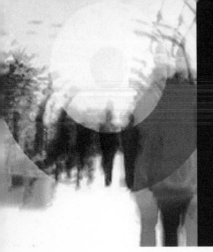

4

MANAGING TEAMS
Leading and Developing Work Teams That Are Efficient, Focused, and Flexible

Starting Point

Go to www.wiley.com/college/Lombardi to assess your knowledge of the basics of team management.
Determine where you need to concentrate your effort.

What You'll Learn in This Chapter

▲ Characteristics of strong teams
▲ Five principles of team orientation
▲ Five phases of team development and three key ways that teams develop
▲ Methods of enhancing individual team members and overall team orientation
▲ Pros and cons of team decision making

After Studying This Chapter, You'll Be Able To

▲ Implement the attributes of strong teams
▲ Practice ways to develop individual team players
▲ Practice methods of enhancing teams to higher levels of performance
▲ Demonstrate how managers effectively lead teams
▲ Apply techniques for successful group decision making

Goals and Outcomes

▲ Master the terminology of team management and team development and recognize tools and techniques associated with strong team management
▲ Understand the importance of strong, high-functioning teams
▲ Compare successful and unsuccessful teams
▲ Use tools and techniques to establish and promote positive team orientation, development, and enhancement
▲ Discuss the results, implications, and limitations of specific plans
▲ Collaborate with, encourage, and develop work team members
▲ Apply appropriate developing, enhancing, and leading techniques to real-life work-team situations
▲ Evaluate overall performance and effectiveness of teams

INTRODUCTION

Teams are one of the most popular ways to organize today's health care operation. Effective teams are motivated, respected, progressive, achievement-oriented, and supportive. Managers can help establish a strong team orientation by clearly defining job roles, creating shared goals, setting up open communication systems, and celebrating team diversity and differences. Because most teams go through multiple stages of development, managers need to lay good groundwork in the areas of expected behaviors, task responsibilities, and communication procedures. Leaders who both encourage a team orientation and develop individual members often produce the strongest teams. Teams can be effective decision-making structures, benefiting the entire organization.

4.1 Setting Up High-Functioning Teams

A **team** is a small group of people with complementary skills, who work together to achieve a shared purpose and hold themselves mutually accountable for its accomplishment. **Teamwork** is the process of people working together to accomplish these goals.

The organizational designs and cultures of today's health care organizations require teams, as well as a comprehensive commitment to empowerment and employee involvement. The ability of managers to develop their teams and lead through teamwork requires a special understanding of how teams operate and the commitment to use that understanding to help them achieve high levels of task performance and membership satisfaction.

4.1.1 Team Effectiveness

Teams transform **resource inputs** people and ideas into **product outputs** a finished good or service, or a special report or action recommendation.[1]

On the output side, **task performance**—good, old-fashioned "getting the job done"—is a concrete result that adds value to the organization. See Figure 4-1.

Also on the output side, you can see that member satisfaction is essential. Unless team members are satisfied with their accomplishments and with their experiences working together, the team is unlikely to retain long-term performance viability.

An effective team is one that achieves and maintains high levels of both task performance and member satisfaction and retains its viability for future action. As shown in Figure 4-1, a team's ability to be effective depends on the strength of its internal operations and on the quality of its inputs.

▲ **Group process:** The way the members of any team actually work together as they transform inputs into outputs. This includes how well

Figure 4-1

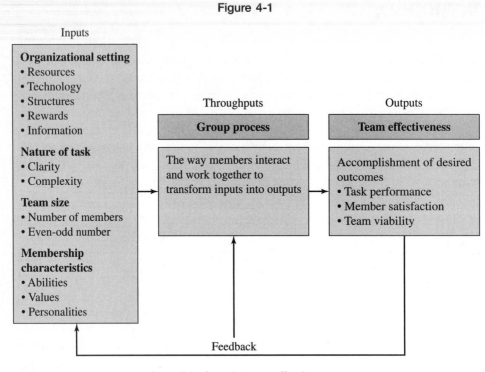

Inputs

Organizational setting
• Resources
• Technology
• Structures
• Rewards
• Information

Nature of task
• Clarity
• Complexity

Team size
• Number of members
• Even-odd number

Membership characteristics
• Abilities
• Values
• Personalities

Throughputs

Group process

The way members interact and work together to transform inputs into outputs

Outputs

Team effectiveness

Accomplishment of desired outcomes
• Task performance
• Member satisfaction
• Team viability

Feedback

A model of work team effectiveness.

team members communicate with one another, make decisions, and handle conflicts.

When the group process breaks down and the internal dynamics fail in any way, team effectiveness can suffer.

In addition to good group processes, the following are also essential to team effectiveness:

▲ The team must have any necessary **resource inputs** to deal best with the task at hand. Among critical input factors, the organizational setting, in particular, can affect how team members relate to one another and apply their skills.

▲ The team must have support in terms of information, material resources, technology, spatial arrangements, organization structures, and rewards.

▲ The nature of the task also affects how well a team can focus its efforts and how intense the group process needs to be.

▲ Clearly defined tasks make focusing work efforts easier. Complex tasks require more information exchange and intense interactions.

Additionally, several compositional factors affect team effectiveness:

▲ **Team size** affects how members work together, handle disagreements, and reach agreements. The number and complexity of interactions can make teams larger than six or seven members difficult to manage. When voting is required, teams with odd numbers of members are often preferred so as to prevent "ties."

▲ **Membership characteristics** are also important, particularly the blend of competencies, skills, and personalities. While a mix of skills, values, and personalities broadens the resources of a team, it also adds complexity to members' interpersonal relationships.[2]

▲ **Team diversity** is the different values, personalities, experiences, demographics, and cultures among the membership. This can present significant group process challenges. The more **homogeneous** the team—the more similar the members are to one another—the easier it is to manage relationships. As team diversity decreases, so, too, does the complexity of interpersonal relationships among members. The more **heterogeneous** the team—the more diversity among members—the greater the variety of available ideas, perspectives, and experiences that can add value to problem-solving and task performance.

In teamwork, as with organizations at large, the diversity lesson is very clear. Much can be gained when the team (and the entire organization) value and man-

---

FOR EXAMPLE

Integrated Care Management at University of Minnesota Health System

The Integrated Care Management program at the University of Minnesota Health System utilizes a team-oriented approach for patient care that combines the processes and talents of the institution's Surgical Intensive Care Unit and its Patient Care Services. In Integrated Care Management, clinical professionals and case managers collaborate on surgery cases, using processes and tools they've developed together. Although the two groups share tools for patient assessment, transition, and discharge, the arrangement allows multiple opportunities for decision making, assigns clear responsibility for various decisions, and permits discussion of alternative treatments. Following implementation of the Integrated Care Management program, the unit achieved positive results, including shorter hospital stays, fewer medication errors, and a cost savings of nearly $10 million.

age diversity. The process challenge is to maximize the advantages of team diversity while minimizing its potential disadvantages.

4.1.2 Identifying Characteristics of Strong Teams

As a health care manager, establishing a team orientation is important in order to build a progressive work environment.

As a new health care manager, you are most likely inheriting a ready-made team. Your department may have been working together under the leadership of your predecessor. (Even if you are forming a brand-new team, the following guidelines can help establish the standards you wish to incorporate into your team-building and team-orientation efforts.) The following are key qualities consistent in all winning teams:

▲ A **motivated** team attains its stated mission successfully and effectively. Motivation can come from a variety of sources, the first of which should be the department manager. Motivation can be positive, emphasizing encouragement and progressive action, or negative, emphasizing less-than-satisfactory consequences due to failure to meet team objectives. Motivation also must come from the work group itself. Individuals must inspire one another to greater performance and support the efforts of all team members. Also, each team member must be self-motivated. See section 10.1 for more information on motivation.

▲ A **credible and respected** team is known for getting the job done. The team earns credibility and commands the respect of patients and other departments. Strong teams have a wide base of technical knowledge and can readily provide whatever level of assistance is needed. Such teams are self-perpetuating, as they attract and retain other strong members.

▲ A **progressive** team grows continuously and develops expertise in an ongoing effort to enhance quality. Teams become progressive by valuing individual contribution, constantly attaining new technical knowledge, and experimenting with and implementing new methods of practices. Conversely, a **regressive** team loses ground and fails to participate positively in organizational activities, and its members are labeled as losers throughout the organization.

▲ An **inspired** team is fueled by their will to win. Individual members are success driven, and their leaders reinforce the importance of succeeding. This combination is the basis for inspiration. So that teams remain inspired, clear goals must be established, outcomes must be defined, and methods of attaining success should be delineated by the leader with the participation of all members.

▲ A **talented and seasoned** team has the skills and abilities needed to achieve a desired end, even if surprises pop up along the way. **Talent** encompasses technical knowledge, performance ability relative to current health care mandates, and awareness of business objectives within the context of those mandates.

▲ An **achievement-oriented** team wants success on an individual, group, and organizational level. In making their contribution, team members must be challenged to become the best they can be. As a manager, you must foster educational development, training opportunities, open communication, and goal attainment for each staff member.

▲ A **spirited** team is supportive, positive, results-oriented, and winning. These adjectives relate not only to the perceptions others have of the team, but also to something perhaps more important: the team's perception of itself. Losing teams are characterized as whiners, dysfunctional, or negative.

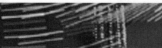

SELF-CHECK

- Identify and define **team, teamwork, resource input,** and **product output.**
- Cite the three compositional factors of any team.
- List the main characteristics of a strong team.

4.2 Establishing a Team Orientation

As first-time manager, you might generate a sense of team orientation by defining the policies—either implicitly or explicitly through staff meetings—that define how the team gets work done. Or perhaps you can establish a team orientation by having your staff brainstorm lists of principles by which they should be guided.

The following five basic principles of team orientation provide a foundation to assist you in formulating a policy of team action.

4.2.1 Clearly Defined Roles

Team members should know their role on the team, and the team itself should have a defined role throughout or within the organization. **Role definition** is essential so that individuals can identify with their work role and with the overall mission of their work group.

Some departments, by virtue of preexisting job descriptions or work group objectives, already have clearly established roles for every team member. If the

---

FOR EXAMPLE

Three Common Team Personalities

Even if a team doesn't have defined job descriptions or roles for each member, health care consultant Donald N. Lombardi contends that most teams have one or more of the three common team personalities. Star players are typically outspoken, have been on the team a long time, and have credibility with other team members. Lombardi recommends that managers seek out the allegiance of star players from day one. Steady players usually make up the majority of the team, producing average to above-average results. Managers should deal with steady players individually to learn their perceptions on how to increase group performance and enhance their contribution to the group. Underachievers are generally disinterested in their work and have no innate drive to improve on their activities. Managers should document their work during performance evaluations, and, if necessary, recommend termination.

---

team you're leading or managing doesn't have clearly defined roles—or if you want to adjust or redefine the roles within your team—take time to review primary work roles with each staff member; compile, refine, or update a job description for each individual; and enlist assistance from your human resources department to establish clearer job descriptions.

In addition to defining the roles of individuals, establish an objective for the entire work group that specifies its relevance to the health care organization's big picture. Compile a departmental mission statement (see section 6.4.7 for more on mission statements). Invite input from your staff and team members by asking, What is it that we contribute to our overall health care organization? What would happen to the hospital if our department was not here?

4.2.2 Strong Interest in Shared Objectives and Goals

A winning team is goal-oriented. Accordingly, upon establishing (or reinforcing) team goals, ensure that all team members are committed to achieving these goals. If they are not, you may want to discuss why, either individually or in a group setting.

Individuals may not be committed to department goals for a number of reasons. For example, a worker may not understand the goals, may be misplaced in his or her work role, or may simply be apathetic.

Hopefully your entire team can be motivated by the goals and objectives. If not, check performance documentation (see section 5.4). You may find that individuals who are not committed to the goals may not be contributing according to the organization's performance standards. If this is the case, consider placing them elsewhere in the organization or perhaps even terminating their position.

4.2.3 Open Communication System

Maintaining open communications with all team members is essential. The easiest way to go about this is to hold regular staff meetings (biweekly or monthly) in which you discuss department objectives, recent events, and organizational information. A roundtable discussion in which all team members describe their current activities and other essential information can be helpful. (Section 4.3.4 explores different types of formal communication systems.)

Also, consider less-formal methods of communication to encourage cooperation and communication among all team members. Take time to discuss work dynamics with each member as frequently as possible—for example, by engaging in a one-on-one "coffee conference" once a week or simply by walking around the department and asking each person how his or her day is going.

4.2.4 Resilience

Great teams are not defeated by adversity—they bounce back. No team is perfect, but you must remember that no team operates under perfect conditions every day. As a result, adverse situations arise that can have negative and demotivating effects. When these situations occur, call a staff meeting to ask these questions:

▲ What went wrong?
▲ How could it have been avoided?
▲ What have we learned from this?
▲ What will we do next time given the same circumstances?

By following this sequence, you give everyone an opportunity to learn from their mistakes, avoid reactive (as opposed to proactive) behavior in tough situations, and become more effective in their everyday work activities.

As manager, take the lead in this discussion by admitting any mistake you may have made and acknowledging whatever may have caused a problem that was outside your department's power to remedy. This process provides a basis on which to generate progressive discussion, which can help turn negative situations into positive future action.

4.2.5 A Variety of Talents, a Diversity of Perspectives

The individual team members in any health care team have various types and levels of experience and different viewpoints and opinions on work activity. Wise health care managers celebrate this diversity by being open and perceptive to a variety of ideas and encouraging staff to share their ideas and perspectives.

Many new managers, in particular, make the mistake of trying to force individuals into one perspective or one common viewpoint. Unfortunately, eliminating diversity sabotages creativity and cuts off individual initiative before it has a chance to blossom.

Ask your team members for their opinions, encourage them to share their opinions in meetings and other group communication forums, and reward creative behavior by giving individuals the opportunity to pursue ideas that might enhance effectiveness and efficiency within the department, thus contributing to the entire organization.

SELF-CHECK

- Explain the importance of clearly defined work roles and shared objectives within teams.
- Identify common tools and methods for open communication.
- List the four questions for dealing with adverse or negative situations.
- Discuss the positive aspects of having teams with diverse backgrounds, skills, and perspectives.

4.3 Developing Teams

Great work teams rarely just happen. Generally, a manager or team leader, who understands the stages of team development, helps build a strong team by establishing norms (see section 4.3.2), task and maintenance needs (4.3.3), and communication networks (4.3.4).

4.3.1 Team Development Process

Research on small groups suggests that there are five distinct phases in the life cycle of any team: forming, storming, norming, performing, and adjourning.[3] Health care managers need to be aware of these phases, identify where their teams are in the development process, and assist their teams in moving on to the next phase, when appropriate.

▲ The **forming stage** involves the initial entry of individual members into a team.

This is a stage of initial task orientation and interpersonal testing. As individuals come together for the first time or two, they ask a number of questions: "What can or does the team offer me?" "What am I asked to contribute?" "Can my needs be met while I serve the task needs of the team?"

In the forming stage, people begin to identify with other members and with the team itself. Team members are concerned about getting acquainted, establishing interpersonal relationships, discovering what is considered acceptable behavior, and learning how others perceive the team's task. This may also be a time when some members rely on or become temporarily dependent on another member who appears powerful or especially knowledgeable. Such things as prior experience with team members in other contexts and individual impressions of organization philosophies, goals, and policies may also affect member relationships in new work teams.

Difficulties in the forming stage tend to be greater in more culturally and demographically diverse teams.

▲ In the **storming stage** of team development, tension often emerges between members over tasks and interpersonal concerns.

This is a period of high emotionality. Team members may experience periods of outright hostility and infighting. Coalitions or cliques may form around personalities or interests. Subteams form around areas of agreement and disagreement involving group tasks or the manner of operations. Conflict may develop as individuals compete to impose their preferences on others and to become influential in the group's status structure.

Important changes occur in the storming stage as task agendas become clarified and members begin to understand one another's interpersonal styles. Here attention begins to shift toward obstacles that may stand in the way of task accomplishment.

Efforts are made to find ways to meet team goals while also satisfying individual needs. Failure in the storming stage can be a lasting liability, whereas success in the storming stage can set a strong foundation for later team effectiveness.

▲ In the **norming stage,** members of the team begin to become coordinated as a working unit and tend to operate with shared rules of conduct.

Cooperation is an important theme for teams in the norming stage. The team feels a sense of leadership, with each member starting to play useful roles. Most interpersonal hostilities give way to a precarious balancing of forces as norming builds initial integration. Harmony is emphasized, but minority viewpoints may be discouraged.

In the norming stage, members are likely to develop initial feelings of closeness, a clearer division of labor, and a stronger sense of shared expectations. These developments help protect the team from disintegration. At this stage, holding the team together may become even more important than successful task accomplishment.

▲ In the **performing stage,** team members are able to deal in creative ways with both complex tasks and interpersonal conflicts. The team operates with a clear and stable structure, and members are motivated by team goals.

Teams in the performing stage are more mature, organized, and well function-ing. The primary challenges of teams in the performing stage is to continue refining the operations and relationships essential to working together as an integrated unit. Such teams need to remain coordinated with the larger organi-zation and adapt successfully to changing conditions over time.

▲ The **adjourning stage** is the final stage of team development, and is one in which team members prepare to disband.

It is especially common for temporary groups that operate in the form of com-mittees, task forces, and projects to have an adjourning stage. Ideally, the team disbands with a sense that important goals have been accomplished. Members are acknowledged for their contributions and the group's overall success.

The adjourning stage may be an emotional time. For members who have worked together intensely for a period of time, breaking up the close relationships may be painful. The ideal is for a team to disband with members feeling they want to work with one another again in the future, should the need or opportunity arise.

4.3.2 Establishing Norms and Cohesiveness

A **norm** is a behavior expected of team members.[4] It is a rule or standard that guides their behavior. When violated, a norm may be enforced with reprimands and other sanctions. In the extreme, violation of a norm can result in a member being expelled from a team or socially ostracized by other members. Groups and teams typically operate under a host of norms—some clearly communicated, others unspoken but powerfully understood.

▲ The **performance norm** defines the level of work effort and performance that team members are expected to contribute.

This important norm can have positive or negative implications for team per-formance and organizational productivity. In general, work groups and teams with positive performance norms are more successful in accomplishing task objectives than are teams with negative performance norms.

Other important norms relate to such things as helpfulness, participation, timeliness, and innovation. Because a team's norms are largely determined by the collective will of its members, a manager or designated leader may not be able to simply dictate which norms are acceptable. Instead, managers must help, sup-port, and encourage team members to develop positive norms. To help build positive norms, team leaders and managers should

▲ act as a role model;
▲ reinforce the desired behaviors with rewards;
▲ control results by performance reviews and regular feedback;

▲ train and orient new members to adopt desired behaviors;

▲ recruit and select new members who exhibit the desired behaviors;

▲ hold regular meetings to discuss progress and ways of improving;

▲ use team decision-making methods to reach agreement.[5]

Cohesiveness is the degree to which members are attracted to and motivated to remain part of a team. This determines the degree of conformity to norms. People in a highly cohesive team value their membership and strive to maintain positive relationships with other team members. They experience satisfaction from identifying and working with the team.

Look at Figure 4-2. When the performance norm of a team is positive and cohesion is high, a best-case scenario results. Competent team members work hard and reinforce one another's task accomplishments while experiencing satisfaction with the team.

But when the performance norm is negative in a highly cohesive team, conformity to the negative norm results in a worst-case scenario—low productivity and restricted work efforts. Between these two extremes are mixed situations of moderate to low productivity.

Managers and team leaders should build and maintain teams with both positive performance norms and high cohesiveness. To help develop positive cohesion, managers should

▲ induce agreement on team goals;

▲ increase membership homogeneity;

Figure 4-2

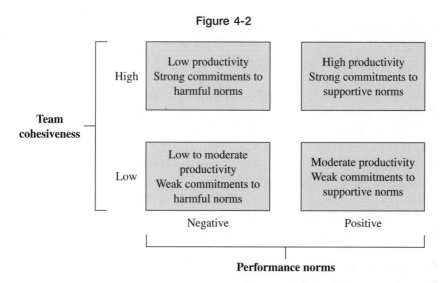

Productivity and the relationship between team cohesiveness
and performance norms.

FOR EXAMPLE

Performance Norms from NRC

For more than 20 years, the for-profit research service National Research Corporation (www.nationalresearch.com) has utilized performance norms to evaluate more than 800 health plans and more than 1,300 hospitals across the United States to create its annually published *Healthcare Market Guide*. In fact, NCR was the first national reviewing organization to utilize performance norms as a way to measure and compare performance by health care providers. Based on its experience in performance measurement research, NRC served as technical advisor to the National Committee for Quality Assurance (www.ncqa.org) during the development of the HEDIS 3.0 Member Satisfaction Survey and to the Joint Commission on Accreditation of Healthcare Organizations (www.jcaho.org).

▲ increase interactions among members;
▲ decrease team size;
▲ introduce competition with other teams;
▲ reward team rather than individual results.

4.3.3 Taking Care of Task and Maintenance Needs

Two types of activities are essential if team members are to work well together over time.[6]

▲ **Task activities** contribute directly to the team's performance purpose.
▲ **Maintenance activities** support the emotional life of the team as an ongoing social system.

All team members share responsibility for both activities. In this sense, any member can help lead a team by taking actions that satisfy its task and maintenance needs. This concept of **distributed leadership** in teams is explained further in Figure 4-3.

Leading through task activities involves such behavior as initiating agendas, sharing information, and summarizing. Leading through maintenance activities involves such things as gatekeeping, encouraging others, and reducing tensions.

Both task and maintenance activities stand in distinct contrast to the dysfunctional activities also described in the figure. Self-serving activities such as withdrawing and horsing around detract from, rather than enhance, team effectiveness.

4.3.4 Instituting Communication Networks

Figure 4-4 shows three interaction patterns and communication networks that teams commonly use.[7] As expected, the best teams use com-

Figure 4-3

**Distributed leadership
roles in teams**

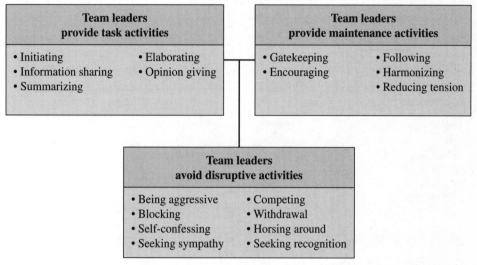

Distributed leadership helps a team meet its task and maintenance needs.

munication networks in the right ways, at the right times, and for the right tasks.

▲ In a **centralized communication network,** sometimes called a *wheel* or *chain structure,* activities are coordinated and results pooled by a central point of control. Most communication flows back and forth between individual members and "the hub," or center point. Centralized networks tend to work best on simple tasks that require little creativity, information processing, and problem-solving.

▲ In a **decentralized communication network,** sometimes called the *all-channel* or *star structure,* all members communicate directly with one another. The decentralized networks work best for more complex tasks because these networks are able to support more intense interactions and information sharing.

▲ In a **restricted communication network,** subgroups within a team experience issue-specific disagreements, such as a temporary debate over the best means to achieve a goal, and the result is a breach in communication. Communication between the subgroups is often limited and biased, with the result that problems can easily occur. When various factions become polarized, the subgroups often engage in contests and even antagonistic relations.

Figure 4-4

Pattern	Diagram	Characteristics
Interacting Group Decentralized communication network		High interdependency around a common task Best at complex tasks
Coacting Group Centralized communication network		Independent individual efforts on behalf of common task Best at simple tasks
Counteracting Group Restricted communication network		Subgroups in disagreement with one another Slow task accomplishment

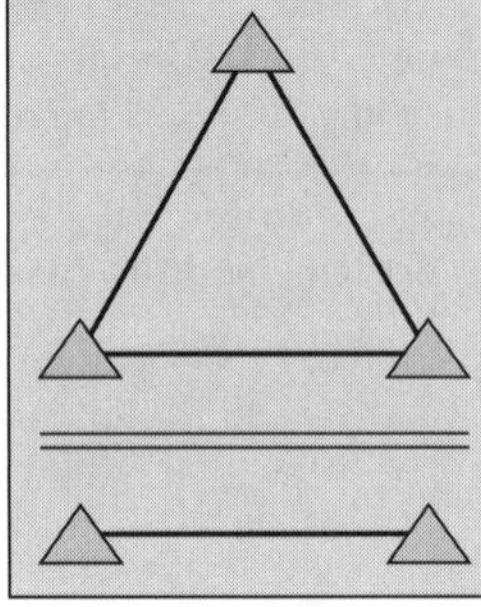

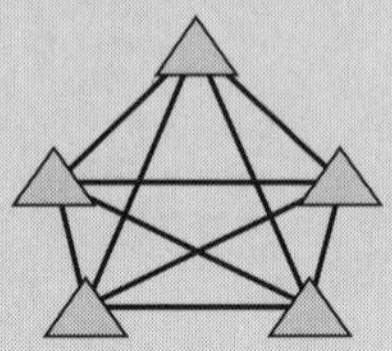

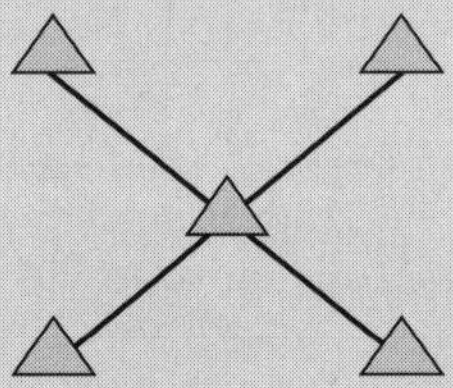

Interaction patterns and communication networks in teams.

SELF-CHECK

- Define **norm, performance norm, cohesiveness, task activity, maintenance activity,** and **distributed leadership.**
- Identify and define the five stages of team development.
- Compare the characteristics of centralized, decentralized, and restricted communication networks.
- Describe how positive and negative norms can affect teams.
- Compare and contrast task activities and maintenance activities.

4.4 Enhancing Teams

Most health care managers first work within an established team—or at least an established team structure. The decisions of your management predecessor(s) have a significant impact on the team you work with, but you always have the opportunity to evaluate and refine the group you're responsible for and lead them toward your personal vision of a healthy, functional, dynamic, high-performing team.

4.4.1 Building—and Rebuilding—Teams

Even the most mature work team is likely to experience problems over time. When such difficulties arise, team-building activities, often led by the team leader or manager, can help.

Team building is a sequence of planned activities used to gather and analyze information on how a team functions. Managers then strive to implement constructive changes to increase the team's operating effectiveness.[8] Most systematic approaches to team building follow the steps described in Figure 4-5. The cycle begins with the awareness that a problem may exist or may develop within the team. Team members then work together, gathering and analyzing data, so the problem is finally understood.

Figure 4-5

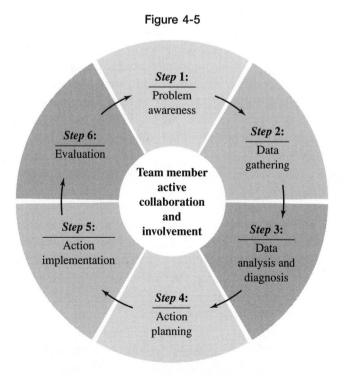

Collaboration and involvement in the team-building process.

Action plans are made by members and collectively implemented. Results are evaluated in similar fashion by team members working together. Any difficulties or new problems that are discovered serve to recycle the team-building process.

The ultimate goal of team building is to create more and better teamwork among group members. This is accomplished as members work together to conduct careful and collaborative assessments of the team's inputs, processes, and results. It is also accomplished as they collectively decide to take action to resolve and/or prevent problems that interfere with team effectiveness.

4.4.2 Encouraging Strong Team Players

Strong health care team members possess eight critical characteristics. As a manager or team leader, you should identify these characteristics (and the work-related behaviors associated with them), as well as encourage your team members to further develop.

▲ **Drive:** Each team member must have a certain amount of drive to attain individual and group goals. He does not need to be jump-started every morning or at the beginning of each shift. The drive toward performing strongly, learning and growing every day, being a motivator for others purely by example, expending energy and applying on-the-job initiative all characterize a stellar team player.

▲ **Confidence:** All team members should feel self-assured about their technical abilities, as well as their resilience to perform under changing and critical circumstances. A strong player usually radiates confidence about departmental goals and everyday work activities. Patients and fellow workers pick up on this attitude and therefore feel comforted by this individual's presence. They have the conviction that the job will get done and that when the going gets tough—an everyday occurrence in health care—the job will still get done.

▲ **Discipline:** Good workers are disciplined. They steadily make exact determinations and seek all facts necessary to making a decision. They get the job done correctly the first time and do not cause little problems that can add up to big problems. Good team members know intrinsically what has to be done and how to do it; that is, they set their own objectives and determine a course of action for achieving those objectives with excellence. Their sense of discipline is self-perpetuating throughout the entire department.

▲ **Desire:** A hunger to get better all the time is a constant motivator for team players. An individual with desire wants to help others and has a strong need to learn and grow on the job. Team members who possess desire do not need to be "hand-fed" with the promise of educational opportunities, promotions, or raises; rather, they seek out learning opportunities every day and are perpetually fueled by this desire to become better at their jobs and stronger in their daily contributions to the organization, team, and patient's health.

▲ **Dedication:** Strong team members emanate dedication to a common goal for all health care workers—to provide stellar health care to all patients. They are equally dedicated to all team goals, departmental objectives, and one another in providing help, guidance, and technical assistance.

▲ **Acumen:** Every health care employee has a certain amount of technical acumen and expertise that they bring to the job. Whether that expertise lies in conducting a good lab assay, filling a prescription correctly, or cleaning a patient's room quickly and efficiently, strong team members bring their unique, essential ability to the workplace every day.

▲ **Loyalty:** Team loyalty is critical in any workplace, especially in the health care industry. Each team member's first loyalty, of course, is to the health care institution and its mission of providing care to its patient community. The second loyalty is to the department manager or team leader and is demonstrated by following set objectives, providing feed-back, and accomplishing team goals. The third loyalty is to the work group, to act as a positive participant who contributes to group goals. Fourth, the team members maintain a dedication to escalating their individual strong performance and progressive development on the job.

▲ **Development:** Each team member should desire to grow and develop on the job. This development expands beyond the parameters of basic technical growth: Strong health care team members seek to learn more about the health care industry and understand the changing dimensions of the business. They know how to interpret the impact of change in the social environment and their communities, and they understand how these changes may affect their particular duties and the institution's mission.

An often-overlooked aspect of team member development is **interpersonal skills.** A strong team member seeks to learn more about others' personalities and professional preferences, relative to job performance. Developing interpersonal skills contributes significantly to an ever-expanding knowledge base from which an employee can grow, prosper, and continuously improve the quantity and quality of their work contribution.

4.4.3 Maintaining and Reinforcing a Strong Team Orientation

Just as establishing a team orientation is not an exact science, keeping a work group committed to and engaged with a team orientation for many months—and perhaps years—is a day-to-day challenge that health care managers face.

Numerous strategies are available to help health care managers constantly reinforce a team concept within their department. Many hospitals or health care organizations have ongoing training programs to help managers continually refine how they motivate their teams and improve efficiency. The following are some of the most useful strategies:

▲ **Point team members back to established, common objectives.** All team members need to know the objectives and mission of the department as well as the organization. Remember that management involves asking the right questions. Question your staff about their perceptions as to the main objectives of the department and the common goals toward which individuals should be striving as members of the team.

▲ **Recognize individual talents and ask for suggestions on how each individual's talent can be applied to the team.** Be a manager who asks team members for individual, unique suggestions and recommendations. The best source for learning how to create synergism between individual talent and group contribution is the individual department member.

▲ **Maintain two-way feedback.** In addition to providing feedback to your staff on ways they can become better team members, ask team members their opinions on your management style within the team and on the way that the team is progressing toward stated goals.

▲ **Identify changing dynamics or factors affecting your department as proactively as possible.** While good teams have the ability to handle change, aware managers make the process of responding to change less painful. Again, elicit ideas from your staff about what is changing relative to their jobs and, more important, how they can best prepare to handle that change successfully.

▲ **Be unafraid to reassign.** A team's ability to bounce back from adversity is a hallmark of success. As a health care manager, you may have to reassign individuals occasionally to help team members who require extra assistance. Rely on veterans and stronger players to provide assistance. Reassigning not only helps a team achieve objectives, but it can increase team allegiance and individual motivation.

▲ **Provide opportunities to grow, learn, and develop.** Present as many in-service exercises as possible, and use the expertise within your department to present new ideas to the group. One strategy in this area is to have show-and-tell sessions in which team members explain to each other new principles, strategies, and methods of accomplishing technology-based ends.

▲ **Establish new goals.** Hold meetings at least once a quarter (or even monthly) to set new goals for the department for continuous improvement. Review past goals and accomplishments, seek explanations for why goals were either achieved or not achieved, and seek input from the group concerning their perceptions as to the achievement of these goals. Make this a group process to ensure credibility as well as maximum input and opportunities for shared knowledge.

4.4.4 Accepting the Challenge of Team Leadership

Harnessing the full potential of teams in today's health care organizations involves special leadership challenges. High-performing teams generally share common characteristics, including a clear goal, a task-driven and results-oriented structure, competent and committed members who work hard, a collaborative climate, high standards of excellence, external support and recognition, and strong and principled leadership.[9]

This last characteristic, the need for strong and principled leadership, may be the key to them all. Outstanding teams are built with the efforts of strong and principled leadership. The best team leaders

▲ **establish a clear vision of the future.** This vision serves as a goal that inspires hard work and the quest for performance excellence. It creates a sense of shared purpose;

▲ **help to create change.** They are dissatisfied with the status quo, influence team members toward similar dissatisfaction, and infuse the team with the motivation to change in order to become better;

▲ **unleash talent.** They make sure the team is staffed with members who have the right skills and abilities. And they make sure these people are highly motivated to use their talents to achieve the group's performance objectives.

FOR EXAMPLE

The Delphi Technique

The Delphi technique, refined and promoted by consultant and meeting facilitator Bruce Withrow (www.facilitators.com), puts team members in charge of the group's future goals and direction. The Delphi technique assumes that team members are experts on their workplace functions and as such can provide better forecasts than upper management or outside consulting gurus. The technique focuses on three phases. During the first phase, a leader asks the team to individually forecast a specific goal for the team (for example, how the team will improve the results of customer feedback surveys by 10% in the next year). The manager then compiles and summarizes the forecasts. In phase two, team members individually evaluate the summarized list of forecasts, critique forecasts, and each prepares a revised forecast. In the third and final phase, the team meets face-to-face and discusses only revised forecasts. Through discussion and voting, the team develops a unified revised forecast, which it can present to management and use as a planning and goal-setting tool for the next year.

Clearly, you don't get a high-performing team by just bringing a group of people together and giving them a shared name or title. Leaders of high-performance teams create supportive climates in which team members know what to expect from the leader and each other, and know what the leader expects from them. The best team leaders empower team members. By personal example, they demonstrate the importance of setting aside self-interests to support the team's goals. And they use team building on a relatively continuous basis, viewing it as an ongoing leadership responsibility.

SELF-CHECK

- Identify and define **team building** and **interpersonal skills**.
- Cite the eight characteristics of strong individuals within a team.
- Discuss strategies for further enhancing and developing high-functioning teams.
- Describe essential traits for leading a team.

4.5 Making Decisions in Teams

Decision making is one of the most important group processes, and decisions in teams can be made in several different ways. Edgar Schein, a respected scholar and consultant, notes that teams make decisions by at least six methods: lack of response, authority rule, minority rule, majority rule, consensus, and unanimity.[10]

▲ In **decision by lack of response,** one idea after another is suggested without any discussion taking place. When the team finally accepts an idea, all others have been bypassed and discarded by simple lack of response rather than by critical evaluation.

▲ In **decision by authority rule,** the leader, manager, committee head, or some other authority figure makes a decision for the team. This can be done with or without discussion and is very time efficient. Whether the decision is a good one or a bad one, however, depends on whether the authority figure has the necessary information and on how well other team members accept this approach.

▲ In **decision by minority rule,** two or three people are able to dominate or "railroad" the team into making a mutually agreeable decision. This is often done by providing a suggestion and then forcing quick agreement by challenging the team with such statements as "Does anyone object? Let's go ahead, then."

▲ In **decision by majority rule,** formal voting may take place, or members may be polled to find the majority viewpoint. Majority rule is perhaps the most common way teams make decisions, especially when early signs of disagreement arise. Although this method parallels the democratic political system, it is often used without awareness of its potential problems. The very process of voting can create coalitions; that is, some people will be "winners" and others will be "losers" when the final vote is tallied. Those in the minority—the "losers"—may feel left out or discarded without having had a fair say. They may be unenthusiastic about implementing the decision of the "majority," and lingering resentments may impair team effectiveness in the future.

▲ In **decision by consensus,** discussion leads to one alternative being favored by most members and the other members agreeing to support it. When a consensus is reached, even those who may have opposed the chosen course of action know that they have been heard and have had an opportunity to influence the decision outcome. Consensus, therefore, does not require unanimity. But it does require that team members be able to argue, engage in reasonable conflict, and yet still get along with and respect one another.[11] And it requires that there be the opportunity for any dissenting members to feel they have been able to speak—and that they have been listened to.

▲ In **decision by unanimity,** all team members agree on the course of action to be taken. While decision by unanimity may sound like the ideal state of affairs and method for decision making in teams, it is also extremely difficult to attain in actual practice. One of the reasons that teams sometimes turn to authority decisions, majority voting, or even minority decisions, in fact, is the difficulty of managing the team process to achieve consensus or unanimity.

The best teams don't limit themselves to just one decision-making method. Instead, they change methods to best fit the problems at hand. An important team leadership skill for managers is helping a team choose the most appropriate decision method—one that provides for a timely and quality decision to which the members are highly committed.[12]

4.5.1 Assets and Liabilities of Team Decisions

In order to manage teams effectively, team leaders must understand both the potential assets and potential liabilities of team-based decisions.[13]

Team decisions are highly desirable whenever time and other circumstances permit. They bring greater amounts of information, knowledge, and expertise to bear on problems. They expand the number of action alternatives that are examined, and they help to avoid tunnel vision and consideration of only limited options. Team decisions increase the understanding and acceptance of outcomes by members. And, importantly, they increase the commitments of members to work hard to implement final plans.

The potential disadvantages of team decision making trace largely to possible difficulties in group process. In a team decision, there may be social pressure to conform. Individual members may feel intimidated or compelled to go along with the apparent wishes of others. There may be minority domination, where some members feel forced or "railroaded" to accept a decision advocated by one vocal individual or small coalition. Also, the time required to make team decisions can sometimes be a disadvantage. As more people are involved in the dialogue and discussion, decision making takes longer. This added time may be costly, even prohibitively so, in some circumstances.

4.5.2 Avoiding Groupthink

Among the risks of team decision making is a phenomenon called **groupthink,** the tendency for highly cohesive groups to lose their critical evaluative capabilities.[14] Members of very cohesive teams may publicly agree with actual or suggested courses of action while privately having serious doubts about them. Strong feelings of team loyalty can make it hard for members to criticize and evaluate one another's ideas and suggestions. Desires to hold the team together and avoid disagreements may result in poor decisions.

Symptoms that groupthink may be occurring include[15]

- ▲ **having illusions of invulnerability:** Members assume the team is too good for criticism or beyond attack;
- ▲ **rationalizing unpleasant and disconfirming data:** Members refuse to accept contradictory data or consider alternatives thoroughly;
- ▲ **believing in inherent group morality:** Members act as though the group is inherently right and above reproach;
- ▲ **stereotyping competitors as weak, evil, and stupid:** Members refuse to look realistically at other groups;
- ▲ **pressuring others to conform to group wishes:** Members refuse to tolerate anyone who suggests the team may be wrong;
- ▲ **self-censorship by members:** Members refuse to communicate personal concerns to the whole team;
- ▲ **having illusions of unanimity:** Members accept consensus prematurely, without testing its completeness;
- ▲ **mind guarding:** Members protect the team from hearing disturbing ideas or outside viewpoints.

FOR EXAMPLE

Good Group Decision Making at FutureThink

What will the delivery of care look like in the year 2013? Rather than blindly follow a vision handed down by upper management, members of the Ohio Hospital Association (OHA) and the Ohio Organization of Nurse Executives (OONE) decided to collaborate and establish as an independent advisory team known as FutureThink. Over the course of 12 strategic brainstorming sessions, the team evaluated best practices of team-based organizational structures throughout Ohio (as well as technological innovations and preventive care measures) and through consensus building developed an integrated model for delivering health care to Ohioans now—and well into the future. You can review FutureThink's proposed solution at www.futurethink.org.

Team leaders and managers can help identify and minimize the effects of groupthink by keeping the following tips in mind:

▲ Assign the role of *critical evaluator* to each team member; encourage a sharing of viewpoints.

▲ Don't, as a leader, seem partial to one course of action; do absent yourself from meetings at times to allow free discussion.

▲ Create subteams to work on the same problems and then share their proposed solutions.

▲ Have team members discuss issues with outsiders and report back on their reactions.

▲ Invite outside experts to observe team activities and react to team processes and decisions.

SELF-CHECK

- Identify and define **groupthink** and its associated symptoms.
- Describe the six types of decision-making processes for groups.
- Discuss pros and cons of making group decisions.
- List strategies for avoiding negative aspects of group decision making.

SUMMARY

Working with and developing teams is a major daily responsibility for most of today's health care managers. Knowing the characteristics of successful teams helps managers identify weaknesses, improve interactions, and further develop their own work teams. Clearly defined job roles, goals, and communication procedures—along with mutual respect—are all critical components for effective teams. Although teams naturally change over time, established expectations, responsibilities, and procedures provide long-term structure and benefit. Strong team leaders must develop both individual members as well as the overall team orientation. Making decisions as a team is a challenging but effective way to enhance the overall effectiveness of a health care organization.

KEY TERMS

Adjourning stage	The final stage of team development, and is one in which team members prepare to disband.
Cohesiveness	The degree to which members are motivated to remain part of a team.
Distributed leadership	A team in which all members share responsibility for both task and maintenance activities.
Forming stage	The first stage of team development; involves the initial entry of individual members into a team.
Group process	The way the members of a team actually work together.
Groupthink	The tendency for highly cohesive groups to lose their critical evaluative capabilities.
Heterogeneous team	A team comprised of a more diverse array of members.
Homogeneous team	A team comprised of same or similar kinds of members.
Interpersonal skills	Ability to learn more about others' personalities and professional preferences, relative to job performance.
Maintenance activities	Work activities that support the emotional life of the team as an ongoing social system.
Norm	A behavior expected of team members.
Norming stage	The third stage of team development; members begin to become coordinated as a work-

	ing unit and tend to operate with shared rules of conduct.
Performance norm	Any behavior expectation that defines the level of work that team members are expected to contribute.
Performing stage	The fourth stage of team development; the team operates with a clear and stable structure, and members are motivated by team goals.
Product outputs	The finished good or service that a team produces.
Resource inputs	The people and ideas that teams use to create outputs.
Role definition	Helps individuals identify with their work role and with the overall mission of their work group.
Storming stage	The second stage of team development; tension often emerges between members over tasks and interpersonal concerns.
Task activities	Work activities that contribute directly to the team's performance purpose.
Task performance	The act of getting a job done.
Team	A small group of people with complementary skills who work together to achieve a shared purpose and hold themselves mutually accountable for its accomplishment.
Team building	A sequence of planned activities used to gather and analyze information on how a team functions.
Team diversity	The different values, personalities, experiences, demographics, and cultures among the members of a team.
Teamwork	The process of people working together to accomplish goals.

ASSESS YOUR UNDERSTANDING

Go to www.wiley.com/college/Lombardi to evaluate your knowledge of the basics of team management.
Measure your learning by comparing pretest and post-test results.

Summary Questions

1. Teams transform resource inputs into product outputs. Which of the following is not an example of a product output from a health care organization?
   (a) A medicated heart catheter
   (b) A bill detailing health insurance claims
   (c) A malignant mole
   (d) An office visit

2. A group process is the way teams actually work together as they transform inputs into outputs. Patient charges are an example of a group process. True or false?

3. Strong teams are usually progressive, which means the team members can join or leave the team with considerable freedom and frequency. True or false?

4. If a team member is not committed to a team objective or goal, a reasonable initial managerial response might be to discuss the objective and expectation with the worker in a one-on-one setting. True or false?

5. All of the following methods are forms of open communication, except
   (a) sticky notes with constructive feedback placed on a team member's work station.
   (b) a biweekly team meeting.
   (c) a 10-minute status roundup at the start of a shift.
   (d) a work-related chat by a team member by the coffee machine.

6. Which of the following is an appropriate question to ask after a team experiences adversity?
   (a) How could the negative situation have been avoided?
   (b) What have we learned from this situation?
   (c) What went wrong?
   (d) All of the above

7. During the norming stage of team development, tensions often emerge between members over tasks and interpersonal concerns. True or false?

8. Rather than dictate performance norms to a team, managers should do all the following except
   (a) hold regular team meetings to discuss progress and ways of improving.
   (b) give individual team members quarterly minireports on whether they're meeting norms.
   (c) act as a role model.
   (d) recruit and select new team members who exhibit desired behaviors.

9. The strongest team combines positive performance norms with low cohesiveness. True or false?

10. The ultimate goal of team building is to
    (a) establish close interpersonal connections between team members.
    (b) encourage open dialogue between leaders and team members.
    (c) introduce new tools and technique for working together.
    (d) create more and better teamwork among group members.

11. Technical acumen is job expertise that relies on scientific understanding and the ability to use technology effectively in the workplace. True or false?

12. The best team leaders
    (a) establish a clear vision of the future.
    (b) help to create change.
    (c) unleash others' talents.
    (d) All of the above

13. Upper management reviews three possible staffing plans and selects the plan your team will follow for the next year. What sort of decision making is happening here?
    (a) Decision by minority rule
    (b) Decision by priority rule
    (c) Decision by authority rule
    (d) None of the above

14. When a team protects itself from information, outside viewpoints, or disturbing ideas, the team is engaging in mind guarding. True or false?

15. Managers can avoid the effects of groupthink on their teams by assuming the role of critical evaluator and carefully weighing each member's viewpoint. True or false?

Review Questions

1. What are the three main compositional factors that affect team effectiveness?
2. Strong teams are typically achievement-oriented. Define *achievement-oriented*.
3. Contrast homogeneous and heterogeneous teams.

4. Why is role definition important to the overall health of a team?

5. What are Lombardi's three most common team personalities?

6. What are some common forms of open communication between manager and team members?

7. During what development stage does a team deal in creative, effective ways with complex tasks and interpersonal conflicts, guided by stable team structure and clear team goals?

8. Distributed leadership allows all team members to share responsibility for both task and maintenance activities. What are some examples of task and maintenance activities?

9. Which type of communication network features subgroups with limited communication opportunities?

10. Loyalty is a characteristic of a strong team player. What are the four key loyalties?

11. Team goals should be established by the group rather than the leader or manger. Why?

12. A team leader who is dissatisfied with the status quo and motivates his or her team to change in order to become better is exemplifying which characteristic of a strong leader?

13. A team that requires all members to agree on the course of action taken is using which kind of decision-making process?

14. Decision-making as a group can be effective when the process is utilized at the right time. When are team decisions most effective?

15. What are signs that your team may not be thinking clearly about problems—and possibly engaging in groupthink?

Applying This Chapter

1. The team of nurses you manage is consistently not meeting its team goals because of a lack of motivation. As the manager, you can motivate team members positively and negatively to achieve goals. What might be an example of a positive and negative motivation?

2. Your team gathers for two short status meetings every week. During meetings, team members present their problems and questions and other team members offer suggestions. As team leader, you sometimes offer recommendations as well, but you generally let the team come to its own solutions. What team-based strengths is your team exhibiting?

3. As team leader, you set the team rule that all patient charts must be up-to-date and submitted to you by noon each workday. Members who don't comply receive a note in their ongoing performance log. What sort of norm are you setting?

4. You manage a treatment team at a daytime hospitalization program for adults with severe mental illnesses. Your treatment team, which includes a consulting psychiatrist, a nurse, a social worker, a physical therapist, and several aides, works directly with 20 patients, facilitating socialization activities for clients. Which of the three most common types of communication networks—centralized, decentralized, or restricted—would be most appropriate in this situation?

5. During last week's team meeting, several team members complained openly about having to complete a new, highly detailed form to request the services of a social worker. The unhappy workers claimed that "paperwork is a waste of time and not in their job descriptions." Which of the strategies for maintaining and reinforcing a strong team orientation might be useful in dealing with these team members?

6. You would like all nurses on your staff, regardless of their professional degree, to do four to six hours of preoperation counseling each week. Most RNs on the team feel that they're too busy to spend time in preoperation counseling. What sort of group decision-making process could you initiate to achieve your goal?

7. During weekly staff meetings for the communication and education department at a large teaching hospital, all staff members recommend potential stories for the hospital's monthly newsletter. One staffer recommended devoting an entire issue of the newsletter to diabetes-related programs at the hospital; another staff member countered that the newsletter should focus on something "exciting and controversial like stem-cell research." Although a diabetes-focus was more appropriate for the newsletter's intended audience (urban, largely African American, and elderly), the staffer in favor of stem-cell research persuaded the director of communications that the next newsletter had to cover stem-cell research. On their joint recommendation, the diabetes-focused newsletter was shelved for a later date. What decision-making process is at work here?

Your Dream Team?

Ideally, successful teams exhibit each of the seven qualities listed in section 4.1.2. However, in the real world, each team has different strengths and weaknesses. Also, as a manager, you have limited time to encourage and develop the seven qualities. As the manager of a communications team that produces a monthly newsletter to patients and family members served by a national conglomeration of nursing care facilities, which three of the seven qualities would you *most* want to encourage and develop within your team member?

Catching a Star Player

The patient-care team you lead at a nursing care facility includes Shirley, a physical therapist with more than 20 years PT experience and nearly 12 years working at your facility. Everyone has considerable respect for Shirley, but she can sometimes be very outspoken in team meetings, convincing other team members to agree with her point of view or complaint. What approach can you take to maximize Shirley's contributions to the team?

Forming Activities for a New Team

You're the leader of a newly established cross-functional team that combines social workers, case managers, custom-service representatives, occupational therapists, and physical therapists at a large, suburban hospital. In the past, each functional group has been very isolating, developing its own culture and procedures. Your new cross-functional team has the goal of sharing information and resources more quickly and efficiently, providing improved care for patients. What are some "forming activities" that would be appropriate for your new team?

Team Building as Problem-Solving

Your team of social workers and case managers has seen a significant increase in cases of pediatric AIDS over the last 5 years, despite extensive public education about preventing the disease. Following the six-step process depicted in Figure 4-5, how might your team utilize a formalized team-building process to collaborate effectively and possibly solve the problem?

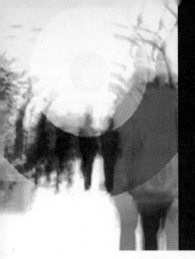

5

MANAGING RESOURCES
Getting the Most from Today's Workforce

Starting Point

Go to www.wiley.com/college/Lombardi to assess your knowledge of basic resource management.
Determine where you need to concentrate your effort.

What You'll Learn in This Chapter

▲ Legal and labor issues that impact human resource management
▲ Ways organizations recruit new employees
▲ Six steps for hiring new employees
▲ Performance appraisals for individuals and teams
▲ Methods of keeping, developing, and terminating employees
▲ Characteristics of office politics and interdepartmental conflict

After Studying This Chapter, You'll Be Able To

▲ Practice ways to find and hire high-quality employees
▲ Examine training techniques for new employees
▲ Examine types of performance-appraising tools
▲ Compare ways of dealing with underperforming employees
▲ Practice techniques for dealing with office politics and conflict

Goals and Outcomes

▲ Master the terminology of resource management and recognize tools and techniques associated with employee recruitment, hiring, training, evaluating, and terminating
▲ Understand laws and processes that affect hiring and developing employees
▲ Identify the negative effects of office politics and conflict
▲ Contrast methods of attracting and selecting employees
▲ Use tools and techniques to appraise employee performance
▲ Solve issues of office politics and conflict
▲ Assess employee training and performance
▲ Determine whether to terminate an employee
▲ Evaluate and select strong job candidates and employees

INTRODUCTION

As a health care manager, no resource is more vital to your department—or, indeed, your organization as a whole—than your human resources, your employees. In today's competitive career marketplace, utilizing strong recruitment techniques goes hand in hand with understanding the latest legal policies and labor practices. The process of selecting quality employees requires managers to go through six distinct phases before hiring. Orientation, training, and performance appraising are all activities managers engage in to develop strong employees. Turnover and termination compel managers to continually engage in the hiring and training process. Managers who respond appropriately to office conflict and politics shape a more productive workplace for themselves and their staffs.

5.1 Meeting Today's Human Resources Demands

People, in all of their diversity, are essential in health care organizations. No one's talents can be wasted in the quest for high performance or greater efficiency. In principle, at least, the following slogans say much about the importance of the human beings that make up today's organizations:

▲ "People are our most important asset."
▲ "It's people who make the difference."
▲ "It's the people who work for us who determine whether our company thrives or languishes."

The basic building blocks of any high-performance health care organization are talented workers with relevant skills and great enthusiasm for their work. One manager summed up the situation as such: "If you hire the right people . . . if you've got the right fit . . . then everything will take care of itself."[1]

5.1.1 Human Resource Management

Human resource management (HRM) involves attracting, developing, and maintaining a talented and energetic workforce to support organizational mission, objectives, and strategies. In order for strategies to be well implemented, workers with relevant skills and enthusiasm are needed. The task of human resource management is to make workers available.

▲ **Attracting** a quality workforce involves human resource planning, recruitment, and selection.
▲ **Developing** a quality workforce involves employee orientation, training and development, and career planning and development.
▲ **Maintaining** a quality workforce involves management of employee retention and turnover, performance appraisal, and compensation and benefits.

Additionally, human resource management must be accomplished within the framework of government regulations and laws. All managers are expected to act within the law and follow equal opportunity principles. Failure to do so is not only unjustified in a free society, but it can also be a very expensive mistake resulting in fines and penalties.

The American legal and regulatory environment covers human resource management activities related to discrimination, pay, employment rights, occupational health and safety, retirement, privacy, vocational rehabilitation, and related areas. It is also constantly changing as old laws are modified and new ones are added.

5.1.2 Laws against Employment Discrimination

Employment discrimination is when someone is denied a job or a job assignment for reasons that are not job relevant. It is against federal law in the United States to discriminate in employment.

A sample of major U.S. laws prohibiting job discrimination is provided in Figure 5-1.

An important cornerstone of legal protection for employee rights to fair treatment is found in Title VII of the Civil Rights Act of 1964, as amended by the

Figure 5-1

Equal Pay Act of 1963	Requires equal pay for men and women performing equal work in an organization.
Title VII of the Civil Rights Act of 1964 (as amended)	Prohibits discrimination in employment based on race, color, religion, sex, or national origin.
Age Discrimination in Employment Act of 1967	Prohibits discrimination against persons poverty; restricts mandatory retirement.
Occupational Safety and Health Act of 1970	Establishes mandatory health and safety standard in workplaces.
Pregnancy Discrimination Act of 1978	Prohibits employment discrimination against pregnant workers.
Americans with Disabilities Act of 1990	Prohibits discrimination against a qualified individual on the basis of disability.
Civil Rights Act of 1991	Reaffirms Title VII of the 1964 Civil Rights act; reinstates burden of proof by employer, and allows for punitive and compensatory damages.
Family and Medical Leave Act of 1993	Allows employees up to 12 weeks of unpaid leave with job guarantees for childbirth, adoption, or family illness.

A sample of U.S. laws influencing human resource management.

Equal Employment Opportunity Act (EEOA) of 1972 and the Civil Rights Act of 1991.

▲ **Equal employment opportunity (EEO):** the right to employment without regard to race, color, national origin, religion, gender, age, or physical and mental ability. The intent is to ensure all citizens have a right to gain and keep employment based only on their ability to do the job and their performance once on the job.

EEO is federally enforced by the Equal Employment Opportunity Commission (EEOC), which has the power to file civil lawsuits against organizations that do not provide timely resolution of any discrimination charges lodged against them. These laws generally apply to all public and private organizations employing 15 or more people.

Under Title VII, organizations are also expected to show **affirmative action.**

▲ **Affirmative action** gives preference in hiring and promotion to women and minorities, including veterans, the aged, and the disabled. Affirmative action ensures that women and minorities are represented in the workforce in proportion to their actual availability in the area labor market.[2]

▲ **Affirmative action plans** may also be adopted by or required of organizations to show that they are correcting previous patterns of discriminatory activity and/or are actively preventing its future occurrence.

FOR EXAMPLE

The U.S. Equal Employment Opportunity Commision

Founded in 1965, the Equal Employment Opportunity Commission has as its mission "the elimination of illegal discrimination from the workplace." Although the definitions of *illegal, discrimination,* and even *workplace* have all evolved over the last 40+ years, the Commission continues to be the final word on appropriate hiring and firing policies for all workplaces in the United States. For example, for the year 2004 alone, the EEOC received 15,376 new charges of disability discrimination and resolved 16,949 disability discrimination charges (recovering more than $47 million for charging parties and other aggrieved individuals, not including monetary benefits obtained through litigation). Find what does and does not constitute discrimination (including age, disability, equal pay, nationality, religion, and sex) at its Web site www.eeoc.gov.

The pros and cons of affirmative action are debated at both the federal and state levels, and controversies often make the news. Criticisms tend to focus on the use of group membership (for example, female or minority) instead of individual performance in employment decisions. The issues raised include the potential for members of majority populations to claim discrimination.[3] White males, for example, may claim that preferential treatment given to minorities in a particular situation interferes with their individual rights.

As a general rule, EEO legal protections do not restrict an employer's right to establish **bona fide occupational qualification.**

▲ **Bona fide occupational qualification:** criteria for employment that can be clearly justified as being related to a person's capacity to perform a job.

The use of bona fide occupational qualifications based on race and color is not allowed under any circumstances; those based on sex, religion, and age are very difficult to support. Years ago, for example, airlines tried to use customer preferences to justify the hiring of only female flight attendants. It didn't work; today men and women serve in this capacity.[4]

In addition to race and gender, which get a lot of attention in the news, other areas of legal protection against discrimination also deserve a manager's concern. Listed below are four examples and brief summaries of their supporting laws. The complexities of these laws would require further research into the context of any possible case to which the laws may be applied.

▲ **Disabilities:** The Americans with Disabilities Act of 1990 prevents discrimination against people with disabilities. The law forces employers to focus on abilities and what a person can do. Increasingly, persons with disabilities are gaining employment opportunities.

▲ **Age:** The Age Discrimination in Employment Act of 1967 (amended in 1978 and 1986) protects workers against mandatory retirement ages. *Age discrimination* occurs when a qualified individual is adversely affected by a job action that replaces him or her with a younger worker.

▲ **Pregnancy:** The Pregnancy Discrimination Act of 1978 protects female workers from discrimination because of pregnancy. A pregnant employee is protected against termination or adverse job action because of the pregnancy and is entitled to reasonable time off work.

▲ **Family matters:** The Family and Medical Leave Act of 1993 protects workers who take unpaid leaves for family matters from losing their jobs or employment status. Workers are allowed up to 12 weeks' leave for childbirth, adoption, personal illness, or illness of a family member.

5.1.3 Current Legal Issues in HRM

Legal issues in human resource management are continually before the courts. The more prominent among them are frequently in the news. Committed health care managers and human resource professionals need to stay informed on the following issues of legal and ethical consequence[5]

▲ **Sexual harassment:** Sexual harassment occurs when a person experiences conduct or language of a sexual nature that affects his or her employment situation. According to the EEOC, sexual harassment is behavior that creates a hostile work environment, interferes with their ability to do a job, or interferes with their promotion potential.

▲ **Equal pay:** The Equal Pay Act of 1963 provides that men and women in the same organization should be paid equally for doing equal work in terms of required skills, responsibilities, and working conditions. However, a lingering issue involving gender disparities in pay involves **comparable worth,** the notion that persons performing jobs of similar importance should be paid at comparable levels. Why should a long-distance truck driver, for example, be paid more than an elementary teacher in a public school? Does it make any difference that the former is a traditionally male occupation and the latter a traditionally female occupation? Advocates of comparable worth argue that such historical disparities are due to gender bias. They would like to have the issue legally resolved.

▲ **Part-time and temporary workers:** The legal status and employee entitlements of part-time workers and independent contractors are also being debated. In today's era of downsizing, outsourcing, and projects, more and more people in all industries—including health care—are being hired as temporary workers who work under contract to an organization and do not become part of its official workforce. They work only "as needed." Problems occur when these individuals are engaged regularly by the same organization and become what many now call *permatemps.* Even though regularly employed by one organization, they work without benefits such as health insurance and pension eligibilities. If they were legally considered employees, these independent contractors would be eligible for benefits, and the implications for their employers would be costly. A number of legal cases are now before the courts seeking resolution of this issue.

▲ **Labor-management relations:** Union representation for health care workers is becoming increasingly common, particularly in larger cities where sizable groups of professionals with similar skills and employment opportunities exist. Nurses of various levels, lab technicians, and even office managers can belong to unions. Health care labor unions are frequently involved in contract negotiations and unfair employment practices investigations. Labor-management issues and their legal foundations are discussed later in the chapter.

5.1.4 Labor-Management Relations

Another aspect of human resource management relates to the influence of organized labor.

▲ **Labor unions** are organizations to which workers belong that deal with employers on the workers' behalves. Labor unions act as bargaining agents, negotiating legal contracts that affect many aspects of human resource management.

Labor contracts typically include the rights and obligations of employees and management with respect to wages, work hours, work rules, seniority, hiring, grievances, and other aspects of employment.

▲ The foundation of any labor and management relationship is **collective bargaining,** which is the process of negotiating, administering, and interpreting labor contracts.

Labor contracts and the collective bargaining process are governed closely in the United States by a strict legal framework.

▲ The Wagner Act of 1935 protects employees by recognizing their rights to join unions and engage in union activities.
▲ The Taft-Hartley Act of 1947 protects employers from unfair labor practices by unions and allows workers to decertify unions.
▲ The Civil Service Reform Act Title VII of 1978 clarifies the rights of government employees to join and be represented by labor unions.

Often, labor and management are viewed as win-lose adversaries, destined to be in opposition and possessed of certain weapons with which to fight one another. If labor-management relations take this form, a lot of energy on both sides can be expended in prolonged conflict.

This model is, to some extent, giving way to a new and more progressive era of greater cooperation.[6] Today's union leaders and corporate leaders appear to recognize that labor-management relations must adapt to changing conditions if they are to survive and prosper.

5.1.5 Human Resource Planning

Any health care organization should at all times have the right people available to do the required work.

▲ **Strategic human resource planning:** a process of analyzing staffing needs and planning how to satisfy these needs in a way that best serves the organizational mission, objectives, and strategies.[7]

The foundations for human resource planning are set by job analysis conducted by human resource professionals with significant input from managers at various levels.

▲ **Job analysis:** The orderly study of just what is done, when, where, how, why, and by whom in existing or potential new jobs.

Job analysis—which often includes human resource personnel observing and interviewing employees who do a specific job and then collaborating with managers to write a comprehensive description of all that a job entails—provides useful information that can then be used to write and/or update **job descriptions** and **job specifications**, which can then be shared with employees and potential job applicants.

▲ **Job descriptions:** Written statements of job duties and responsibilities.
▲ **Job specifications:** Lists of the qualifications—such as formal education, prior work experience, and skill requirements—that should be met by any person hired for or placed in a given job.

The elements in strategic human resource planning are shown in Figure 5-2. The five-step process outlined in the figure begins with a review of organizational mission, objectives, and strategies, which establishes a frame of reference for forecasting human resource needs. Ultimately, the planning process helps

Figure 5-2

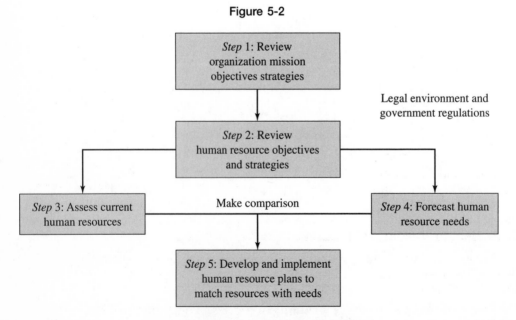

Steps in strategic human resource planning.

managers identify staffing requirements, assess the existing workforce, and determine what additions or replacements are required to meet future needs. The entire process, of course, must be implemented in a manner consistent with the legal environment.

5.1.6 Attracting a Quality Workforce

Attracting and selecting new members of your team can easily spell the difference between success and failure as a health care manager. When you select a top performer, you have an individual from whom the entire team can draw inspiration and rely on for steady or stellar performance. Conversely, when you select an individual who is not a top performer, the negative results can be staggering.

Although far from being an exact science, the process of hiring and selecting new employees can take on some structure, complete with strategies and proven approaches for success. After a human resource plan is prepared, the process of attracting a quality workforce can systematically begin.

▲ **Recruitment** is a set of activities designed to attract a qualified pool of job applicants to an organization. Emphasis on the word *qualified* is important.

Effective recruiting should bring employment opportunities to the attention of people whose abilities and skills meet job specifications.

The three basic steps in a typical recruitment process are

1. advertise a job vacancy;
2. establish preliminary contact with potential job candidates;
3. perform an initial screening to identify all qualified applicants.

In recruiting potential nursing candidates soon to graduate from a health care training school, for example, advertising is done by a hiring hospital by posting short job descriptions in print or on Web sites through the campus placement center. Preliminary contact is made after candidates register for interviews with hospital recruiters on campus. Preliminary interviews typically run 20 to 30 minutes, during which time the candidate presents a written resume and briefly explains his or her job qualifications. To further screen the candidates, the hospital recruiter shares interview results and resumes with key decision makers at the hospital. They choose a final pool of candidates to be invited for further interviews during a formal visit to the organization.

Recruitment is certainly one of the most difficult endeavors for the modern-day health care manager. The reason for this is the ongoing shortage of qualified personnel in virtually all health care positions. This means you must work assiduously toward generating a good roster of candidates and use as many recruitment sources as possible.

External versus Internal Recruitment

Recruitment can be either internal or external:

▲ **External recruitment,** in which job candidates are sought from *outside* the hiring organization. Newspapers, employment agencies, colleges, technical training centers, personal contacts, walk-ins, employee referrals, and even competing health care organizations are all sources of external recruits.

▲ **Internal recruitment** seeks applicants from *inside* the organization. This involves notifying existing employees of job vacancies. Most health care organizations have a procedure for announcing vacancies through newsletters, electronic bulletin boards, and the like. They also rely on managers to recommend high-performing workers as candidates for advancement.

Both recruitment strategies offer potential advantages. External recruiting brings in outsiders with fresh perspectives and provides access to specialized expertise or work experience not otherwise available from insiders. Internal recruitment is usually less expensive and involves people whose performance records are well established. A history of serious internal recruitment can also be encouraging to employees; it shows that one can advance in the organization by working hard and achieving high performance at each point of responsibility.

Recruitment Tactics

Health care managers rely on several tried-and-true methods to recruit quality job candidates. Although organizations have specific techniques and resources (consult with your human resources department), the following tactics are all useful:

▲ **Job fairs:** Whenever possible, try to attend job fairs in your specific technical area. Although many job fair attendees are simply shopping around and aren't interested in immediate employment, collecting resumes and obtaining information on potential candidates is a continuous process for proactive health care managers.

▲ **School liaisons:** Many health care professionals maintain contact with the schools they graduated from. Contact the school's placement office or a favorite teacher, and ask whether any up-and-coming talent may be suitable for your open position. School liaisons may also know alumni in the field who may be suitable candidates as well. If you are trying to fill an entry-level position, contact a guidance counselor at a local high school or vocational school and inquire about likely candidates.

▲ **Employment referral systems:** Most organizations have an employee referral system in which employees refer qualified individuals to human resources for openings in the organization. If your organization does not have an employee referral system, or if you work in a small health care organization, discuss with your supervisor the possibility of providing a monetary reward to an employee who recommends a candidate for an open position who is subsequently hired.

▲ **Professional contacts:** Contact former colleagues or institutions and discuss the availability of potential candidates. If you belong to a professional organization, contact a representative within that organization to generate a list of potential candidates.

▲ **Agencies:** Many health care recruiters frown on placement and search agencies because recruitment services are costly and often yield less than satisfactory results. Contact an agency only with the assistance of your human resource department or your immediate supervisor. When you work with an agency, spend as much time as possible with the primary recruiter in developing a list of expectations and revised job descriptions.

▲ **Advertising:** Employment ads in print and online media can be somewhat expensive, and unfortunately they can provide inconsistent results. If you run an ad, work with your human resource director and supervisor to craft the ad. Make certain the ad receives good placement within the newspaper or magazine, has a catchy logo, and contains a three-to-five-sentence depiction of the job, the salary range, and the name of a specific contact person. These elements will eliminate people who are simply job shopping or who are not in the salary range established for the position.

▲ **Team/staff referrals:** Members on your own team may know someone qualified for an open position. However, unless they are asked, your team members may assume you're not interested in their recommendations.

Community-Based Recruitment

Smaller health care providers, particularly in rural areas or in distinct neighborhoods (of large East Coast cities, for example) use community-based recruitment. These institutions write a three-to-five-sentence depiction of the open position, the point of contact, and salary range, and make copies on their organization's stationery. They post these copies on bulletin boards in key areas within the community: supermarkets, convenience stores, libraries, community centers, post offices, and places of worship.

When using community-based recruitment, be sure to get permission from the appropriate authority at each posting area. Getting their permission is also an opportunity for you to gain their support and participation in the search effort by reviewing the contents of your notice and discussing any potential applicants they might know among their customers or congregation. The business and religious anchors in the community are typically positive allies in the health care recruitment process.

SELF-CHECK

- Identify and define **human resource management, discrimination, Equal Employment Opportunity, sexual harassment, labor union, collective bargaining, recruitment,** and **affirmative action.**
- List the three main activities of human resource management.
- Describe key laws and legal issues that affect hiring employees.
- Discuss the role of labor unions in hiring and managing employees.
- Explain ways human resource departments can plan for the future.
- Compare typical employee recruitment techniques.

5.2 The Selection Process

To avoid the negative aspects of hiring a poor performer, you need to understand the selection process. **Selection** is the process of choosing from a pool of applicants the person or persons who offer the greatest performance potential.

Health care managers who successfully master the selection process not only diminish the chance that they have to terminate poor performers or address performance problems, but they also enhance all their management responsibilities by having the luxury of working with well-motivated, talented people.

FOR EXAMPLE

Using a Targeted Selection System

The Shore Health System in Maryland (www.shorehealth.org) uses the CARE factors (community, accountability, respect, and excellence) as its organizational standards during all hiring processes. Hiring managers and HR professionals at Shore Health System utilize a structured selection system with a set of 75 open-ended questions and interpretive guides to make sound decisions about recruiting, interviewing, and selecting top job candidates.

Figure 5-3

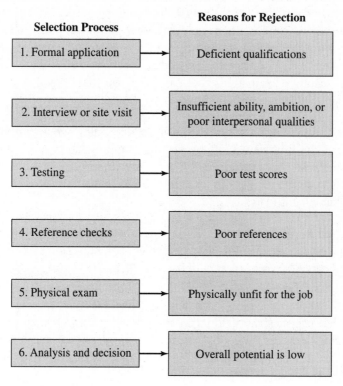

Steps in the typical selection process and possible reasons for rejection.

Figure 5-3 shows the six typical steps in the selection process, including

▲ completion of a formal application form;

▲ interviewing;

▲ testing;

▲ reference checks;

▲ physical examination;

▲ final analysis and the decision to hire or reject.

The following six sections explore each step of the selection process in greater detail.

5.2.1 Reviewing Applications and Resumes

Applicants typically use two forms to apply for jobs:

▲ The **application form** declares the individual to be a formal candidate for a job. It documents the applicant's personal history and qualifications.

The application should only request information that is directly relevant to the job and the applicant's potential job success.

▲ The **personal resume** is often included with the job application and should accurately summarize an applicant's special qualifications. As a recruiter and hiring manager, you need to learn how to screen applications and resumes for insights that can help you make good selection decisions.

Your main objective in reviewing resumes is to determine whether the person can do the job. (The interview is where you determine what type of person the candidate is and how they would do the job.) Try to sort the resumes by your criteria, and organize the candidates into three basic categories: unqualified, possible, and probable candidates.

▲ **Unqualified applicants** simply do not have the quantitative skills established on the job description. For example, they either do not have the required degree or years of experience required.

▲ **Possible candidates** have the quantitative skills sought and may have additional factors that merit consideration. For example, for the position of staff pharmacist, an individual in the possible category may have all the necessary degrees, including the specific professional accreditation to prepare for state compliance reviews, and a good range of years of professional experience.

▲ **Probable candidates** are individuals who seem almost perfect for the position. This is typically the smallest group of applicants.

Establish a short list of candidates, beginning with the probable group and including applicants from the possible group until you have approximately seven or fewer candidates. However, do not fall into the seductive trap of reading too much into a resume. Try to take the information at face value; remember that the resume is simply a summary of qualifications, not an in-depth insight into the applicant's personality.

5.2.2 Interviewing

Interviews are extremely important in the selection process because of the information exchange they allow. The interview is a time when both the job applicant and potential employer can learn a lot about one another.

However, interviews are also recognized as potential stumbling blocks in the selection process. To avoid them, keep these general pointers in mind when you conduct a job interview:

▲ **Plan ahead:** Review the job specifications and job description as well as the candidate's application; allow sufficient time for a complete interview.

▲ **Create a good interview climate:** Allow sufficient time, choose a quiet place, be friendly and show interest, and always give the candidate your full attention.

▲ **Conduct a goal-oriented interview:** Know what information you need and get it. Look for creativity, independence, and a high energy level.

▲ **Avoid questions that may imply discrimination:** Focus all questioning on the job applied for and the candidate's true qualifications for it.

Proceed with caution when asking questions of job candidates in an interview situation. The following list covers some potentially illegal areas of job interviewing and suggests legal alternatives.

▲ **National origin:** *Illegal*—Are you a U.S. citizen? *Legal*—Are you authorized to work in the United States?

▲ **Family:** *Illegal*—Are you married? *Legal*—Would you be willing to relocate?

Illegal—Do you plan to have children? *Legal*—Are you willing to travel as needed?

Illegal—Who lives with you? *Legal*—This job requires occasional overtime; is that okay?

▲ **Age**: *Illegal*—How old are you? *Legal*—Are you over 18?

▲ **Arrest record:** *Illegal*—Have you ever been arrested? *Legal*—Have you ever been convicted of a crime relevant to job performance?

▲ **Military service:** *Illegal*—Were you honorably discharged from the military? *Legal*—What type of training did you receive in the military?

▲ **Disability:** *Illegal*—Do you have any disabilities? *Legal*—Can you perform (some specific task) as an essential part of the job?

In **traditional recruitment,** the emphasis is on selling the organization to job applicants. Human resource professionals and hiring managers communicate only the most positive features of the job and organization to potential candidates.

Traditional recruitment may create unrealistic expectations that are difficult to fulfill, and dissatisfied new hires may quickly leave. The cost of job turnover, including lost productivity, search fees, and recruiting costs, can be very high.

Realistic job previews, by contrast, try to provide the candidate with all pertinent information about the job and organization without distortion and *before* the job is accepted.[8] Instead of selling only positive features of a job, this approach tries to be realistic and balanced in the information provided.

With more realistic job expectations, new employees may be less prone to premature turnover and often experience higher levels of initial job satisfaction.

5.2.3 Employment Tests

Whenever tests are used and in whatever forms, the goal should be to gather information that helps predict the applicant's eventual performance success. Like any selection device, an employment test needs to measure exactly what it intends to relative to the job specification—for example, written communication skills or computer literacy. The test should also meet the criterion of reliability by yielding approximately the same results over time if taken by the same person. Furthermore, any employment test used in the selection process should be legally defensible on the grounds that it actually measures an ability required to perform the job.

New developments in testing allow for actual demonstrations of job-relevant skills and personal characteristics. Numerous larger health care organizations and hospitals now have assessment centers that help evaluate candidates' potential by observing their performance in experiential activities designed to simulate daily work.

Another form of testing is work sampling, which directly assesses a person's performance in the job. Here, applicants are asked to work on actual job tasks while being graded by observers on their performance.

5.2.4 Reference Checks

Reference checks are inquiries to previous employers, academic advisors, co-workers, and/or acquaintances regarding the qualifications, experience, and past work records of a job applicant.

Although they may be biased if friends are prearranged "to say the right things if called," reference checks can be helpful. The Society for Human Resources Management (SHRM), for example, estimates that 25% of job applications and resumes contain errors.[9] Use a reference simply as a validation of what you may already have decided about a candidate, not as a revelation; certainly, in no case should a reference be the main factor in your decision.

Realize that U.S. labor law severely restricts the reference-checking process. Fundamentally, individuals who provide references are only required to provide limited information: the person's name, position, length of employment, and approximate salary range.

5.2.5 Physical Examinations

Many health care organizations ask job applicants to take a physical examination. This health check helps ensure that the person is physically capable of fulfilling job requirements. It may also be used as a basis for enrolling the applicant in health-related fringe benefits such as life and health insurance programs.

A recent and controversial development in this area is the emerging use of substance-abuse testing. This has become part of preemployment health screening and is a basis for continued employment at some organizations. At a minimum, care must be exercised that any required test is job relevant and does not discriminate in any way against the applicant.

5.2.6 Final Decision to Hire or Reject

The best selection decisions are most likely to be those involving extensive consultation among the manager or team leader, potential co-workers, and human resource staff.

The emphasis in selection must always be comprehensive and focus on all aspects of the person's capacity to perform in a given job. Just as a "good fit" can produce long-term advantage, a "bad fit" can be the source of many and perhaps long-term problems. Of course, you should also always remember that you're not seeking the perfect person or perfect match for the position; you're simply seeking the best-qualified person given the criteria for the job.

SELF-CHECK

- Identify and define **selection, realistic job preview, traditional job recruitment,** and **reference check.**
- List the six typical steps in the selection process.
- Describe three useful categories for sorting potential job candidates.
- Discuss techniques to make job interviews effective and questions/topics to avoid for legal reasons.
- Explain appropriate uses of employment tests, reference checks, and physical examinations during the selection process.

5.3 Developing a Quality Workforce

When people join any organization, they must "learn the ropes" and become familiar with the way things are done. **Socialization** is the process of influencing the expectations, behavior, and attitudes of a new employee in a way considered desirable by the organization.[10] The intent of socialization in the human resource management process is to help achieve the best possible fit between the individual, the job, and the organization.

5.3.1 Employee Orientation

Socialization of newcomers begins with *orientation*. **Orientation** is a set of activities designed to familiarize new employees with their jobs, co-workers, and key aspects of the organization as a whole. This includes clarifying the organizational mission and culture, explaining operating objectives and job expectations, communicating policies and procedures, and identifying key personnel.

The first 6 months of employment are often crucial in determining how well someone is going to perform over the long run. During this time, original expectations are tested, and patterns are set for future relationships between an individual and employer.

If orientation is neglected, newcomers are left to fend for themselves during this critical period. On their own or through casual interactions with co-workers, otherwise well-intentioned and capable people may learn inappropriate attitudes and/or behaviors.[11] Good orientation, by contrast, enhances a person's understanding of the organization and adds a sense of common purpose as a member.

5.3.2 Training and Development

Training is a set of activities that provides the opportunity to acquire and improve job-related skills. Training is appropriate and necessary for both new and established employees (particularly those who desire to upgrade or improve their skills to meet changing job requirements).

Training can take many forms:

- ▲ **On-the-job training** takes place in the work setting while someone is doing a job.
- ▲ **Job rotation** allows people to spend time working in different jobs and thereby expand the range of their job capabilities.
- ▲ **Coaching** occurs when an experienced person gives technical advice to someone else. This can happen on a formal basis by supervisors or co-workers. It can also occur more informally in the form of help spontaneously offered in teams.
- ▲ **Apprenticeship** is a work assignment as understudy or assistant to someone who already has the desired job skills. Through this relationship, an apprentice learns a job over time and eventually becomes fully qualified to perform it.
- ▲ **Modeling** occurs when someone demonstrates through personal behavior what is expected of others.
- ▲ **Mentoring** occurs when new or early career employees are formally assigned as protégés to senior employees who then coach, model, and otherwise assist them to develop job skills and get a good start in their careers.

FOR EXAMPLE

Mentoring for Diagnostic Imaging Professionals

In response to ongoing shortages of qualified job candidates in the diagnostic-imaging professions, including radiography and cardiovascular interventional technologists, the American Association of Cardiovascular and Pulmonary Rehabilitation (www.aacvpr.org) established a year-long mentoring program in 2004. The program pairs new and senior members in the organization, based on application responses. Although much of the mentoring occurs via phone or e-mail, members both new and senior have been very pleased with the program and the new connections they've made—35 pairs participated in 2004, and that number nearly doubled the following year. For more information about the AACVPR's mentoring program, visit www.aacvpr.org/membership/mentorship.cfm.

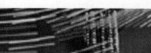

SELF-CHECK

- Identify and define **socialization, orientation,** and **training.**
- Explain the importance of orientation and training in the managing of employees.
- Describe common training tools and techniques.

5.4 Performance Appraisal

One of the most difficult responsibilities of a health care manager is the assessment and conduct of **performance appraisals.** Taking qualitative, subjective perceptions of performance and ascribing a quantitative, objective rating is generally a difficult and complex task. This task becomes important specifically as most performance evaluations are tied to the individual staff member's salary and potential salary increases.

Performance appraisals serve two basic purposes in the maintenance of a quality workforce:

▲ The **evaluation purpose** is intended to let people know where they stand relative to performance objectives and standards.

▲ The **development purpose** is intended to assist in their training and continued personal development.[12]

FOR EXAMPLE

Criterion-based, Values-driven Performance Evaluation Systems

A major motivational tool for both the marginal performer and the superstar employee is the annual performance evaluation. However, when the performance evaluation is merely a checklist review of the existing job description, distinguishing between great and merely adequate employees becomes difficult. At Jane Phillips Medical Center in Bartlesville, Oklahoma (www. jpmc.org), managers use a performance evaluation that measures how an individual performs relative to job specifications; assesses the CARE or PACT factors of attitude orientation, people skills, and team orientation; *and* recognizes contributions made beyond the set job description. This standard, multidimensional evaluative tool has been a key reason for a recent upswing in employee morale at this urban, nonprofit facility.

Performance appraisals should meet the criteria of reliability and validity. To be *reliable,* the method should consistently yield the same result over time and for different raters. To be *valid,* it should be unbiased and measure only factors directly relevant to job performance. These criteria are especially important in today's complex legal environment. A manager who hires, fires, or promotes someone is increasingly called upon to defend such actions—sometimes in specific response to lawsuits alleging that the actions were discriminatory. At a minimum, written documentation of performance appraisals and a record of consistent past actions is required to back up any contested evaluations.

5.4.1 Appraisal Methods

The following are performance appraisal methods commonly used in organizations:

▲ **Graphic rating scales** offer checklists of traits or characteristics thought to be related to high performance outcomes in a given job. A manager rates the individual on each trait using a numerical score. The primary appeal of graphic rating scales is that they are relatively quick and easy to complete. Their reliability and validity are questionable, however, because the categories and scores are subject to varying interpretations.

▲ **The narrative technique** is a written essay description of a person's job performance. The commentary typically includes actual descriptions of performance, discusses an individual's strengths and weaknesses, and provides an overall evaluation. Free-form narratives are sometimes used in combination with other performance appraisal methods, such as the graphic rating scale.

▲ The **critical-incident technique** involves keeping a running log or inventory of effective and ineffective job behaviors. By creating a written record of positive and negative performance examples, this method documents success or failure patterns that can be specifically discussed with the individual.

▲ **Multiperson comparisons** formally compare one person's performance with that of one or more others. Multiperson comparisons can be used on their own or in combination with some other method. They can also be done in different ways.

- In *rank ordering,* all persons being rated are arranged in order of performance achievement, with the best performer at the top of the list and the worst performer at the bottom; no ties are allowed.

- In *paired comparisons,* each person is formally compared to every other person and rated as either the superior or the weaker member of the pair. After all paired comparisons are made, each person is assigned a summary ranking based on the number of superior scores achieved.

- In *forced distribution,* each person is placed into a frequency distribution that requires that a certain percentage fall into specific performance classifications, such as top 10%, next 40%, next 40%, and bottom 10%.

5.4.2 Designing and Implementing a Documentation System

Documentation is the process of objectively recording performance and performance levels. Managers and executives at all levels of a health care organization rely on documentation to provide proof that accepted standards of performance have been met.

Documentation does take time and effort, but without it, the compilation of a comprehensive performance appraisal is next to impossible. Keep the following documentation tips and strategies in mind:

▲ **Set up a performance documentation logbook.** A simple spiral-bound notebook (or organization-specific logsheets) is all that's necessary to record the dates, significant incidents, and critical contributions for each staff member.

▲ **Be specific.** General notes like "has a bad attitude" or "never documents well on charts" have little use in preparing a performance appraisal. Whenever possible, note specific, quantifiable details and refer back to established performance objects. And always date any entry in logbooks.

▲ **Note positive incidents, as well as negative.** Performance appraisals should not be all gloom and doom. Keeping records of what employees do especially well can help your employees recognize their strengths and plan the future paths of their careers.

Finally, realize that whatever form your documentation takes, your professional notes cannot be used or subpoenaed in court. Many health care managers fear their notes may be used against them in a court of law. This is not the case, as the only documentation used in a court labor proceeding is the official performance evaluation filed with the health care organization. You use your professional notes—not anyone else's. Use them to increase employees' constructive performance and in turn provide stellar health care to your patients.

5.4.3 Delivering Performance Appraisals

By maintaining detailed, organized documentation, performance appraisals should be relatively easy to write. Sharing appraisals, however, can be another story entirely. The following guidelines can help you effectively deliver appraisals to your employees.

▲ **Prepare fully for the evaluation.** Ensure you fill out all paperwork correctly and completely. Consider how you want to present the performance evaluation, and simply conduct a review of what you have written on the evaluation.

▲ **Create an appropriate physical environment for delivering an appraisal.** Sit at your desk, a table, or wherever you are most comfortable; close the door; and avoid interruptions while delivering the evaluation. The occasion should be a private interchange between you and the employee.

▲ **Provide the employee with a copy of the evaluation.** The employee can use it as a guide, follow the discussion throughout the entire process, and keep the copy as a planning tool for future performance.

▲ **Manage emotionalism.** If an employee becomes emotional during the evaluation, usually because of a negative reaction, ask whether the employee wants to take a break or reschedule the evaluation. If the employee elects postponement, schedule a follow-up meeting within a week's time and deliver the appraisal fully at that time. If the employee again becomes emotional, either get assistance from your manager or the human resource department, or simply conduct the review in monologue fashion. (Use this last strategy when you suspect the employee is reacting poorly to the performance evaluation as an excuse for poor performance or as a means to avoid the evaluation completely.)

▲ **Use a direct and objective style.** Use clear terms, state your case objectively, and avoid personalizing the evaluation. Try to stay on an even keel, using emotion only as appropriate. At the same time, feel free to express dissatisfaction to an employee who is not performing acceptably or pride in an employee who is performing at an outstanding level.

▲ **Use a point-by-point strategy.** Work through the evaluation from beginning to end. Stop frequently to ask whether the employee has any questions or would like elaboration on any part of the information given so far.

▲ **Set a time limit for the appraisal and stay within it.** For example, an hourly employee may take a half hour to complete a performance appraisal, whereas a skilled worker may need 45 minutes. Try to stay within these parameters, and keep that standard for all employees.

▲ **Give closure.** Ensure that the employee signs the performance-evaluation form and that all questions are answered. Remember, not all employees will be thrilled with their reviews.

5.4.4 Reviewing Group Performance

In addition to individual performance appraisals, many managers conduct team or group performance appraisals. While these appraisals may or may not be required by your specific health care organization, group performance appraisals can be worthwhile endeavors. Gathering together as a team to assess the group's strengths and weakness, as well as discuss future goals can yield significant results in creating a workplace where employees feel part of a team.

To effectively conduct a group performance appraisal, managers must encourage staff to be direct and candid about their assessment of past performance as a group. Focus the conversation on performance, not on personality-based issues. Avoid referring to the personalities of former managers and other team members. In emphasizing performance, you discover areas for improvement and crystallize specific methods on how to improve performance throughout the department and within individual work roles.

Discussion about *what we are doing wrong* also helps establish trust. By acknowledging that the department is not perfect and that you as manager are not perfect, you remind everyone involved that you share the human quality of imperfection. By reviewing mistakes and concentrating on where a problem may exist, your staff will appreciate your commitment to them and therefore feel freer to share their thoughts on areas for improvement.

One way to facilitate a group performance appraisal is to have all team members brainstorm areas for improvement. First list events or work aspects that need improvement. Then, ask your staff to focus in on things they can control or are doing right relative to the problems or challenges cited. Finally, brainstorm situations and circumstances of which the department has either limited or no control.

In later sessions (or perhaps regular department meetings), you can continue to discuss as a group how the team can become stronger. This could include another exercise on how the team can meet the needs of the patient at an even higher level of quality and effectiveness. Use five basic questions to initiate discussions:

▲ Where does communication seem to break down?

▲ When do we operate as a team most efficiently?

▲ When do we operate as a team least efficiently?

▲ On a scale of 1 to 10, how would you rate the level of pride we have in our department (1 = no pride, 10 = great pride)?

▲ What can we do better as a group?

These questions serve to facilitate a group process for discussion of specific areas needing improvement and, more directly, address areas in which the unit can work more strongly as a team.

SELF-CHECK

- Identify and define **performance appraisal** and **documentation**.
- Explain the two purposes of conducting performance appraisals.
- Contrast various appraisal methods.
- Describe techniques for effective documentation and presentation for performance appraisals.
- Discuss the pros and cons of group performance appraisals.

5.5 Maintaining a Quality Workforce

Attracting and developing a qualified workforce is only a portion of a health care manager's responsibilities. For long-term effectiveness, a health care workforce must be successfully nurtured and managed. This requires proper attention to such maintenance issues as career planning and development, work-life balance, retention and turnover, and compensation and benefits.

5.5.1 Career Planning and Development

Career planning is the process of systematically matching career goals and individual capabilities with opportunities for their fulfillment. Career planning involves answering such questions as "Who am I?" "Where do I want to go?" and "How do I get there?"

While some suggest that a career should be allowed to progress in a somewhat random but always opportunistic way, others view a career as something to be rationally planned and pursued in a logical step-by-step fashion. In fact, a

---

FOR EXAMPLE

Ongoing Training, Every Day

At Pascack Valley Hospital in New Jersey, a list of strategies for patient relations—known as the hospital's "Whatever It Takes" customer service program—is printed on the back of the laminated name badges that every employee carries and uses daily. The badges serve as a constant good reminder of the hospital's standard of customer care, as well as the criteria that is used to evaluate all health care-specific workers in annual appraisals. Additionally, outstanding performances in one of the criteria listed on the badges are rewarded with merit bonuses, providing a needed financial incentive for the hospitals ongoing staff-development programs.

---

well-managed career probably includes elements of each. The carefully thought-out plan can point you in a general career direction; an eye for opportunity can fill in the details along the way.

5.5.2 Work–Life Balance

Today's fast-paced and complicated lifestyles bring with them inevitable pressures on the balance between careers and personal time. Human resource policies and practices that support a healthy work-life balance are increasingly valued. Work-life balance concerns include

▲ the needs of single parents, who must balance complete parenting responsibilities with a job;

▲ the needs of dual-career couples, who must balance career needs and opportunities of each partner;[13]

▲ the "family-friendliness" of an employer, including access to on-site day care, medical and dental offices, dry cleaning, and even video rentals.[14]

5.5.3 Retention and Turnover

The several steps in the human resource management process both conclude and recycle with the management of promotions, transfers, terminations, layoffs, and retirements. Proactive health care managers approach any of these *replacement situations* as an opportunity to review human resource plans and ensure that the best people are selected to perform the required tasks.

Some replacement decisions shift people between positions within the organization.

▲ **Promotion** is movement to a higher-level position.

▲ **Transfer** is movement to a different job at a similar level of responsibility.

Another set of replacement decisions relates to retirement, something many people look forward to—until it is close at hand. Then the prospect of being retired often raises fears and apprehensions. Many organizations offer special counseling and other forms of support for preretirement employees, including advice on company benefits, money management, estate planning, and use of leisure time. Downsizing is sometimes accompanied by special offers of early retirement—that is, retirement before formal retirement age but with special financial incentives.

The most extreme replacement decisions involve termination.

▲ **Termination:** the involuntary and permanent dismissal of an employee.

For the person being dismissed, accepting the fact of termination is difficult. The termination notice may come by surprise and without the benefit of advance preparation for either the personal or the financial shock.

5.5.4 Compensation and Benefits

When properly designed and implemented, compensation and benefit systems help attract qualified people to the health care organization and retain them.

▲ **Base compensation** is the form of salary or hourly wages that can make the organization a desirable place of employment.

Unless an organization's prevailing wage and salary structure is competitive, attracting and retaining a staff of highly competent workers is difficult. A basic rule of thumb is to study the labor market carefully and pay at least as much as, and perhaps a bit more than, what competitors are offering.

The organization's employee-benefit program also plays a role in attracting and retaining capable workers.

▲ **Fringe benefits:** the additional nonwage or nonsalary forms of compensation now constitute some 30% or more of a typical worker's earnings. Benefit packages usually include various options on disability protection, health and life insurance, and retirement plans.

Interestingly, the ever-rising cost of fringe benefits, particularly employee medical benefits, is a major worry for health care employers. Some are attempting to gain control over health care costs by becoming more active in employees' choices of health care services and providers. An increasingly common approach overall is flexible benefits, sometimes known as *cafeteria benefits,* which allow the employee to choose a set of benefits within a certain dollar amount. Employees gain when such plans are better able to meet their needs; employers gain from being more responsive to a wider range of needs in a diverse workforce.

5.5.5 Contrasting Probation and Termination

Terminating employees is an unfortunate but necessary part of being a health care manager. Knowing *when* to fire someone can be as difficult as knowing *how*. When individual performance has deteriorated to the point of being counter-productive, it is clearly time for separation. In many cases, individuals are actually relieved when terminated because they have become frustrated and ineffective in their work roles.

Do not expect anyone to thank you for terminating them, however, or to admit that it was their fault for being terminated. Terminating an employee is a very difficult undertaking, and this section offers suggestions to make the termination process as painless and productive as possible.

▲ **Disciplinary probation** is generally acknowledged as a final step before termination. Probation is generally a 3-month process in which poor performers are given the opportunity, usually one last chance, to turn performance around to an acceptable level.

Many health care managers think that probation is a farce because if the individuals "behave" for 3 months, there is no guarantee that they will perform steadily for the rest of the year. In fact, they generally believe that performance will usually regress.

In many cases, employees who are on probation terminate themselves by securing other employment while on probation, thus saving the headache of having to fire them. In this regard, probation is a worthwhile practice and should be used in conjunction with a performance evaluation for an employee who is likely to be terminated eventually anyway.

5.5.6 When to Terminate

When should you fire someone? Each case deals with a unique individual and specific circumstances. You should terminate an employee if most of the following conditions are present:

▲ **Chronic poor attitude:** An employee who regularly appears to be inflexible, overly aggressive or confrontational, irresolute, and tunnel-visioned and displays a poor work ethic and no sense of industry is a candidate for termination. Rarely are individuals who demonstrate these attitudes likely to change. In an industry that requires high adaptability, appropriately assertive behavior, perseverance, and a strong work ethic, these problems, which probably cannot be corrected, are unacceptable.

▲ **Poor interpersonal skills:** An individual who consistently demonstrates interpersonal behavior problems and creates conflicts may be a candidate for termination. In a people-oriented field such as health care, poor interpersonal skills do not make for long-term success.

▲ **Negative effect on others:** When an employee's negative behavior creates intradepartmental conflict and the employee has been counseled several times about the effect caused by these conflicts, termination must be considered.

▲ **Poor performance documentation:** If the employee's pattern of performance documentation over a 1-year period has been largely negative, termination must be considered. Such individuals typically not only fail to grow and develop on the job, but they also usually regress to a level of performance that is less than what was expected for the current year. In short, individuals who have demonstrated a full year of poor performance have probably fallen into a pattern that cannot be remedied by probation or another year on the job. In essence, they are absorbing a salary that can be better spent on a better performer.

▲ **Negative or no reaction to counseling:** After a problem employee has been counseled by you, the human resource department, or other appropriate individuals in your organization and the individual still fails to perform acceptably, chances are the situation is unresolvable.

▲ **Outside negative input:** If patients, peers, or other department members have constructively criticized the individual's performance, most likely the performance is affecting the entire workflow of your department. To keep this problem from festering, termination must be enacted.

▲ **Detrimental effect on the organization:** A poor performer who is in a critical work position can adversely affect the entire organization. If you have clear evidence that this is the case, termination must be enacted quickly to maintain exceptional organizational integrity and performance.

▲ **Regressive patterns, trends, and habits:** A person who consistently demonstrates poor on-the-job behavior, inappropriate work personality, and poor work habits—all substantiated by your own documentation—is a candidate for termination.

5.5.7 How to Terminate

After determining that termination is necessary, you need to act quickly and effectively. The following checklist can help you through this difficult process.

1. **Explain documentation.** All prior appropriate documentation should be on hand for presentation at the time of termination. Explain in 2 to 3 minutes your overriding documentation and the reasons you considered termination as the only possible remedy. Documentation must be used as the basis for any discussion of termination.

2. **Recap performance counseling.** Quickly summarize all efforts made to resolve the performance problem.

3. **Get to the point.** Tell the individual that you are terminating them for cause. If the employee already guessed that he or she is being terminated and says so, simply acknowledge it and move on to the next step.

4. **Have a witness on hand.** If you have never fired an employee, ask a third person (your boss or someone from the human resource department) to be present at the session. This allows you to have support on hand as well as someone to help guide you through the process.

5. **Allow a monologue.** If the person being fired feels like talking or wants to ventilate, allow them 3 to 5 minutes to do so. Then respond that although you respect his or her feelings, the decision has been made.

6. **Get closure.** Instruct the individual to gather his or her belongings and leave the premises. If necessary, call security to escort them off the premises.

7. **Prepare an exit letter.** A letter of termination delineating cause and signed by the former employee should go in the personnel file, along with the person's comments, if any. Any other paperwork that completes the process should be included.

8. **Communicate with your staff.** Notify staff that you have terminated the individual and that you plan to fill the position quickly. You need not disclose the reasons for the termination. If your employees have questions, recommend they come into your office on an individual basis and discuss. (If further discussion is desired, only the future of the department should be discussed, not the terminated employee.)

9. **Reject additional input.** After you terminate an employee, you need not accept further input from another employee. Your focus should be on the future, specifically on employee suggestions for filling the position.

10. **Fill the position quickly.** You have an opportunity to command trust and allegiance from your staff by providing them with a productive, professional new colleague.

Termination is never easy, but by using these techniques and enlisting the support of your superiors and human resource staff, you can move through this difficult situation.

SELF-CHECK

- Identify and define **career planning, promotion, transfer, disciplinary probation, base compensation, fringe benefits,** and **termination.**
- Discuss common work-life balance concerns.
- Contrast typical replacement situations, including promotion, transfer, and termination.
- List typical reasons for probation or termination.
- Describe the steps of probation and termination.

5.6 Dealing with Office Politics and Resolving Conflict

Unfortunately, exercising your talents as a health care manager will probably be tested by overtly political behavior, or at least annoyed by day-to-day dealings of "office politics." It is important that health care managers avoid political quagmires in the workplace in the interest of providing stellar, progressive services to patients and to the health care organization.

Office politics cause several significant problems for the health care manager and the health care organization as a whole.

▲ **Politics inhibit productivity:** Generally speaking, workers are not particularly motivated to perform well for individuals who are more politics-minded than performance-minded. A great deal of time is spent avoiding power plays and preparing for counteractions. Consequently, productivity suffers, and worst of all the patient is deprived of receiving the full range of services the health care organization is capable of providing.

▲ **Politics stifle creativity:** Because politics can promote paranoia, team members may be reluctant to share new ideas or work in a group process that encourages creativity or innovation. As a result, staff growth and development are compromised, or top performers relocate to a less political or, better yet, nonpolitical environment. Again, the patient and the organization suffer.

▲ **Politics cripples teamwork:** Individuals who are suspicious of each other and have limited respect for each other end up resenting one another and avoiding open communication. Politics destroys allegiance and loyalty among team members and the overall objective of the team or organization. Group morale begins to diminish until finally individual employee motivation begins to erode.

▲ **Overt negative politics alters communication:** Overt negative politics include altered messages, altered presentation of messages, or flat-out noncommunication in certain situations. Politics often begin after a third party enters the picture, creating an unbalanced dynamic and opportunity for two people to discuss a third person—often in an uncomplimentary manner.

5.6.1 Signs of Overtly Political Behavior

Whenever a premium is placed on politics as opposed to performance in the health care environment, the team or department finds itself at risk of falling apart—or at least beginning to be much less productive. Five basic indicators that can signal overtly political behavior include

▲ **double-talk.** Individuals who tell one story to one person and an entirely different story to another are double-talkers. Their motives may be to cover the bases on a particular issue, deliberately create disharmony, or simply try to pit two people against each other;

▲ **backstabbing.** Backstabbers overtly pledge allegiance to you and your ideas but covertly downplay them and insult your intelligence;

▲ **power mongering.** Power mongers try to control everything. These individuals are also called *turf protectors* or *empire builders* because they often use resources and territory as the principal focus of their subversive efforts. As a health care manager, you may fall prey to a power monger's claim of being in charge of something that in fact he or she has no control of;

▲ **victim role.** Some individuals claim that the organization is out to get them and that you had better watch yourself. People with this mind-set are more interested in their own survival than in assisting fellow workers through the health care mission;

▲ **game playing.** Game players use phony behavior in trying to engender support. They play games with fellow staff as well.

5.6.2 Dealing with Overtly Political Behavior

As a manager, how do you deal with politics? Whether the politician is a member of your staff or a colleague, these five strategies may be useful:

▲ **Avoidance** is easy. Simply try to stay out of the way of political behavior whenever possible. If avoidance is not feasible on a daily basis, keep all contact on a business level and discuss only business issues. If someone tries invariably to shift the focus to a politically oriented level, firmly return them to the issue at hand. Remember that your primary managerial responsibility is to bolster staff motivation and productivity while contributing to your facility's goal of high-quality patient care.

▲ **Confront the person** and let her know that you are aware of her political intent. For example, if you are asked a loaded question, simply counter by asking another question such as, "Why are you asking me that?" You risk incurring wrath, but you at least discourage overtly political behavior.

▲ **Disclosure and support** works if the troublesome individual is someone on the management team or someone who reports to your own manager. Simply present evidence of the political behavior to your supervisor, without judgment or opinion. Use objective reporting. For instance: "You know, a funny thing happened the other day. I was talking to (name), who seemed persistent in wanting to discuss (topic)." This approach indicates your apprehension in dealing with this individual and signals your need for specific assistance.

▲ With **direct input** from your own manager, you can actively enlist support. Simply tell your supervisor about the problem, review the evidence, and ask directly for assistance: "What would you do if you had this situation?" (If you perceive your boss to exhibit excessively political behavior, you may want to request the help of another mentor within the organization in dealing with this behavior.)

▲ **Gather documentation** as evidence of political behavior by colleagues or staff. The more examples you collect, the better case you can make for termination (if the person is staff) or for limited contact (if the source is a colleague). Record evidence or examples of notable political behavior, and be sure to handle reports tactfully.

5.6.3 Symptoms of Intradepartmental Conflict

Despite a health care manager's best efforts to establish trust throughout her work group and to avoid potential conflict, human nature unfortunately creates occasions for intradepartmental conflict. **Intradepartmental conflict** is any conflict that takes place within a single department or work group.

Initially, intradepartmental conflict takes place on an *interpersonal basis*. Interpersonal conflict, particularly within a work group, is potentially the most damaging type of problem a health care manager can deal with. If interpersonal conflict exists within a department and is not abated and healed, eventually it can have drastic negative consequences for the entire department—even implosion.

Numerous indicators signal intradepartmental conflict. Use your instincts and observations to examine the conflict in a cause-and-effect fashion. Following is a list of potential symptoms, causes, and effects on your department.

▲ **Anger:** Interpersonal adversity, loss of temper, lack of patience, or flat-out confrontational behavior may all be exhibited in certain kinds of interpersonal conflict.

▲ **Avoidance:** When an individual declines to work with someone or simply avoids contact with that person, work may not be done and the team processes may be compromised. Avoidance is more subtle than anger and often more common.

▲ **Blame:** One individual may claim another person is entirely responsible for a mistake. Often the person blaming is attempting to cover for his own inability or failure to perform. Blaming creates hostility among team members and betrays basic trust and pride in the organization.

▲ **Excuse making:** One individual uses another's behavior as a reason for not performing a particular task. The individual may focus specifically on a personality nuance as being the problem that gets in the way of accomplishment. Another form of making excuses is to rationalize the negative behavior of others.

▲ **Isolation and fragmentation:** Certain team members may exclude one or more players because of personality conflict. Isolation jeopardizes the group-participation process, and ultimately, one or more individuals may withdrawal the resources needed to get a job done. Extreme isolation may lead workers to organize into factions. This fragmentation can become particularly detrimental in any group process, especially one that requires quick, efficient response.

▲ **Confrontation:** Argumentative personality types use intimidation and confrontation to disrupt process, waste time, and demoralize others.

▲ **Criticism:** Continuous nit-picking severely diminishes morale. Ironically, others often respond to constant criticism by becoming defensive and in turn critical of the chronic criticizer.

▲ **Erosion of performance:** The quality and efficiency of work diminishes, resulting in ill feelings and costly overtime. Some staff begin to look for another workplace if the situation is not corrected by the manager.

▲ **Regression:** A performance continues to erode, worker may do less and less, bringing work process to a grinding halt. In an era in which health care must be progressive, every employee's performance must contribute to its maximum potential.

5.6.4 Resolving Intradepartmental Conflict

Many organizations have recommended approaches to dealing with interdepartmental conflict. As you gain more experience as a manager and see what does (and doesn't) work, you're sure to develop your own ways of resolving disagreements between staff members. The following six-step process can adapt well to a multitude of situations and organizationally recommended processes:

1. **Go on a fact-finding mission.** Begin any effort to resolve intradepartmental conflict by performing thorough fact finding every step of the way. *Fact finding* is the process of collecting information from all involved parties before arriving at a decision. For example, when an intradepartmental conflict takes place between two individuals, you may want to investigate by discussing the situation with both parties separately and by asking them the same two questions: what they think the problem and root cause may be, and how the situation can be resolved. At that point, bring both parties together, present both ideas for resolution, and once again state your optimism for correction as well as your refusal to tolerate further interpersonal conflict.

2. **Separate issues into two categories.** First identify business-related attributes of the problem—business outcomes, performance dimensions, and technical areas. Then list personal issues that may bear on the conflict. Review this information completely with the involved party and reach consensus on

the facts of the issues. If no one acknowledges the facts, you may have to state more directly your belief in their validity and supplement that statement with the pledge that you will not accept this behavior any longer.

3. **Move the discussion to performance.** Focus specifically on the business effects from the conflict. Cite work that is not being done; explain how the employee's (or group's) behavior affects other department members and how this behavior interferes with others' getting their jobs done. Discuss further how this behavior affects other departments and, most important, patients.

4. **Ask why this behavior has taken place and how it might be corrected.** Try to get to the bottom of what the parties believe is contributing to the problem and how the cause can be alleviated. Following this discussion, present your own ideas on why the problem exists; however, spend most of your discussion on how the problem must be remedied.

5. **State clearly, concisely, and resolutely your expectations, standards, and policies for future action.** Explain what you accept as satisfactory behavior and what you consider poor performance or interpersonal conflict. Future actions may include probation or other disciplinary action, including termination.

6. **Express your confidence that the situation will be corrected and ask whether particular assistance is needed to do so.** Try to strike a delicate balance between expressing optimism that the situation can be corrected and underscoring the fact that continued poor performance and intradepartmental conflict will not be tolerated under any conditions.

Interpersonal conflict is complex and can hinder progressive action. As a manager, you must deal with it resolutely and in a timely fashion so that the majority of your department is not adversely affected.

FOR EXAMPLE

Alternative Dispute Resolution

Alternative dispute resolution (ADR) is a term that includes a wide range of techniques—conflict management, arbitration, mediation, and more—for resolving workplace conflict without involving expensive, time-consuming, and often unsatisfying legal professionals. Updated daily, ADRWorld.com (www.adrworld.com) collects and publishes news stories on alternative dispute resolution in the workplace. Membership in the community is free, and members can receive a weekly e-newsletter that has top stories and court decisions related to conflict resolution. Members also have access to a free searchable database of summarized news stories and legal rulings involving ADR in all 50 U.S. states.

SELF-CHECK

- Identify and define **office politics** and **intradepartmental conflict**.
- List four negative impacts of office politics.
- Identify five common types of political behavior.
- Discuss five ways to respond to political behavior.
- Describe five common responses to intradepartmental conflict.
- Detail a six-step response to intradepartmental conflict.

SUMMARY

Human resources—your staff, employees, and team members—are the most valuable resources in a health care organization. Human resource management requires adherence to employment and discrimination laws, as well as savvy recruiting, thorough interviewing and selection, and efficient training and development. Regular performance appraisals—both of individuals and work teams—provides feedback and improves the overall function of the organization. Promoting, transferring, and terminating are all potential responses to retention and turnover in the workplace. Proactive managers monitor and effectively respond to office politics and conflict before their work environments begin to suffer.

KEY TERMS

Affirmative action	Preference in hiring and promotion to women and minorities, including veterans, the aged, and the disabled.
Base compensation	An employee's salary or hourly wage.
Bona fide occupational qualification	Criteria for employment that can be clearly justified as being related to a person's capacity to perform a job.
Career planning	The process of systematically matching career goals and individual capabilities with opportunities for their fulfillment.
Collective bargaining	The process of negotiating, administering, and interpreting labor contracts.
Comparable worth	The notion that persons performing jobs of similar importance should be paid at comparable levels.

Disciplinary probation	The final step before termination, generally a 3-month process in which poor performers are given the opportunity to turn performance around to an acceptable level.
Documentation	The process of objectively recording performance and performance levels.
Employment discrimination	Situation in which someone is denied a job or a job assignment for reasons that are not job relevant.
Equal employment opportunity (EEO)	The right to employment without regard to race, color, national origin, religion, gender, age, or physical and mental ability.
Fringe benefits	The additional nonwage or nonsalary forms of compensation workers receive, including disability protection, health and life insurance, and retirement plans.
Human resource management (HRM)	Attracting, developing, and maintaining a talented and energetic workforce to support organizational mission, objectives, and strategies.
Intradepartmental conflict	A conflict that takes place within a single department or work group.
Job analysis	The orderly study of just what is done, when, where, how, why, and by whom in existing or potential new jobs.
Job descriptions	Written statements of job duties and responsibilities.
Job specifications	Qualifications (educational level, prior experience, or skills) that should be met by any person hired for a given job.
Labor unions	Organizations to which workers belong that deal with employers on the workers' behalves.
Orientation	A set of activities designed to familiarize new employees with their jobs, co-workers, and key aspects of the organization as a whole.
Performance appraisal	Taking qualitative, subjective perceptions of performance and ascribing a quantitative, objective rating.
Promotion	Movement of an employee to a higher-level position.
Realistic job previews	Opportunities during the selection process that provide candidates with all pertinent information

	about the job and organization without distortion before the job is accepted.
Recruitment	A set of activities designed to attract a qualified pool of job applicants to an organization.
Reference checks	Inquiries to previous employers, academic advisors, co-workers, and/or acquaintances regarding the qualifications, experience, and past work records of a job applicant.
Selection	The process of choosing from a pool of applicants the person or persons who offer the greatest performance potential.
Sexual harassment	Situation in which a person experiences conduct or language of a sexual nature that affects his or her employment situation.
Socialization	The process of influencing the expectations, behavior, and attitudes of a new employee in a way considered desirable by the organization.
Strategic human resource planning	A process of analyzing staffing needs and planning how to satisfy these needs in a way that best serves organizational missions, objectives, and strategies.
Termination	The involuntary and permanent dismissal of an employee.
Training	A set of activities that provides the opportunity to acquire and improve job-related skills.
Transfer	Movement of an employee to a different job at a similar level of responsibility.

ASSESS YOUR UNDERSTANDING

Go to www.wiley.com/college/Lombardi to evaluate your knowledge of resource management.

Measure your learning by comparing pretest and post-test results.

Summary Questions

1. Equal employment opportunity (EEO) is the right to employment without regard to race, color, national original, religion, gender, age, or physical and mental ability. True or false?

2. Collective bargaining allows unions to
   (a) establish the base wage for specific jobs.
   (b) purchase benefits for union members.
   (c) negotiate and interpret labor contracts on behalf of union members.
   (d) None of the above

3. Effective recruitment tactics include all of the following except
   (a) staff referrals.
   (b) sales forces.
   (c) school liaisons.
   (d) advertising.

4. Hiring managers need to be careful when asking job candidates questions on the topic of
   (a) military service.
   (b) age.
   (c) national origin.
   (d) All of the above

5. During a reference check, a hiring manager may attempt to verify an applicant's qualifications, experience, and past work record; however, references are only required to verify the candidate's name, position, length of employment, and approximate salary range. True or false?

6. Currently, it is legal to ask a job candidate to submit to a physical exam prior to extending a job offer to ensure that the candidate is physically capable of fulfilling job requirements. True or false?

7. The purpose of socialization on the job is to help the team form personal connections with one another, thereby improving productivity. True or false?

8. For a new employee, an appropriate and effective method of training and development would be
   (a) manuals.
   (b) modeling.

(c) lectures.

(d) projects.

9. Performance appraisals have two basic purposes: evaluation and promotion. True or false?

10. If you wanted to conduct an appraisal that evaluates an employee's performance against another employee's performance, you could use which of the following appraisal methods?

    (a) Graphic rating scale

    (b) Critical incident technique

    (c) Narrative technique

    (d) Multiperson comparisons

11. Group or team appraisals are most effective when the emphasis is on personalities rather than performance. True or false?

12. Effective career-planning requires managers to help workers balance work priorities and life demands. Today's work-life concerns include

    (a) child care.

    (b) two-career households.

    (c) single parent families.

    (d) all of the above.

13. Disciplinary probation is often an ineffective tool for improving an employee's work output or attitude. Many individuals simply behave during probation and return to old habits after. True or false?

14. When terminating an individual, do all the following, except

    (a) have your boss or an HR professional present during the termination meeting.

    (b) hold an open question-and-answer session with remaining staff after the termination.

    (c) allow the terminated individual to vent his or her frustrations for 3 to 5 minutes.

    (d) summarize quickly efforts made to resolve performance problems.

15. Office politics ultimately have a negative effect on a workplace for all of the following reasons, except

    (a) office politics stifle individuality.

    (b) office politics cripple teamwork.

    (c) office politics inhibit productivity.

    (d) office politics alter communications.

16. Isolation in the workplace can lead workers to organize into separate factions, a process known as *fragmentation*. True or false?

17. The first step to resolving intradepartmental conflict is to ask yourself why a behavior has taken place and how it might be corrected. True or false?

Review Questions

1. When an organization legally establishes and justifies criteria for employment, the organization is relying on what legal principle?

2. How do job descriptions differ from job specifications?

3. In internal recruitment, an organization looks within its staff for perspective job candidates. What are some benefits of utilizing internal recruitment?

4. A manager assigns more responsibility to a single nurse because she doesn't have to worry about the family obligations that married staff do. Which Equal Employment law does this violate?

5. At what stage during the six-step selection process would an applicant be asked to perform a work task while an observer watches and grades their performance?

6. Realistic job previews for job candidates are gaining popularity even though previews take time and have some costs associated with them. What benefits do realistic job previews offer?

7. After you sort job applicants into the three recommended categories, which applicants should you interview first?

8. You have an experienced team member give technical advice to a less experienced member. What sort of on-the-job training are you encouraging?

9. What are some appropriate topics to include as part of employee orientation?

10. Graphic rating scales are popular tools for performance appraisals because they are quick and easy to use. However, what is their main downside?

11. What should you do if an employee begins crying or shouting during a performance appraisal?

12. In addition to wages or salary, fringe benefits play a major role in attracting and retaining quality employees. What are some examples of common fringe benefits an organization can offer?

13. After you terminate an employee, what are some things you should do in regards to remaining employees?

14. Although employees on probation rarely change their behaviors permanently, it can still be an effective tool. In what way?

15. Backstabbing and game playing are two indicators that your team may be struggling with office politics. What behaviors are involved in these activities?

16. Step 2 in the recommended process for resolving intradepartmental conflict recommends separating issues into two categories. What are these categories and how do they differ?

Applying This Chapter

1. Roberto is encouraged by his manager to transfer to a less-demanding part-time position because he's 55 and will probably be thinking about retirement in the next 5 to 10 years. Roberto feels somewhat uncomfortable with his manager's suggestion. What type of discrimination might be underlying the manager's recommendation?

2. During an interview, you ask a candidate whether she's ever been denied health insurance. You ask the question because you know your organization is having difficulties managing the cost of employees' medical services and prescriptions. Why is your question most likely illegal?

3. As the clinic manager of a student-health center, you lead a team of eight nurses and nursing aides, many of whom are working their first health care job. Describe two ways you can incorporate coaching as a training and development technique in your role as the manager of a student-health clinic.

4. Upper management has requested that you quickly evaluate the performances of 20 staff members for report on the progress of implementing new charting requirements. You need to conduct and present your evaluation in 1 week's time. What sort of performance appraisal tools would be fast and effective to evaluate your staff?

5. Because of his consistently poor attitude, confrontational actions with patients, and lack of response to counseling efforts, you decide to terminate Randall, a nurse on the team you manage at a pediatric hospital. What are some things you should do within your team after the termination?

6. Cameron says that other nurses in his department don't respect him because they're female and are only interested in helping other women. He comes to you, as his manager, and asks you to overlook the fact that he's late to work once or twice a week because the stress of working in a hostile environment makes coming in on time difficult. What type of political behavior is Cameron engaging in?

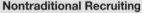

Nontraditional Recruiting

The medical laboratory you manage is consistently running short on entry-level lab assistants to help the staff of four experienced technicians set up, execute, and clean up tests. Employees with post-college education are typically unsatisfied working in the lab assistant position. How might you engage various individuals and organizations in your community to attractive appropriate job candidates?

Worthwhile Testing

As the hiring manager for a multiphysician convenience clinic, you decide that you'd like to incorporate some form of job testing for all office-management candidates. Several past new hires had very weak computer, organizational, and/or customer service skills—and traditional interviewing didn't reveal these deficiencies. What are some useful tests you might include in future interviews?

Cost-Effective Training

As the office manager of a multiphysician, suburban medical clinic, you manage a group of 10 "specialists," including a scheduler, several billing/accounting technicians, two insurance provider liaisons, and several customer-service representatives. You also have five administrative assistants who float among the specialists, assisting the specialists on an as-needed basis. You've identified that the high turnover rate in administrative assistants is connected to a lack of good training and career development opportunities. What are some cost-effective training and development programs you can put in place to improve the work experience (and job retention) of the administrative assistants in your office?

Dutiful Documentation

The manager of a nursing team at a nursing care facility documents the following performance note in an individual performance logbook for Emily, a health aide who's been with the organization for less than a year: "On March 31, Emily didn't do her job today and got huffy with me. She claims she was busy helping transfer patient Leonard Crelborne to another facility. Crelborne's family was upset about the transfer and Emily was able to calm them down by explaining the situation." In what way is this an effective piece of documentation? In what way is this an ineffective piece of documentation?

Salary Comparisons

While people are drawn to health care careers for many reasons, salary is an undeniably important motivation for many workers. Do you know the range of base compensation you can anticipate in your chosen health care career? While no resource or professional can tell you definitely the hourly wage or salary you'll receive, several print and online resources can give you a range of salaries that your base compensation should fall within. Get started on comparing salaries by visiting Monster.com's frequently updated, nationwide salary calculator at http://content.salary.monster.com/. The easy-to-use tool compares potential salaries in hundreds of health care careers, in thousands of geographic regions across the United States.

Choosing Your Response

Jayne, a pediatric nurse with more than 10 years of patient-care experience at several hospitals, frequently refers to herself as the "top dog" in the department. She uses her experience as reason to trade off less-appealing patients with other nurses in the department. Jayne claims that she's the only nurse in the department who knows how to operate several pieces of high-tech equipment and refuses to teach other staffers how to use the equipment. No one wants to work with Jayne because she's condescending, yet nearly everyone must beg Jayne for help on a daily basis because they don't know how to do certain procedures she's always responsible for. As Jayne's manager, how would you choose to respond to the situation: avoid, confront, disclose/seek support, rely on direct input, or gather documentation?

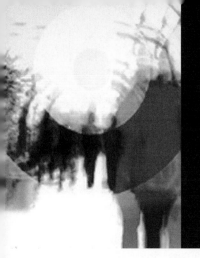

6

MANAGERIAL AND SUPERVISORY PLANNING
Preparing for the Road Ahead

Starting Point

Go to www.wiley.com/college/Lombardi to assess your knowledge of the basics of planning.
Determine where you need to concentrate your effort.

What You'll Learn in This Chapter

- ▲ The benefits of planning
- ▲ Common types of plans
- ▲ The five steps of the planning process
- ▲ Widely used planning tools and techniques
- ▲ The importance of SWOT analysis

After Studying This Chapter, You'll Be Able To

- ▲ Demonstrate how organizations can improve by using planning
- ▲ Analyze the critical factors that distinguish different plans
- ▲ Distinguish the importance of each step of the planning process
- ▲ Compare the relative merits of planning tools and techniques
- ▲ Examine how plans can be adapted to account for uncertainty and change

Goals and Outcomes

- ▲ Master the terminology, understand the steps, and recognize the tools of the planning process
- ▲ Distinguish among types of plans based on their time horizon, scope, and focus
- ▲ Organize planning activities around the planning process
- ▲ Use tools and techniques to analyze parts of the planning process
- ▲ Discuss the results, implications, and limitations of specific plans
- ▲ Collaborate with others to carry out a SWOT analysis
- ▲ Apply proper planning techniques to real-life situations
- ▲ Evaluate real plans and use planning tools to produce on-going process improvement

INTRODUCTION

While all managers must monitor the day-to-day flow of work and resources, good managers are also always looking ahead. A thorough plan, based on an accurate understanding of the current workplace and focused on achievable goals for the future, helps everyone in an office, department, or workgroup to work effectively, meeting today's demands and tomorrow's challenges. Plans can vary in length and scope, depending on the needs of the organization. A five-step planning process often yields the strongest plans. Organizations utilize numerous standard tools and techniques to create high-quality plans, including the popular and effective tool of SWOT analysis.

6.1 Why Plan?

Successful managing requires thorough planning. **Planning** is the process of deciding exactly what you, your team, or your department wants to accomplish and how to best go about meeting your goals. Planning is the foundation on which all other managerial responsibilities rest.

6.1.1 Successful Plans

All successful plans have four components. They

▲ organize processes, procedures, and staff for efficient and effective work.

▲ influence and lead team members or employees who report to you.

▲ monitor work progress, schedules, and budgets.

▲ identify problems and suggest corrective actions.

The following explores the importance of planning, the basic types of plans health care managers work with, the step-by-step way plans are created, and a host of special tools and techniques that can make plans more effective and efficient for everyone who utilizes them.

In today's demanding health care workplace, your department, team, or workgroup needs to consistently meet goals both large and small to help improve the overall company as well your specific group. Meeting—and, hopefully, exceeding these goals and expectations—enables your department and company to become ever better at what they do, staying one step ahead of the competition.

Health care organizations face pressures and challenges from many sources, all of which increase the importance of good planning. External forces include competition, increased government regulations, ever-more complex technologies, the uncertainties of a global economy, and rising labor and resource costs. Internal forces include the demand for greater efficiency, increased diversity in the workforce, and the introduction of new processes, structures, and work arrange-

FOR EXAMPLE

Paying Attention to ADD

Cincinnati Children's Hospital Medical Center (www.cincinnatichildrens.org) recently decided to address an increasingly common behavior disorder for U.S. kids and teens: attention deficit hyperactivity disorder (ADHD). Swamped with referrals for pediatricians and family physicians outside Cincinnati Children's, a new task force developed evidence-based mental health guidelines for diagnosing and treating ADHD outside of Cincinnati Children's Mental Health Clinic. In addition to helping local pediatricians and family practice physicians make accurate diagnoses, the guidelines also help reduce wait time for patients otherwise being referred to Cincinnati Children's for their condition. For 1 year following the introduction of the guidelines, trained Cincinnati Children's staff will be available for phone and on-site consultation, supporting the guidelines and empowering local physicians.

ments. In today's ever-changing work environment, good planning offers a number of benefits and advantages for your employees, your teammates, and even your own career.

6.1.2 Greater Focus and Flexibility

Good planning improves focus and flexibility for both you and your organization.

▲ **Focus:** An organization with focus knows what it does best, knows the needs of its customers or patients, and knows how to serve them well. An individual with focus knows where he or she wants to go in a career or situation and is able to keep that objective in mind, even in difficult circumstances.

▲ **Flexibility:** An organization with flexibility is willing and able to change and adapt to shifting circumstances and operates by looking toward the future (rather than the past or present). An individual with flexibility balances his or her career plans with the problems and opportunities posed by new and developing circumstances—both personal and organizational.

6.1.3 Improved Coordination

Good planning improves coordination, or the way in which various people and departments interact and work together. Most health care organizations are buzzing hives of activity with many different individuals, groups, and departments each pursuing different tasks and objectives. However, everyone's accomplishments must collectively meet the needs of the organization as a whole.

Figure 6-1

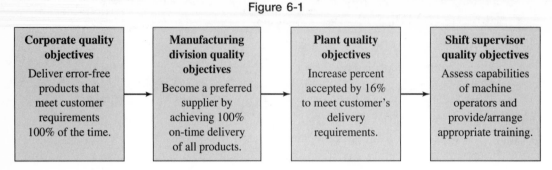

Corporate quality objectives	Manufacturing division quality objectives	Plant quality objectives	Shift supervisor quality objectives
Deliver error-free products that meet customer requirements 100% of the time.	Become a preferred supplier by achieving 100% on-time delivery of all products.	Increase percent accepted by 16% to meet customer's delivery requirements.	Assess capabilities of machine operators and provide/arrange appropriate training.

A sample hierarchy of objectives for a medical records management group.

A comprehensive plan creates a **hierarchy of objectives** in which the goals for each area of the organization are linked together, scheduled chronologically, or ranked in terms of importance. Figure 6-1 shows a hierarchy of objectives in a large health care organization. The objective for the Records Management group in a health insurance provider is "to store, organize, retrieve, and share vital patient data efficiently and appropriately." This objective fits within the insurance provider's corporate objective to "facilitate timely and cost-effective health-care treatment for our clients 100% of the time." This objective also translates down the hierarchy to the level of the patient-interaction representative, where the specific job objective becomes a formal commitment to "assist patients in locating and better utilizing their medical records to receive superior medical treatment."

6.1.4 Enhanced Control

Control means meeting the desired outcomes as efficiently as possible (on bud-get, on time, etc.). Good planning facilitates control. Without planning, the control process lacks a framework for measuring how well things are going and determining what can be done to make them go better.

A good plan clearly defines the desired objectives and performance results, and identifies specific ways and actions to reach these goals. If results are less than expected, you can evaluate the original objectives, the actions being taken, or both and then adjust the objectives and actions to improve future accomplishments. Good plans help you compare results with original expectations, suggest actions improve future accomplishments, and refine future objectives.

6.1.5 Better Time Management

Good planning helps with time management. You've probably experienced the difficulties of balancing your available time with numerous commitments, opportunities, and obligations. Each day, health care workers are bombarded by a multitude of tasks and demands in a work setting that abounds in interruptions, crises, and unexpected events. A manager's job is especially subject to such complications. Managers can easily fall prey to "time wasters," such as allowing others to dominate your time or completing nonessential procedures and reports.

"Basically, the whole day is a series of choices" says Lewis Platt, former chairman of Hewlett-Packard. Platt offers a philosophy for dealing with the dilemmas many managers face: you must make choices that allocate your time to the most important priorities. Platt encourages you to be "ruthless about priorities," continually adjusting what you're doing and how you're doing it to maximize your efficiency.

6.1.6 Solution-Focused

Good planning provides managers with more than a set of processes and procedures. A good plan offers immediate solutions that managers can utilize quickly. As a manager, you should expect certain problems to arise fairly often. Most problems can be classified as structured or unstructured.

▲ **Structured problems:** familiar situations; the information needed to resolve these problems is straightforward and clear. You can plan ahead and develop specific ways to deal with structured problems, or even take action to prevent their occurrence. In the workplace, "personnel" problems are common whenever decisions are made on pay raises and promotions, vacation requests, committee assignments, and the like. Knowing this, proactive managers plan ahead so they can handle complaints effectively when they arise. A well-crafted plan offers prepared responses (based on successful past experience, of course) that are appropriate for specific problems.

▲ **Unstructured problems:** unexpected and ambiguous situations that lack critical information. Unstructured problems require novel solutions. Proactive managers can get a jump on unstructured problems by recognizing situations that may be susceptible to problems and then making plans that can be implemented if unfavorable results occur. Taken to the extreme, an unstructured problem can become a **crisis:** an unexpected and demanding problem that can result in disaster. In today's post-9/11 world, no one can avoid or even anticipate all potential crises. However, managers at many progressive organizations now anticipate that crises will, unfortunately, occur and have developed early warning systems and crisis-management plans to deal with problems in the best possible ways.

6.1.7 Ready for Action

Good planning helps create an **action orientation,** which means you and your organization act and react confidently and quickly to new situations. When you're working from a well-crafted plan, you don't need to spend hours lamenting what went wrong or assigning blame. Instead, you can refer to your plan as a resource and determine next steps or possible solutions.

Additionally, a plan helps you and your organization avoid the "complacency trap" of simply being carried along by the flow of events or being distracted by the successes or failures of a given moment. When you're always looking toward the future, you have clear performance targets and you can often anticipate decisions that need to be made before difficult situations or problems arise.

SELF-CHECK

- Identify and define **focus, flexibility, hierarchy of objectives,** and **unstructured problem.**
- Cite the characteristics of successful plans.
- Explain the main benefits of successful planning.

6.2 Types of Plans

Health care organizations utilize a wide variety of plans. These plans vary in terms of time spans, scope, and level of application. In all cases, plans must be both well made and well implemented for success. You can describe most plans as either short-range or long-range, and strategic or operational.

6.2.1 Short-Range versus Long-Range

Short-range plans cover 1 year or less, **intermediate-range plans** cover 1 to 2 years, and **long-range plans** look 3 or more years into the future. For best results, plans at each time range mesh together, with short-range goals and activities helping to satisfy some portion of intermediate and long-range goals. Top management usually sets long-range plans and provides general direction for lower-level managers. In turn, lower managers formulate and execute short-range plans, while still keeping mindful of the organization's long-term objectives.

6.2.2 Strategic versus Operational

Plans throughout an organization differ in terms of scope. **Strategic plans** address long-term needs and set comprehensive action directions for an organization. Top-level managers typically offer strategic plans, determining objectives for the entire organization and then deciding on the actions and resource allocations to achieve them. By contrast, **operational plans** define what needs to be done in specific areas to implement strategic plans. Operational plans frequently found in the health care industry include

- ▲ **product plans:** methods and technology needed to create valuable goods or services;
- ▲ **financial plans:** dealing with the money required to support various operations;
- ▲ **facilities plans:** buildings, major equipment, and work layouts required to support business activities;
- ▲ **marketing plans:** activities and efforts required to sell and distribute goods or services;
- ▲ **human resource plans:** recruitment, selection, and placement of people into various jobs.

Working in the health care field, you encounter dozens of different types of plans. Policies, procedures, schedules, and budgets are some of the common plans that managers work with, refer to, and enforce on an almost daily basis.

6.2.3 Policies and Procedures

Organizations typically operate with many policies and procedures. These standing plans are used over and over again to direct behavior in certain types of situations. However, a policy and procedure have distinct differences:

- ▲ **Policy:** communicates broad guidelines for making decisions and taking action in specific circumstances. To cite an example, human resource policies cover matters such as alcohol and substance abuse or sexual harassment. These guidelines help ensure that all employees' daily actions and decisions are consistent with organizational values, strategies, and objectives.
- ▲ **Procedure:** describes exact rules for dealing with specific situations. Procedures are often published in employee handbooks or manuals as standard operating procedures, or SOPs. Clearly written procedures ensure that everyone receives fair, equal, and nondiscriminatory treatment.

To cite an example: A sexual harassment policy sets expectations for employee behavior; sexual harassment procedures define precise actions to be taken when someone believes he or she has been harassed on the job. Both policy and procedure need to be clearly documented and agreed to by all.

6.2.4 Schedules and Budgets

Increasingly, today's workplace focuses on **projects,** specific goals that can be accomplished by teams working under tight deadlines. Good plans are essential

> ## FOR EXAMPLE
>
> ### Setting Priorities at the National Cancer Institute
>
> The overarching mission of the National Cancer Institute is to "reduce the incidence of cancer and integrate early detection through the development and effective delivery of medical approaches and the promotion of effective, evidence-based public health interventions and policies." To better pursue this worthy goal, the NCI in 2003 realigned its efforts to focus first and foremost on cancer prevention and early detection. While NCI continues to fund state-of-the-art biological research and technological development, the organization's renewed emphasis on prevention and detection affects a greater portion of the population and identifies cancer early on, when it is most curable. Visit http://plan.cancer.gov for a comprehensive listing of NCI's numerous initiatives, goals, and programs.

in order to manage resources (time, money, materials, workers, and so on) and to accomplish defined tasks.

▲ **Project schedules:** identify the activities required to accomplish a specific major project. In a health care organization, project schedules may guide the shift of a medical office staff from paper-based patient files to electronic files or rollout and integration of new federal regulations on patient privacy. In either case, a project schedule defines specific task objectives, activities, due dates, and resource requirements. A good project schedule sets priorities so everyone involved knows not only what needs to be done but also in what order so that the entire project gets finished on time.

▲ **Budgets:** plans that commit resources to activities, projects, or programs. They are powerful tools that allocate scarce resources among multiple and often competing uses. Good managers are able to bargain for and obtain adequate budgets to support the needs of their work groups or teams. They are also able to achieve performance objectives while keeping resource expenditures within the allocated budget.

Projects and departments sometimes have **fixed budgets** that allocate a set amount of resources that can be used, but not exceeded, for a specified purpose. If the department head allotted you a $25,000 budget for equipment purchases for the year, you couldn't spend more on equipment unless you had approval.

A **flexible budget,** by contrast, allocates resources based on the need level of various departments or activities. A project leader's budget may increase to allow for hiring temporary workers during a time of transition for a customer service center. However, in subsequent years, the project leader's budget may decrease because new computer systems and improved processes should eliminate the need for costly temporary workers.

In a **zero-based budget,** a project or activity is budgeted as if it were brand-new. All projects must compete anew for available funds in each budget cycle. Managers operating within a zero-based budget cannot assume that resources previously allocated will simply continue in the future. Dynamically changing businesses, government agencies, and other organizations use zero-based budgets to ensure that the most desirable and timely programs receive the most funding.

SELF-CHECK

- Identify and define **plans, policies, procedures, schedules, and budgets.**
- Name the specific characteristics of the different types of operational plans.
- Explain the relationship between policies and procedures.
- Identify and compare the different types of budgets.

6.3 The Planning Process

At its most basic, planning is decision making. When you plan, you use information to make plans that address significant problems and opportunities. Figure 6-2 shows a typical approach to decision making as applied during the **planning process.** The planning process begins with identification of a problem and ends with evaluation of implemented solutions. This section covers each step of the planning process in detail, addressing the key responsibilities of managers at each phrase. The following are five steps in the planning process:

Step 1: Identify and define the problem.

Step 2: Generate and evaluate possible courses of action.

Step 3: Choose a preferred solution.

Step 4: Implement the solution.

Step 5: Evaluate results.

6.3.1 Identify and Define the Problem

During the first step of planning and decision making—finding and defining the problem—you gather information, evaluate information, and deliberate. Problem symptoms usually signal the presence of a performance deficiency or opportunity.

Figure 6-2

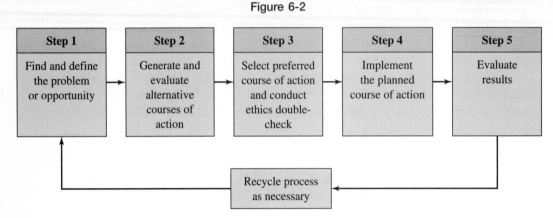

Making decisions during the planning process.

During this step, you need to assess the situation properly by looking *beyond* symptoms to find out what is really happening. Take special care to not just address a symptom while ignoring the true problem. The way you define a problem originally can have a major impact on how you go about resolving it. Poor problem definition can lead to poor or ineffective plans. The following are three common mistakes:

▲ **Focusing on symptoms instead of causes.** Symptoms indicate that problems may exist, but don't mistake them for the problems themselves. Most managers can spot problem symptoms (like a drop in an employee's performance). Instead of treating symptoms (such as simply encouraging higher performance), good managers need to address the symptom's root causes (in this case, discovering that the worker's need for additional training in how to use a complex new computer system).

▲ **Defining the problem too broadly or too narrowly.** To take a classic example, the problem stated as "build a better mousetrap" can be more broadly defined as "get rid of the mice now." That is, managers should define problems so as to give themselves the best possible range of planning options.

▲ **Choosing the wrong problem to deal with.** Managers need to set priorities and make plans that deal with the most important problems first. Focusing on several small, less-important initiatives divides you and your team's focus. Your efforts may not yield the greatest possible benefit to your department or organization. By contrast, managers also need to give planning priority to problems that are truly solvable. While many health care managers may want to overhaul the Medicare system, focusing on streamlining the Medicare billing processes for your department is a much more doable goal for you and your teammates.

A variety of tools and techniques help managers identify and define problems. Section 6.4 discusses several commonly used tools and techniques for planning.

6.3.2 Generate and Evaluate Possible Courses of Action

After you define the problem, you can begin formulating one or several potential solutions. At this stage of planning and decision making, you may need to gather more information, evaluate data, analyze internally and externally gathered statistics, and weigh the pros and cons of each possible course of action. Involving others during this planning stage is critical in order to develop a range of solutions, get the most out of available information, and build future commitment for the plan.

Your plan will only be as good as the quality of the alternative solutions you generate during this step. The better the pool of alternatives, the more likely a good solution can be achieved. A very basic evaluation used at this step is

▲ **cost-benefit analysis,** which compares alternative costs (time, money, resources, human capital, etc.) to the expected benefits. At a minimum, the benefits of a preferred alternative should be greater than its costs. Although cost-benefit analysis is often quantitative (based on measurable facts and figures), the results need to be tempered by your subjective, qualitative judgments to ensure full evaluation of the options.

6.3.3 Choose a Preferred Course of Action

At this stage in the planning process, you must make a decision and select a particular course of action. Exactly how you make a decision and who may need to weigh in on the decision varies for each planning situation. In some cases, you may determine the best alternative by using cost-benefit analysis criterion; share this choice with your manager, and then proceed with executing your plan. Other times, numerous criteria may come into play, and you may need to present the case for your decision to multiple committees and managers, gradually getting others to buy into your solution. However, after you generate and evaluate the alternatives, you must make a final choice to continue on in the planning process.

You should test any decision to follow a particular plan of action by performing an ethics check. This evaluation ensures that you properly consider the ethical aspects of working in today's complex, fast-changing work environment.

6.3.4 Implement the Planned Course of Action

After you select the preferred solution to a problem, you next establish and implement appropriate actions to meet your final goal. This is the stage at which you finally set directions and initiate problem-solving actions.

Nothing new can happen according to the plan unless action is taken. Managers not only need the determination and creativity to make a plan, but they also need the ability and willingness to implement it. Additionally, most successful plans require managers *and others* to take some sort of action. Many plans fail at this stage because a manager didn't adequately involve others and gain their support. Managers who use participation wisely get the right people involved in decisions and problem-solving from the beginning. When they do, plans are more likely to be implemented quickly, smoothly, and to everyone's satisfaction.

6.3.5 Evaluate Results

Planning and decision making are not complete until you evaluate the results. In this final stage, you compare your accomplishments with your original objectives. If the desired results are not achieved, the process must be reviewed and renewed to allow for corrective actions.

Remember to examine both the positive and negative consequences of a chosen course of action. If the original solution appears inadequate, a return to earlier steps may be required to generate a modified or new plan. Evaluation is also made easier if the original plan includes objectives with measurable targets and timetables.

FOR EXAMPLE

Office of Minority Health, U.S. DoHHS

As the U.S. population becomes increasingly diverse, health care organizations must respond with sensitivity to the needs of patients from diverse cultural backgrounds and languages. In 1997, the Office of Minority Health undertook the developments of national standards to provide consistent and comprehensive health care for all Americans. After reviewing and analyzing existing procedures throughout the United States, an advisory committee drafted new standards. The standards were published in the *Federal Register* in December of 1999, and the committee requested feedback from any organizations, agencies, or individuals affected by the standards. By means of three regional public meetings, an interactive Web site, and extensive mailings, the committee incorporated feedback from 413 individuals or organizations over a 4-month period. By working carefully and gradually building consensus, the final version of the Culturally and Linguistically Appropriate Service (CLAS) standards effectively combines the input of a broad range of stakeholders. You can review the final standards by visiting www.omhrc.gov

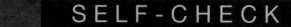

SELF-CHECK

- Cite the five steps of the planning process.
- Name the three common mistakes of problem definition.
- Define **cost-benefit analysis**.
- Explain how you might determine the ethical implications of the decision you plan to adopt.
- Describe how a plan is put into effect.
- Explain how a plan's effectiveness is determined.

6.4 Planning Tools and Techniques

Planning is challenging in any circumstances, and the difficulties increase as the work environment becomes more uncertain. To help master these challenges, managers make use of a number of useful planning tools and techniques during the planning process and after a plan is put into place. Some of the most common planning tools and techniques include

- ▲ forecasting;
- ▲ contingency planning;
- ▲ scenario planning;
- ▲ benchmarking;
- ▲ participation;
- ▲ strategic planning.

6.4.1 Forecasting

Forecasting is the process of making assumptions about what will happen in the future. A *forecast* is a specific vision of the future. All good plans involve forecasts, particularly during Steps 1 and 2 of the planning process.

Some forecasts are *qualitative* and use expert opinions to predict the future. In this case, a single person of special expertise or reputation or a panel of experts may be consulted. Other forecasts are *quantitative* and use mathematical and statistical analysis of data to predict future events.

In the final analysis, forecasting always relies on human judgment. Even the results of highly sophisticated quantitative forecasting still require interpretation and are subject to error. Forecasting is not planning—it is a planning tool. Treat forecasts cautiously, reviewing all information with a critical and questioning eye.

6.4.2 Contingency Planning

Planning always involves thinking ahead. But the more unstructured the problems and more uncertain the planning environment, the more likely that your original assumptions, predictions, and intentions may prove to be in error. Even the most carefully prepared plans may prove inadequate as experience develops. Unexpected problems and events frequently occur. When they do, plans have to be changed.

As a manager, you are better off anticipating problems than being surprised by them. **Contingency planning** is the process of identifying alternative courses of action that you can implement if and when an original plan proves inadequate because of changing circumstances. Sometimes contingency plans are created by good forward thinking on the part of managers and staff. At other times, a devil's advocate method, in which you formally assume the worst-case forecasts of future events and brainstorm responses can yield effective contingency plans.

Whatever methods you use to establish contingency plans, remember that the earlier the need for changes can be detected, the better. Look for "trigger points" in regular processes and procedures that can indicate that your existing plan is no longer desirable and needs to be closely monitored.

6.4.3 Scenario Planning

Scenario planning is a popular and long-term version of contingency planning. Scenario planning involves identifying several alternative future states of affairs that may occur. Managers and staff then deal hypothetically with each situation and formulate possible plans.

The creative brainstorming process helps organizations operate more flexibly in dynamic environments. Royal Dutch/Shell has been doing scenario planning for many years. The process began years ago when top managers asked themselves a perplexing question: "What would Shell do after its oil supplies ran out?" The question was approached by creating alternative future scenarios while remaining sensitive to the nature of growing environmental changes. Although recognizing that planning scenarios can never be inclusive of all future possibilities, a Royal Dutch/Shell planning coordinator once said that scenarios help "condition the organization to think" and remain better prepared than its competitors for "future shocks."

6.4.4 Benchmarking

Another important influence on the success or failure of planning is the frame of reference used as a starting point. All too often, managers and planners have limited awareness of what is happening outside their immediate work setting. Successful planning must challenge the status quo; it cannot simply accept things the way they are.

Benchmarking is a technique that uses external comparisons to evaluate one's current performance and identify possible future actions; it is one tool that broadens a work group and organization's field of view. The purpose of benchmarking is to find out what other people and organizations are doing very well and plan how to incorporate these ideas into your own operations. Health care-specific benchmarking programs and Web sites—such as www.healthdatacheck.com—have emerged as useful tools to help health care managers track and compare performance.

6.4.5 Participation and Group-Involvement

Participation is critical to the planning process. **Participative planning** involves the people who are affected by a plan or who are required to help implement the plan to aid in the planning process. Participation can increase the creativity and information available for planning. It can also increase the understanding, acceptance, and commitment of people to final plans. Indeed, planning in organizations should rarely, if ever, be done by individuals. To create and implement the best plans, others must be genuinely involved during all planning steps. Even though participative planning takes more time, it can improve results by improving implementation.

6.4.6 Strategic Planning

A **strategy** is a comprehensive action plan that identifies long-term direction and guides managers and staff in ways to best utilize the organization's resources. Successful strategic plans using resources focus an entire organization's energies on a clear target or goal. Usually strategic plans originate in the uppermost management and executive levels of a company. Smaller, more specific plans in departments, teams, or work groups need to mesh with and build on the overarching strategic plans.

6.4.7 Missions, Values, and Objectives

Mission statements, core values statements, and **objectives** are all strategic planning tools that help managers create plans that fit the organization's vision for the future of its business endeavors.

▲ **Mission:** an organization's reason for existence as a supplier of goods and/or services to society. A good mission statement is precise in identifying where the organization intends to operate, who the organization serves, and what products or services it provides. The best organizations have clear and compelling missions. At the Breast Cancer Program of the Dana-Farber-Harvard Cancer Center, the mission is "to reduce death due to breast cancer and lengthen and improve the quality of life of women with this disease." At Merck it is "to preserve and improve human life."

FOR EXAMPLE

Mission and Core Values

The mission of the Massachusetts Consortium for Children with Special Health Care Needs (CSHCN) is "to improve systems of care for children with special health care needs and their families throughout the Commonwealth of Massachusetts." To further explain how the Massachusetts Consortium goes about achieving its mission, it promotes eight specific core values in all its endeavors: diversity of membership, flexible participation, respect for differences of opinion, an informal welcoming atmosphere, collaboration across organizations and patient families, building connections across organizations, shared leadership, and big-picture thinking. To find out more about the Massachusetts Consortium's programs, visit www.neserve.org/maconsortium/index.

▲ **Core values:** affect and guide the action of an organization. Often posted along with the organization's mission statement, these values reflect the organization's broad beliefs about what is and is not appropriate. The presence of strong core values gives character to an organization, backs up the mission statement, and helps guide the behavior of members in meaningful and consistent ways. For example, core values at Merck include corporate social responsibility, science-based innovation, honesty and integrity, and profit from work that benefits humanity.

▲ **Objectives:** direct activities toward key and specific results. Whereas a mission statement sets forth an official purpose for the organization, objectives are usually shorter-term targets against which actual performance can be measured. Examples of business objectives may include producing at a certain level of profit, gaining and holding a specific share of a market, recruiting and maintaining a high-quality workforce, or making a positive contribution to society.

SELF-CHECK

- Cite six common planning tools and techniques.
- Define **contingency planning**.
- Describe the purpose of benchmarking.
- Define **strategic planning**.
- Compare mission, core values, and objectives.

6.5 SWOT Analysis

In order to produce effective plans, managers and staff must have a clear picture of what's happening within the organization and within its greater business environment. SWOT analysis (strengths, weaknesses, opportunities and threats) is a common tool used to analyze strengths and weaknesses inside the organization, and opportunities and threats outside the organization.

6.5.1 Internal Factors

A **SWOT analysis** begins with a systematic evaluation of the organization's resources and capabilities. A major goal is to identify **core competencies** in the form of special strengths that the organization has or does exceptionally well in comparison with competitors. Simply put, organizations need core competencies that do important things better than the competition and that are very difficult for competitors to duplicate. Core competencies may be found in special knowledge or expertise, outstanding technologies, unique products, or superior distribution systems, among many other possibilities.

▲ **Strengths:** the resources and capabilities an organization can use to develop competitive advantage.
▲ **Weaknesses:** the absence of strengths.

A major strategic goal of any organization is to create processes that highlight core competencies for competitive advantage by building upon organizational strengths and minimizing the impact of weaknesses.

6.5.2 External Factors

A SWOT analysis is not complete until opportunities and threats in the external environment are also analyzed.

▲ **Opportunities:** include possible new markets, a strong economy, weaknesses in competitors, and emerging technologies.
▲ **Threats:** include the emergence of new competitors, scarce resources, changing customer demands, and new government regulations, among other possibilities.

For the purpose of a SWOT analysis, the external environment includes macro environment factors such as technology, government, social structures, population demographics, the global economy, and the natural environment. The external environment also encompasses developments in the industry or business environment, which includes resource suppliers, competitors, customers, and patients.

In a stable and predictable external environment, you can more successfully implement a strategy for a longer period of time. By contrast, in a more dynamic and uncertain environment, you must choose flexible strategies that can change and evolve over time. Given the nature of competitive environments today, strategic management must be considered an ongoing process in which strategies are formulated, implemented, revised, and implemented again in a nearly continuous manner.

SELF-CHECK

- Define **SWOT**.
- Identify the internal and external factors of a SWOT analysis.
- Define **core competencies**.
- Cite important macro environmental factors.

SUMMARY

Planning is the process of deciding exactly what you want to accomplish and how to best go about doing it. Successful plans have common characteristics, and good planning helps improve an organization's focus, coordination, control, time management, and attitude. Plans can be classified as short or long term, and strategic or operational. They comprise policies, procedures, schedules, and budgets. The five steps of the planning process are: (1) identify and define the problem, (2) generate and evaluate possible courses of action, (3) choose a preferred solution, (4) implement the solution, and (5) evaluate results. Planning tools and techniques make the difficult task of planning more manageable. SWOT analysis systematically compares the internal and external factors affecting an organization.

KEY TERMS

Action orientation	A state of mind in which you and your organization act and react confidently and quickly to new situations.
Benchmarking	Using external comparisons to evaluate an organization's current performance and identify possible future actions.
Budget	Financial plans that commit resources to activities, projects, or programs.

Contingency planning	The process of identifying alternative courses of action that you can implement if and when an original plan proves inadequate because of changing circumstances.
Control	Meeting the desired outcomes as efficiently as possible.
Core competencies	Special strengths that an organization has or does exceptionally well in comparison with competitors.
Core values	Principles that affect and guide the action of an organization.
Cost-benefit analysis	Comparing alternative costs (time, money, resources, human capital, etc.) to the expected benefits.
Crisis	An unexpected and demanding problem that can result in disaster.
Fixed budget	A financial plan that allocates a set amount of resources that can be used, but not exceeded, for a specified purpose.
Flexibility	The willingness or ability to change and adapt to shifting circumstances.
Flexible budget	A financial plan that allocates resources based on the need level of various departments or activities.
Focus	Knowing what an organization does best, knowing the needs of customers and patients, and knowing how to serve customers and patients well.
Forecasting	The process of making assumptions about what will happen in the future.
Hierarchy of objectives	Plans in which the goals for each area of the organization are linked together, scheduled chronologically, or ranked in terms of importance.
Intermediate-range plan	A plans that covers 1 to 2 years.
Long-range plan	A plan that looks 3 or more years into the future.
Mission statement	Precisely worded declaration that identifies where an organization intends to operate, who it serves, and what products or services it provides.
Objectives	Short-term targets that direct activities toward key and specific results.
Operational plan	A plan that defines what needs to be done in specific areas to implement a strategic plan.
Opportunities	External factors of a SWOT analysis that include possible new markets, a strong economy, weaknesses in competitors, and emerging technologies.

Participative planning	Involves the people who are affected by a plan or who are required to help implement the plan to aid in the planning process.
Planning process	Deciding exactly what you, your team, or your department wants to accomplish and how to best go about meeting your goals.
Policy	Formal statements that communicate broad guidelines for making decisions and taking action in specific circumstances.
Procedure	Statement that describes exact rules for dealing with specific situations.
Projects	Specific goals that can be accomplished by teams working under tight deadlines.
Project schedules	Time-focused places that identify the activities required to accomplish a specific major project.
Scenario planning	Identifying alternative future states of affairs that may occur and then dealing hypothetically with each situation and formulating possible plans.
Short-range plan	Plan that covers 1 year or less.
Strategic plan	Action plans, usually from uppermost management or executive management, that focus an entire organization's energies on a clear target or goal.
Strategy	A comprehensive action plan that identifies long-term direction and guides managers and staff in ways to best utilize the organization's resources.
Strengths	Internal factors of a SWOT analysis.
Structured problem	Familiar situations.
SWOT analysis	A common planning tool used to analyze strengths and weaknesses inside an organization, and opportunities and threats outside the organization.
Threats	External factors of a SWOT analysis that include the emergence of new competitors, scarce resources, changing customer demands, and new government regulations, among other possibilities.
Unstructured problem	Unexpected and ambiguous situations that lack critical information.
Weaknesses	Internal factors of a SWOT analysis.
Zero-based budget	A budget in which all projects or activities must compete anew for available funds in each budget cycle.

ASSESS YOUR UNDERSTANDING

Go to www.wiley.com/college/Lombardi to evaluate your knowledge of the basics of planning.

Measure your learning by comparing pretest and post-test results.

Summary Questions

1. Successful plans help organizations organize processes and influence employees. True or false?

2. Well-run organizations use plans to monitor work progress, set schedules, and prepare budgets. True or false?

3. Plans are rarely used to identify problems and suggest corrective actions. True or false?

4. Plans can address both structured problems and unstructured problems. Which of the following is true?

   (a) Unstructured problems are highly predictable.

   (b) Structured problems don't require planning.

   (c) Structured problems often involve many unknowns.

   (d) Unstructured problems typically arise in unexpected or ambiguous situations.

5. Short-range plans cover 1 year or less, intermediate-range plans cover 1 to 2 years, and long-range plans look 3 or more years into the future. True or false?

6. Strategic plans address the direction of an organization; operational plans define specific actions that help move the organization in the right direction. True or false?

7. The planning process begins with identification of a problem and ends with evaluation of implemented solutions. True or false?

8. Which of the following is NOT a common error when identifying problems?

   (a) Focusing on symptoms instead of causes

   (b) Defining the problem too broadly or too narrowly

   (c) Choosing the wrong problem to deal with

   (d) Defining the problem in quantifiable terms

9. An important part of the planning process is evaluating the results. This step is made easier if

   (a) the plan includes objectives that are certain to be achieved.

   (b) the plan includes objectives that are intangible.

(c) the plan includes objectives with measurable targets and timetables.

(d) the plan doesn't define objectives.

10. Common planning techniques include forecasting, scenario planning, and benchmarking. True or false?

11. Contingency planning is the process of identifying alternative courses of action in anticipation of

(a) accurate forecasting.

(b) playing devil's advocate.

(c) changing circumstances.

(d) successful completion of the plan.

12. SWOT is a common method of comparing internal analyses with external analyses. True or false?

13. Core competencies are

(a) an organization's opportunities.

(b) an organization's ability to plan.

(c) an organization's ability to overcome weaknesses.

(d) an organization's special strengths.

Review Questions

1. Good planning improves organizational focus. Define *focus*.

2. How does good planning improve coordination?

3. Enhanced control and better time management are characteristics of good planning. How are they related?

4. How does good planning help you resolve problems?

5. How do policies relate to procedures?

6. What are the most important attributes of a good project schedule?

7. Budgets are plans that commit resources to activities, projects, or programs. There are fixed, flexible, and zero-based budgets. What is a fixed budget?

8. Put the five steps of the planning process in proper order.

9. What is cost/benefit analysis?

10. The third step of the planning process entails making decisions about the particular course of action you need to take. Who should participate in these decisions?

11. Good plans include forecasts, particularly during which steps of the planning process?

12. What is the key element of a successful strategic plan?

13. In general terms, what are an organization's objectives?

14. What is one of the main objectives of a SWOT analysis?
15. What can a SWOT analysis help an organization do?

Applying This Chapter

1. Members in the billing and customer-service groups at your organization are going to spend one afternoon a week "cross-training" so customer-service representatives know more about billing procedures and billing employees learn more about working directly with customers. What benefit of planning is in effect here?

2. You need to introduce new organization-wide procedures for online processing of invoices to the other employees in your department. What benefits of planning might you highlight for your teammates in order to get them in favor of the new procedures?

3. The Johnson Country Health Foundation holds an off-site brainstorming session in which staff discusses ways it can increase its public awareness by 15% over the next 2 years. Which of the five planning steps does this activity best relate to?

4. You manage a patient referral helpline in which callers receive recommendations for physicians who treat special conditions or who have special training or skills. In the last year, the number of calls your helpline receives has doubled. While you don't have the budget to hire additional staff, you have an additional $20,000 to spend on your department to improve efficiency and customer satisfaction. Using the five-step planning process in this chapter as your guide, discuss how you will improve efficiency and customer satisfaction in your organization.

5. The Colorado Eldercare Initiative recently conducted a patient satisfaction survey for its in-state patients as well as patients from more than 300 nursing care facilities across the United States. What planning tool or technique might the Colorado Eldercare Initiative be attempting to use?

6. As a project manager at a not-for-project public health organization, you've been selected to lead the development of a new Web site to encourage teens to avoid or quit smoking. What tools and techniques would be essential to include in your planning for the Web site?

Is Your Plan up to Par?

Plans are in place just about everywhere—in workplaces, schools, public building, churches, and more. Many plans detail how work should be performed or what to do in specific situations. Visit the Web site for St. Cloud (MN) hospital at www.centracare.com and click the patient safety link (or go directly to www.centracare.com/sch/quality/judge_quality.html) to examine St. Cloud (MN) Hospital's patient safety and quality plan. Consider the following questions:

- Does the plan deliver on the promises outlined in section 6.1?
- Specifically, will the plan help someone work with greater focus or flexibility?
- Does the plan improve time management or control of resources?
- Does the plan offer solutions and inspire action?
- How can the plan be improved?

Locate another formal plan by reviewing an employee or student handbook, a committee's bylines and charter, or an official Web site.

Centers for Disease Control and Prevention Budget

Go to www.cdc.gov/fmo/fmofybudget.htm to review the current operating budget of the Centers for Disease Control and Prevention.

- What is the total operating budgeting of the CDC?
- What are the three top-funded programs at the CDC?

Symptom and Problems

What might be some possible problems causing the symptoms described in this following scenario: A small dental office waiting room fills with patients most afternoons. Patients tend to get restless and irritated because most must wait 45 to 60 minutes past their scheduled appointment times before seeing the dentist.

Minding Mission Statements

A mission statement should identify *where* the organization intends to operate, *who* the organization serves, and *what* products or services it provides. Evaluate the following mission statements and see whether each covers all the bases:

1. "To achieve and maintain full immunization protection for each child in San Francisco in order to promote community health and wellness." (San Francisco Immunization Coalition)
2. "To ensure the quality of life at the end of life through compassionate care for all individuals and their families in Central Iowa." (Hospice of Central Iowa)
3. "To provide balanced, credible information about public policy issues that affect healthcare coverage." (Blue Cross/Blue Shield HealthIssues.com)

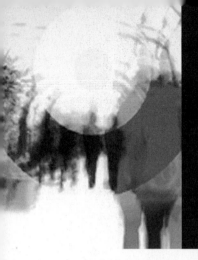

7

KEEPING THINGS IN CHECK
Controls and the Control Process

Starting Point

Go to www.wiley.com/college/Lombardi to assess your knowledge of the basics of the control process.
Determine where you need to concentrate your effort.

What You'll Learn in This Chapter

▲ Four steps of the control process
▲ Characteristics of effective controls
▲ Three main types of controls
▲ Specific control techniques for discipline, information, and finances
▲ Operational control strategies, including purchasing, inventory, and quality
▲ Ways to successfully manage by objectives (MBO)
▲ Traits of internal control and self-management

After Studying This Chapter, You'll Be Able To

▲ Practice the control process
▲ Compare internal and external controls
▲ Differentiate among discipline, information, and financial controls
▲ Examine the three aspects of operational controls
▲ Apply management by objective techniques

Goals and Outcomes

▲ Master the terminology and tools related to controls and the control process
▲ Explain how control fits with other management-process responsibilities
▲ Recognize common ethical dilemmas and responses
▲ Contrast the three main types of controls
▲ Use controls to assess performance, improve processes, and boost quality
▲ Choose appropriate controls to manage employees, schedules, budgets and quality
▲ Design effective control processes
▲ Evaluate the effectiveness of controls and control processes

INTRODUCTION

Control plays a positive and necessary role in the management process. By regularly following the four-step control process, managers can make their departments more effective and productive. The three categories of controls can be utilized to monitor employee discipline, manage schedules, and enforce budgets. Controls are particularly useful and important in discussions of purchasing, inventory, and quality. Management by objectives is a classic control-based tool that encourages internal control and self-management.

7.1 Understanding the Control Process

As section 1.5 points out, **controlling**—the process of measuring performance and taking action to ensure desired results—is a basic function for health care managers, on par with organizing, planning, and leading. The purpose of controlling is straightforward—to make sure that plans are fulfilled and that actual performance meets or surpasses objectives.

▲ **Planning** sets the directions and allocates resources.
▲ **Organizing** brings people and material resources together in working combinations.
▲ **Leading** inspires people to best utilize these resources.
▲ **Controlling** checks that the right things happen, in the right way, and at the right time. It helps ensure that the performance contributions of individuals and groups are consistent with strategic and operational plans. It helps ensure that performance accomplishments throughout an organization are well integrated in means–ends fashion. And it helps ensure that people comply with organizational policies and procedures.

Figure 7-1 shows how controlling fits in with the rest of the management process.

Figure 7-1

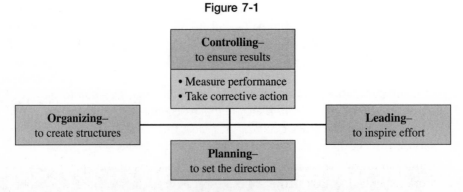

The role of controlling in the management process.

Figure 7-2

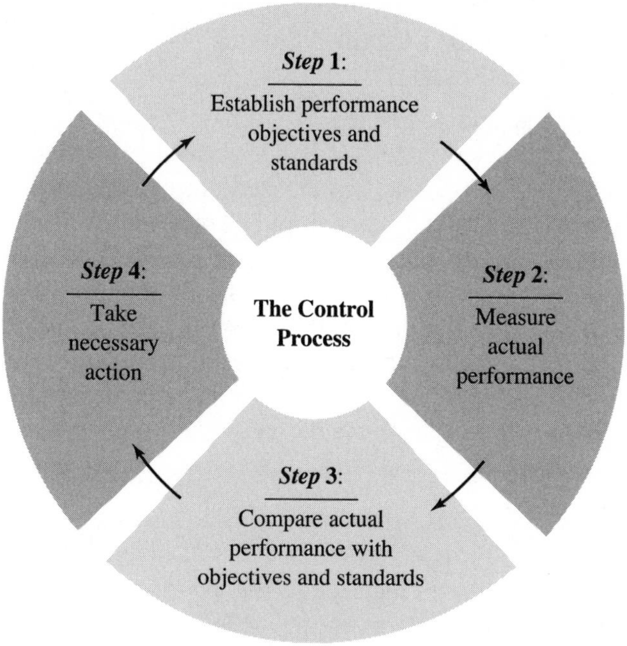

Step 1:
Establish performance
objectives and
standards

Step 2:
Measure
actual
performance

**The Control
Process**

Step 3:
Compare actual
performance with
objectives and standards

Step 4:
Take
necessary
action

Four steps in management control.

The **control process,** as shown in Figure 7-2, involves four steps: establishing objectives and standards, measuring actual performance, comparing results with objectives and standards, and taking corrective action as needed.

7.1.1 Step 1: Establishing Objectives and Standards

The control process begins when performance objectives and standards are set through planning (see section 6.3 for more on the planning process). The objectives provide the performance targets, and the standards provide the yardstick for assessing actual accomplishments.

Two types of standards can be used for this purpose:

▲ **Output standards** measure results in terms of performance quantity, quality, cost, or time. Examples include percentage error rate, dollar deviation from budgeted expenditures, and the number of patients serviced in a time period.

▲ **Input standards,** by contrast, measure effort in terms of the amount of work expended in task performance. They are used in situations where outputs are difficult or expensive to measure. Examples include conformance

FOR EXAMPLE

Behavioral Standards for Customer Service at Durham Regional Hospital

In 2004, employees and managers at Durham Regional Hospital (www.durhamregional.org) determined that customer-service excellence was one of the facility's greatest strengths and established output standards for customer services. A committee defined seven core customer service behavioral categories, including greetings, telephone behavior, and patient respect. In each behavior category, the committee then listed specific actions or activities that were consistent with outstanding customer service. All employees received training on the behavioral standards and signed formal agreements to abide by the standards. To review the seven categories of behavior standards, visit www.durhamregional.org/team/customerservice.

to rules and procedures, efficiency in the use of resources, and work attendance or punctuality.

7.1.2 Step 2: Measuring Actual Performance

The second step of the control process is to measure actual performance. The measurement must be accurate enough to spot significant differences between what is really taking place and what was originally planned. A common failure in health care organizations is an unwillingness or inability to rigorously measure performance. Often, this involves reluctance by managers to specifically assess the accomplishments of other people at work. Yet without measurement, effective control is not possible. Managers need to get comfortable with the act of measurement, and they need to be consistent in doing it.

7.1.3 Step 3: Comparing Results with Objectives and Standards

Step three in the control process is to compare measured performance with objectives and standards. This establishes whether or not any corrective actions are needed. The **control equation** summarizes this step:

▲ Need for Action = Desired Performance − Actual Performance

You can apply the control equation in an **historical comparison** that uses past performance as a standard for evaluating current performance.[1] Or you can rely on a **relative comparison** that uses the performance achievements of other people, work units, or organizations as evaluation benchmarks. Or you rely on an

engineering comparison that uses standards set scientifically through such methods as time and motion studies.

7.1.4 Step 4: Taking Corrective Action

The last step in the control process is to take any action necessary to correct or improve future performance. Step four allows for a judicious use of **management by exception**—the practice of giving priority attention to situations that show the greatest need for action. This approach can save valuable time, energy, and other resources, while allowing all efforts to be concentrated on the areas of greatest need.

You may encounter two types of exceptions:

▲ In a **problem situation,** actual performance is below the standard. As a manager, you seek to understand the reasons for this type of performance deficiency and then take corrective action to restore performance to the desired level.

▲ In an **opportunity situation,** actual performance is above the standard. As a manager, you also need to understand the reasons for this extraordinary performance and allow for action to continue operating at a higher accomplishment level in the future.

7.1.5 Setting up Effective Controls

One of the problems with the control process is that many managers are too busy and/or unwilling to follow it. Many managers make a decision, take action, and then forget about it as they go on to other tasks. There is no follow-up to make sure things go according to plan.

The best managers, by contrast, are proactive and positive in applying the control process to full advantage. Rather than simply assuming things are going right, they make sure that everything works out as intended.

Effective controls in organizations share the following characteristics:

▲ **Controls are strategic and results-oriented.** The controls support strategic plans and focus on significant activities that make a real difference to the organization.

▲ **Controls are understandable.** They support decision making by presenting data in understandable terms; they do not involve complex reports and hard-to-understand statistics.

▲ **Controls encourage self-control.** They allow for mutual trust, good communication, and participation among everyone involved.

▲ **Controls are timely and exception-oriented.** They report deviations quickly, lending insight into why a performance gap exists and what you can do to correct it.

▲ **Controls are positive in nature.** They emphasize their contribution to development, change, and systems improvement; they deemphasize their role in penalties and reprimands.

▲ **Controls are fair and objective.** They are considered impartial and accurate by everyone; they are respected for one fundamental purpose—performance enhancement.

▲ **Controls are flexible.** They leave room for individual judgment and can be modified to fit new circumstances as they arise.[2]

SELF-CHECK

- Identify and define **control, control process, output standards, input standards,** and **management by exception.**
- Describe the four steps of the control process.
- Compare output standards and input standards.
- Differentiate among historical, relative, and engineering comparisons.
- Explain problem situations and opportunity situations.
- List characteristics of effective controls.

7.2 Types of Controls

Health care managers utilize three major types of managerial controls—feedforward, concurrent, and feedback control.[3] Shown in Figure 7-3, each is relevant to a different aspect of the organization's activities. Each has an important role to play in the quest for long-term productivity and high performance.

Figure 7-3

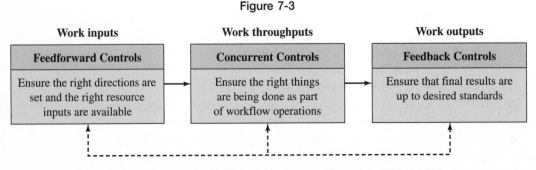

Work inputs	**Work throughputs**	**Work outputs**
Feedforward Controls	**Concurrent Controls**	**Feedback Controls**
Ensure the right directions are set and the right resource inputs are available	Ensure the right things are being done as part of workflow operations	Ensure that final results are up to desired standards

Three types of controls: feedforward, concurrent, and feedback control.

7.2.1 Feedforward Controls

The controls that are accomplished *before* a work activity begins are called **feedforward controls,** or preliminary controls. These controls ensure that objectives are clear, that proper directions are established, and that the right resources are available to accomplish them. By making sure that the stage is properly set for high performance, feedforward controls are preventive in nature. They help eliminate later problems by asking an important but often neglected question: What needs to be done before we begin?

In a student health clinic, for example, preliminary control of examination materials and patient forms play major roles in ensuring the clinic runs smoothly and well. Nurses are responsible for checking on a daily basis that all reusable and disposable tools are stocked and organized; front desk assistants preassemble clipboards that include all necessary patient forms that will be completed during each patient visit.

7.2.2 Concurrent Controls

The controls that focus on what actually happens *during* the work process are called **concurrent controls,** or steering controls. These controls monitor ongoing operations and activities as they take place to make sure things are being done according to plan. In a sense, concurrent controls ask the key question, Now that we've started, what can we do to improve things before we finish?

Consider the student health clinic again. Nurse-practitioners, serving as shift leaders, can provide concurrent control through direct supervision of medical assistants who interact directly with the student-patients. The nurse-practitioners can constantly observe what is taking place in multiple examination rooms and can help out with exams as needed. The nurse-practitioners can intervene immediately when something is not done right and help correct things on the spot.

7.2.3 Feedback Controls

The controls that take place *after* work is completed are called **feedback controls,** or postaction controls. These controls focus on the results achieved rather than on work inputs and activities. They ask the question, Now that we are finished, how well did we do?

A student-health clinic can, for example, send out confidential surveys to students that ask them to assess their experiences. Similarly, a final exam grade tells you how well you performed—after the course is over. A budget summary informs managers of any cost overruns—after a project is completed. In these and other similar cases, the feedback gained is most useful for improving things in the future.

FOR EXAMPLE

Emergency Room Excellence

The emergency room at Robert Wood Johnson University Hospital Hamilton (www.rwjhamilton.org) is a state-of-the-art and award-winning facility that utilizes numerous control processes to establish, measure, and ensure its 15/30 guarantee. The guarantee promises that all emergency room patients see a nurse within 15 minutes and a physician within 30 minutes, or the hospital pays the emergency room bill. To achieve the guarantee, the hospital instituted a PromptCare facility to focus on the needs of non-life-threatening ER patients. The Emergency Department also upgraded its patient tracking and documentation system to not only obtain medical information quickly, but also to measure and compare performance results.

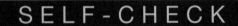

SELF-CHECK

- Identify and define **feedforward control, concurrent control, and feedback control.**
- Compare and contrast the three types of controls.

7.3 Control Strategies

Health care managers have two broad options with respect to control. First, they can rely on people to exercise self-control. This strategy of **internal control** allows motivated individuals and groups to exercise self-discipline in fulfilling job expectations.[4] Second, managers can take direct action to control the behavior of others. This is a strategy of **external control** that occurs through personal supervision and the use of formal administrative systems.

Each component in an organization's control systems should contribute to maintaining predictably high levels of performance. At the same time that internal control is encouraged and supported, external control should be appropriate and rigorous.

Health care organizations with effective controls typically use both strategies to good advantage, but more progressive workplaces seem to have a renewed emphasis on internal and self-controls. This is consistent with trends toward more participation, empowerment, and employee involvement.

7.3.1 Management Process Controls

The discipline of the management process itself facilitates control.

During planning,

▲ **control via strategy and objectives** occurs when work behaviors are initially directed toward appropriate end results. When performance goals are clearly set and understood, lack of performance (because of poor direction in one's work) is less likely to occur;

▲ **control via policies and procedures** operates in similar ways. To the extent that good policies and procedures exist to guide behavior, an organization's members are more likely to act uniformly on important matters;

▲ **control via learning** occurs when past experience is systematically considered and incorporated into future strategies, objectives, policies, and procedures.

Management control is also facilitated by good organizing:

▲ **Control by selection and training** occurs when capable people are hired and given the ongoing training needed to perform their jobs at high levels of accomplishment. The closer the match between individual skills and job requirements, the less need there is for external control and the greater the opportunity for internal control.

▲ **Control via performance appraisal** occurs when individual performance is assessed and evaluated to ensure high performance results. This also helps to identify areas where training and development are needed.

▲ **Control via job design and work structures** operates in a similar fashion, putting people in jobs designed to best fit their talents. When all jobs are well coordinated in workflows and operations, this structures activities and adds substantially to control.

Leadership contributes to control through performance modeling. This occurs as leaders set the examples so that workers have good models to follow in their job activities.

▲ **Control by performance norms** occurs when team or group members share commitments to high performance standards and reinforce one another's efforts to meet them.

▲ **Control via organization culture** occurs in a similar fashion when core values add a shared sense of meaning and add purpose throughout the organization.

7.3.2 Employee Discipline Systems

Absenteeism, tardiness, sloppy work. The list of possible misbehaviors in the workplace can go on to even more extreme actions: falsifying records, sexual harassment, embezzlement, and more. All are examples of behaviors that can and should be formally addressed in employee discipline systems. **Discipline** is the act of

---

FOR EXAMPLE

"Hot Stove" Rules of Discipline

According to classic management author Douglas McGregor,[5] one way for managers to develop a consistent approach to disciplinary situations is to apply the "Hot Stove" rules, which begin with a simple rule: "When a stove is hot, don't touch it." When this rule is violated, you get burned— immediately, consistently, but usually not beyond the possibility of repair. By extension, reprimands should be immediate (a hot stove burns quickly). Reprimands should be directed toward someone's actions, not their personality (a hot stove doesn't hold grudges, doesn't try to humiliate people, and doesn't accept excuses). Reprimands should be consistently applied (a hot stove burns anyone who touches it, and it does so every time). Reprimands should occur in a supportive setting (a hot stove conveys warmth but also operates with the inflexible rule of "don't touch").

---

influencing behavior through reprimand. Ideally, the use of discipline in managerial control is handled in a fair, consistent, and systematic way.

Progressive discipline ties reprimands to the severity and frequency of misbehavior. Under such a system, penalties for employees vary according to how significant the inappropriate behavior is and how often it occurs. The goal is to achieve compliance with organizational expectations through the least extreme reprimand possible.

However, the system should still be strict and rigorous. For example, the progressive discipline guidelines of one hospital state, "The level of disciplinary action shall increase with the level of severity of behavior engaged in and based on whether the conduct is of a repetitive nature." In this particular case, the ultimate penalty of discharge is reserved for the most severe behaviors (for example, any felony crime) or for continual infractions of a less severe nature (being continually late for work and failing to respond to a series of written reprimands and suspensions).

7.3.3 Information and Financial Controls

The pressure is ever present today for all health care organizations to use their resources (human, financial, capital, and more) well and to perform with maximum efficiency.

For control purposes, health care managers need to generally understand the following important financial aspects of organizational performance:

▲ **Liquidity:** The ability to generate cash to pay bills.
▲ **Leverage:** The ability to earn more in returns than the cost of debt.

▲ **Asset management:** The ability to use resources efficiently and operate at minimum cost.

▲ **Profitability:** The ability to earn revenues greater than costs.

These financial aspects of organizational performance are typically assessed using a variety of **financial ratios.** Upper managers often use the ratios to initially set goals, while middle and lower management use the ratios to track actual performance. Ratios are also useful for historical comparisons within the firm or in external benchmarking relative to industry performance.

A number of popular financial ratios are listed here along with up ($\uparrow$) and down ($\downarrow$), which indicate the preferred directions for these ratios to develop over time.

▲ **Liquidity ratios:**
$\uparrow$ Current ratio = Current assets/current liabilities
$\uparrow$ Acid test = (Current assets − inventory)/current liabilities

▲ **Leverage ratios:**
$\downarrow$ Debt ratio = Total debts/total assets
$\uparrow$ Times interest earned = Profits before interest and taxes/total interest

▲ **Asset management ratios:**
$\uparrow$ Inventory turnover = Sales/average inventory
$\uparrow$ Total asset turnover = Sales/total assets

▲ **Profitability ratios:**
$\uparrow$ Net margin = Net profit after taxes/sales
$\uparrow$ Return on investment (ROI) = Net profit after taxes/total assets

SELF-CHECK

- Identify and define **internal control, external control, discipline, progressive discipline,** and **financial ratios.**
- Compare internal and external controls.
- Explain how control fits with the other three components of the management process.
- Discuss characters of effective controls for employee discipline.
- Contrast the tools and techniques of discipline, reprimand, and progressive discipline.
- Explain ways to apply controls to information and financial topics.

7.4 Managing and Controlling Operations

Control is an essential part of **operations management,** the portion of management duties that emphasizes utilizing people, resources, and technology to the best advantage. Among the important aspects of operations management today, purchasing control, inventory control, and, of course, quality control, deserve special attention.

7.4.1 Purchasing Control

Everywhere in today's economy—including throughout the health care industry—the rising costs of materials seem to be a fact of life. Controlling these costs through efficient purchasing management is an important productivity tool. Like an individual, a thrifty organization must be concerned about how much it pays for what it buys.

To leverage buying power, many health care organizations now have centralized purchasing to allow buying in volume. Additionally, many health care organizations now commit to only a small number of suppliers with whom they can negotiate special contracts, gain quality assurances, and get preferred service.

Although first-time health care managers typically have limited ability to control purchasing processes, savvy managers pay attention to the costs associated with any material purchased regularly and try to find the lowest cost, highest quality, and best service possible. Often by sharing purchasing control information with supervising managers and upper management, health care managers can identify significant cost-savings opportunities for their organizations.

7.4.2 Inventory Control

Health care organizations maintain inventories of materials, tools, supplies, equipment, and more. Organizations use their inventories to smooth out periods of excess or undercapacity and meet periods of unusual demand. But because inventories represent costs, they must be well managed. Many health care organizations, particularly those with clinical operations, try to maintain a 4- to 6-week on-hand supply of essential tools and materials.

Some health care inventory controls are quantitative and even computerized. For example, the **economic order quantity (EOQ)** is a quantitative method of inventory control that involves ordering a fixed number of items every time an inventory level falls to a predetermined point. When this point is reached, a decision is automatically made (often now by computer) to place a standard order. The objective is always to have new inventory arrive just as old inventory runs out. This minimizes the total cost of the inventory.

Another approach to inventory control is **just-in-time scheduling (JIT).** Made popular by Japanese industrial productivity, JIT systems are beginning to receive consideration in some cutting-edge health care organizations. JIT systems try to reduce costs and improve workflow by scheduling items to arrive just in time to be used. JIT systems minimize storage costs, often reduce costs, and can maximize the use of space and improve the quality of results. However, finding ways to appropriately adapt JIT systems to health care settings will be an ongoing challenge for many years to come.

7.4.3 Quality Control

In the context of managerial control systems, **quality control** involves checking processes, materials, products, and services to ensure that they meet high standards. Quality control encompasses all aspects of an organization's operations—from the selection of materials and supplies right down to the last task performed as part of a specific service or product.

Although health care organizations rarely have as statistically rigid quality-control plans as automobile parts manufacturers, for example, most health care organizations have detailed processes and procedures in place in which supervising managers or peers evaluate a random sampling of files or charts on an established (often daily or weekly) schedule. At many health care organizations, especially those with clinical operations, managers typically observe and evaluate staff in hands-on activities, such as patient interactions, examinations, laboratory procedures, and so on.

Because the delivery of appropriate health care services is, by necessity, quite individualized, not all service experience can be *exactly* the same. However, a staff member's skills or abilities are typically evaluated against established criteria or expectations.

Often, quality-control evaluations and observations become part of employees' performance appraisals. See section 5.4 for more information on appraising employees.

FOR EXAMPLE

Award-Winning Quality

The Malcolm Baldridge National Quality Awards (www.quality.nist.gov) are presented annually by the president of the United States to leading business, education, and health care organizations that make significant achievement in quality and performance excellence. To review health care-specific award criteria, comprehensive evaluative questions, and detailed profiles of past health care award winners, visit www.quality.nist.gov/HealthCare_Criteria.htm. By reviewing and answering these questions, any health care manager can find useful, proven ideas for establishing patient-focused programs with exceptional quality-assurance procedures.

SELF-CHECK

- Identify and define **operations management, economic order quantity, just-in-time scheduling,** and **quality control.**
- Discuss the importance of purchasing control, inventory control, and quality control in the overall health of a health care organization.
- List ways that managers can make a positive impact on purchasing control.
- Compare and contrast economic order quantity and just-in-time scheduling as inventory control methods.
- Suggest ways that managers can exercise some degree of quality control in today's health care workplace.

7.5 Integrated Planning and Controlling

When planning is done well, control gets better—and vice versa. Without good planning, control lacks a framework for performance measurement. Without good control, planning lacks the follow-through needed to ensure results.

7.5.1 Six Sigma

Six Sigma is a collection of rigorous, systematic control tools that use information and statistical analysis to measure and improve an organization's performance, practices and systems. Six Sigma strives to identify and prevent "defects"—perhaps a faulty car door hinge at an automobile assembly factory or an incorrectly administered dose of painkillers in a health care setting. By carefully monitoring quality and performance, managers can anticipate potential defects, create effective solutions, and exceed expectations of all stakeholders.

Six Sigma techniques first appeared in the manufacturing sector—Motorola and General Electric were two earlier adopters and promoters of the techniques—and have been successfully adapted to health care settings in recent years. For more information about incorporating Six Sigma techniques within a health care organization, visit http://healthcare.isixsigma.com.

7.5.2 Management by Objectives

Management by objectives, or MBO, is a useful technique that helps to integrate planning and controlling. Formally defined, MBO is a structured process of regular communication in which a supervisor and subordinate jointly set performance objectives for the subordinate and review results accomplished.[6]

Figure 7-4

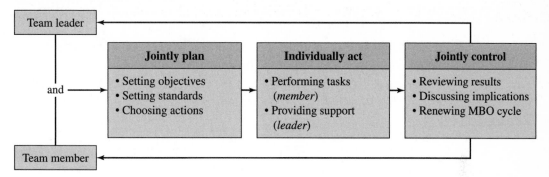

An MBO framework for integrated planning and controlling in a work team.

MBO requires a formal agreement between the supervisor and subordinate concerning

▲ the subordinate's performance objectives for a given time period;
▲ plans through which the objectives will be accomplished;
▲ standards for measuring whether the objectives are accomplished;
▲ procedures for reviewing performance results.

Figure 7-4 shows MBO in a work team structure. Note that the team leader and team member jointly establish plans and jointly control results in any good MBO action framework. They agree on the high-priority performance objectives for the member along with a timetable for their accomplishment and the criteria to be used in evaluating results.

A major advantage of management by objectives is that the process clearly focuses a person's work efforts on the most important tasks and objectives. Another is that it focuses a supervisor's work efforts on areas of support that can truly help the individual meet the agreed-upon objectives.[7]

7.5.3 Steps to Successful MBO

The following process can help managers make MBO as successful as possible:

1. An individual lists key performance objectives for a time period, with target dates for accomplishing them.
2. The supervisor reviews objectives and discusses them with the employee; the supervisor documents the agreed-upon set of objectives.
3. The supervisor and subordinate meet regularly to review progress and make revisions or update objectives as needed.

4. At a specified time, such as after 6 months, the individual prepares a "performance report" that lists major accomplishments and comments on discrepancies between expected and actual results.

5. The supervisor and subordinate discuss the self-appraisal, with an emphasis on its implications for future performance.

6. A new set of objectives is established for the next time period, as in Step 1, and the MBO cycle begins again.

Some things to avoid in MBO include tying the process to pay, focusing too much attention on only those objectives that are easily quantified, requiring excessive paperwork, and having supervisors simply tell subordinates their objectives.

7.5.4 Performance Objectives

Performance objectives are essential to the MBO process, and the ways objectives are specified and established influences how well MBO works. In many organizations, the MBO process emphasizes improvement and personal growth objectives, specifically.

▲ **Improvement objectives** document intentions for improving performance in a specific way and with respect to a specific factor. An example is "to reduce patient complaints by 10%."

▲ **Personal development objectives** pertain to personal growth activities, often those resulting in expanded job knowledge or skills. An example is "to learn the latest version of a computer spreadsheet package."

Effective MBO objectives are

▲ **specific:** targeting a key result to be accomplished;
▲ **time-defined:** identifying a specific date for achieving results;
▲ **challenging:** offering a realistic and attainable challenge;
▲ **measurable:** stating goals in quantitative terms, whenever possible.

One of the more difficult aspects of MBO relates to the last criterion—the need to state performance objectives in quantitative terms. Ideally, you can focus the agreement on a measurable end point—for example, "to reduce office supply expenditures by 5% by the end of the fiscal year."

But some jobs, particularly managerial ones, involve performance areas that are hard to quantify. Rather than abandon MBO in such cases, try to agree on performance objectives that are stated as verifiable work activities. The accomplishment of the activities can then serve as an indicator of progress under the

---

FOR EXAMPLE

MBO at University of Minnesota Hospitals

In 1999, the Social Service Department of the University of Minnesota Hospitals (www.fairview-university.fairview.org) officially adopted an MBO-based employee evaluation system as part of ongoing appraisals and performance reviews. In addition to standard MBO techniques and procedures used throughout the business world, the University of Minnesota program includes a statement of program philosophy and statement of essential program functions. Staff reaction to the system has been mixed, while hospital administration has been uniformly favorable. In the future, the MBO system will be integrated with a management information system.

---

performance objective. An example is "to improve communications with my staff in the next 3 months by holding weekly team meetings." Whereas it can be difficult to measure "improved communications," you can fairly easily document whether the "weekly group meetings" have been held.

7.5.5 Internal Control and Self-Management

Simply defined, **internal control** is self-control. People who are motivated to take charge of their own behavior on the job are exercising internal control. Of course, people are more likely to do this when they participate in setting performance objectives and the standards of measurement. This, of course, is what the notion of management by objectives is all about. Given clear objectives to which they are committed, people are likely to manage themselves in pursuit of performance excellence.

Additionally, because MBO provides structure opportunities for people to participate in decisions that affect their work, the experience can be empowering and motivating. Because it creates enthusiasm to fulfill one's performance obligations, MBO encourages self-management rather than external control.[8]

None of this advice is lost on today's best health care managers. Although they may describe how they manage using differing language, many of the best managers utilize MBO concepts. If you want high performance from individual contributors, you must hire the best people, work with them to set challenging performance objectives, give them the best possible support, monitor their progress, and hold them accountable for results.

SELF-CHECK

- Identify and define **management by objectives, improvement objectives, personal development objectives,** and **internal control.**
- Describe the four critical parts of any management-by-objectives agreement.
- List the six steps of creating a management-by-objectives agreement.
- Compare improvement objectives to personal development objectives.
- Explain four characteristics of effective MBO objectives.
- Discuss the importance of internal control and self-management in the workplace.

SUMMARY

Controlling—the measuring of performance and taking action to ensure desired results—is a vital part of the management process. By establishing standards, measuring performance, comparing results, and taking corrective action, managers can improve the efficiency and productivity of their departments. Controls can be applied at three stages: before, during, and after an action. Establishing effective controls is critical to disciplining employees, as well as monitoring financials, purchasing, inventory, and quality. Management by objectives is an integrated set of tools and techniques in which managers and employees set performance objectives, with the ultimate goal of developing internal control and self-management in the workplace.

KEY TERMS

Asset management	The ability to use resources efficiently and operate at minimum cost.
Concurrent controls	Controls that focus on what actually happens during the work process, also called *steering controls.*
Control equation	Need for Action = Desired Performance − Actual Performance

Controlling	The process of measuring performance and taking action to ensure desired results; a basic function for health care managers.
Control process	A four-step method for measuring performance.
Discipline	The act of influencing behavior through reprimand.
Economic order quantity (EOQ)	A quantitative method of inventory control that involves ordering a fixed number of items every time an inventory level falls to a predetermined point.
Engineering comparison	Comparison that uses standards set scientifically through such methods as time and motion studies.
External control	Attempting to control the behavior of others through personal supervision or formal administrative systems.
Feedback controls	Controls that take place after work is completed, also called *postaction controls*.
Feedforward controls	Controls that are accomplished before a work activity begins, also called *preliminary controls*.
Historical comparison	Comparison that uses past performance as a standard for evaluating current performance.
Improvement objectives	MBO goals that document intentions for improving performance in a specific way and with respect to a specific factor.
Input standards	Control measurements that focus on the amount of work expended in task performance.
Internal control	Allowing motivated individuals and groups to exercise self-discipline in fulfilling job expectations.
Just-in-time scheduling (JIT)	A Japanese model for industrial productivity, JIT systems try to reduce costs and improve workflow by scheduling items to arrive just in time to be used.
Leverage	The ability to earn more in returns than the cost of debt.
Liquidity	The ability to generate cash to pay bills.
Management by exception	The practice of giving priority attention to situations that show the greatest need for action.

Management by objectives (MBO)	A structured process of regular communication in which a supervisor and subordinate jointly set performance objectives for the subordinate and review results accomplished.
Operations management	The portion of management duties that emphasizes utilizing people, resources, and technology to the best advantage.
Opportunity situation	Actual performance is above the standard.
Output standards	Control measurement results that focus on performance quantity, quality, cost, or time.
Personal development objectives	MBO goals that pertain to personal growth activities, often those resulting in expanded job knowledge or skills.
Problem situation	Actual performance is below the standard.
Profitability	The ability to earn revenues greater than costs.
Progressive discipline	A discipline system in which reprimands are tied to the severity and frequency of misbehavior.
Quality control	Checking processes, materials, products, and services to ensure that they meet high standards.
Relative comparison	Comparison that uses the performance achievements of other people, work units, or organizations as evaluation benchmarks.
Six Sigma	A collection of rigorous, systematic control tools that uses information and statistical analysis to measure and improve an organization's performance, practices, and systems.

ASSESS YOUR UNDERSTANDING

Go to www.wiley.com/college/Lombardi to evaluate your knowledge of the basics of the control process.

Measure your learning by comparing pretest and post-test results.

Summary Questions

1. Controlling is an important part of the management process because it ensures that
   (a) the performance contributions of individuals and groups are consistent with plans.
   (b) the right things happen in the right way and at the right time.
   (c) the performance accomplishments throughout the organization are well integrated.
   (d) All of the above

2. The four steps of the controlling process are
   (a) monitoring progress, evaluating results, preparing plans, and responding to change.
   (b) establishing standards, measuring performance, comparing results, and taking corrective action.
   (c) eliminating error, establishing procedures, testing employees, and evaluating teamwork.
   (d) identifying problems, brainstorming solutions, evaluating data, and reporting results.

3. Many managers fail to get the most out of the controlling process because they do not follow up on their decisions. True or false?

4. Feedforward controls are preventative in nature; they ensure that objectives and directions are clear before work begins. True or false?

5. Which of the following is an example of a concurrent control?
   (a) A manager posting a memo in the break room
   (b) A nurse evaluating a supply cabinet based on an inventory checklist
   (c) A manager monitoring a receptionist's phone call with a patient
   (d) All staff receiving training in CPR, regardless of position

6. Anticipating that a nursing aide will need assistance moving a patient is an example of a feedback control. True or false?

7. Internal controls are based within the employee's team or department, while external controls come from the larger organization. True or false?

8. The process of performance modeling makes the management process responsibilities of controlling and leading compatible. True or false?

9. Which of the following is NOT a way to combine the control and organizing responsibilities of management?

   (a) Control via policies and procedures

   (b) Control by selection and training

   (c) Control via job design

   (d) Control via performance appraisal

10. Ratios are used to control financial aspects of an organization's performance. An area that is appropriate for financial control is

    (a) leverage.

    (b) profitability.

    (c) liquidity.

    (d) all of the above.

11. An example of an effective purchasing control technique is

    (a) buying on margin, from alternative sources.

    (b) buying in volume, through a centralized purchasing department.

    (c) keeping inventory quantities limited, to avoid overstocking.

    (d) exchanging goods for services, with a focus on reciprocity.

12. The principle of economic order quantity involves ordering a set amount of an item any time inventory drops below a set point. True or false?

13. All of the following are possible quality-control measures except

    (a) a manager delivering a detailed performance appraisal to an employee.

    (b) a manager randomly evaluating an employee's paperwork.

    (c) a worker logging how many patients he or she worked with during a shift.

    (d) a manager observing an employee's work and providing immediate feedback.

14. MBO objectives require a formal agreement between supervisor and subordinate concerning schedules for completing tasks and tools for developing further skills. True or false?

15. The first step in establishing a successful MBO objective is to

    (a) identify obstacles for completing tasks, as well as available supporting resources.

    (b) list key performance objectives for a time period with target dates for accomplishing them.

    (c) discuss the process of self-appraisal with an emphasis on its implications for future performance.

    (d) None of the above

16. While an improvement objective focuses on bettering one's performance in some specific way, a personal development object focuses on expanding job knowledge or skills. True or false?

17. Which of the following objectives meets all four critical criteria for an effective MBO objective?

    (a) To treat patients with respect and honesty

    (b) To meet with staff and listen to their concerns

    (c) To facilitate an off-site communication team planning to meet every quarter

    (d) To be on time for meetings

Review Questions

1. The first step of the control process is to establish objectives and standards. What are two types of standards?

2. Which type of performance standard focuses on the amount of work expended to complete a task?

3. In Step 3 of the control process, you compare results with objectives and standards. What are the three types of comparisons?

4. What type of control seeks to eliminate later problems by asking what needs to be planned before beginning?

5. A nurse manager notices that an RN is having difficulty administering a shot; the manager assists the RN, retraining him on procedure. What type of control is happening?

6. Rather than focusing on inputs and activities, feedback controls focus on what?

7. What types of controls are related to a manager's leading responsibilities?

8. Progressive discipline bases reprimands on the severity and frequency of the misbehavior. What is the overarching goal of progressive discipline?

9. When capable people are hired and given the ongoing training needed to perform their jobs at high levels of accomplishment, what specific type of control is being utilized?

10. Control is an essential part of operations management. What three work-related aspects fall under the scope of operations management?

11. Team leaders and department managers rarely have the ability to exercise high levels of purchasing control. What can managers at this level do to provide some level of purchasing control?

12. Every month, LPNs at a nursing care facility audit the contents of every resident's storage closet and note the type and quantity of medical supplies. What type of control are the LPNs exercising?

13. Just-in-time inventory control systems try to reduce costs and improve workflow by scheduling items to arrive just in time to be used. What are some benefits of just-in-time systems?

14. In order for an MBO objective to be effective, it must have what four critical characteristics?

15. Although management by objectives takes considerable work on the part of manager and employee, it has several advantages. What is an advantage of utilizing MBO?

16. In the MBO process, after an employee prepares a self-appraisal, what happens next?

Applying This Chapter

1. The manager of a small medical clinic adds several items to a checklist of exam-room preparation responsibilities after finding his staff inconsistently preparing rooms. What step of the control process is the manager enacting?

2. In an effort to establish controls, a new manager decides to spend one afternoon each week double-checking every chart his nursing care staff has completed for the previous week. In what ways is this attempt at control ineffective?

3. After each dialysis session, patients at Mayhaven Kidney Health Center are given evaluation postcards with five multiple-choice questions that they're asked to complete and mail in. The postcards are an example of what type of potentially effective control?

4. The manager of a critical care unit has begun noticing inconsistencies in the charting methods of her nursing staff. What would be examples of an internal and an external control the manager could set up to improve charting?

5. Where in the day-to-day operations of a 100-bed nursing care facility might an economic order quantity system of inventory control be appropriate? Where would a just-in-time inventory control system be appropriate?

6. The medical billing center you manage institutes a new MBO-based performance objective that "customer service representatives will establish person-to-person contact with any caller within 30 seconds." Does this objective meet all four requirements for MBO objectives?

Comparison as Part of the Control Process

Comparing measured performance with objectives and standards (Step 3 in the control process) is critical to determining whether you need to take any corrective action. Evaluate your performance on an important recent exam you took, report you wrote, or presentation you gave. Consider the three types of comparisons as you evaluate your performance. From a *historical comparison* standpoint, how does your performance compare with your previous performances on similar exams, reports, or presentations? From a *relative comparison* standpoint, how does your performance compare with performances of other students in your class? From an *engineered comparison* standpoint, how does your performance compare with standards established by your instructor or professor?

Feedforward Controls

Apply feedforward controls the next time you have a challenging, upcoming event in your life. For example, taking a final exam, interviewing for a job, purchasing a car, or planning a wedding are all major events for which you can utilize feedforward controls before the actual event happens. Set the stage for high performance by asking yourself, What specifically is my goal? Are there any rules, regulations, or directions I need to know about ahead of time? What resources (financial, time, people) are available to me to help me meet by goal?

Job Descriptions as Control Tool

Job descriptions can be effective managerial control tools (control by selection and training, as well as control by job design and work structures). However, for job descriptions to be effective, they must be valid, current, and at least 80% reflective of the major duties of the position. Develop your ability to evaluate job descriptions by reviewing the job description for a job you have currently or had recently. You can locate job descriptions through your human resource department, online, and within company handbooks. To evaluate a job description, compile a top-10 list of the tasks you do on a regular basis, then assign the percentage of time that you spend on each task in a typical workday. Next, assign to each task a *weighted value* between 1 and 100, according to its relative importance. Multiple the percentage of the time and the weighted value to determine the relative importance of each given task. Review the results of your relative importance list against the official job description to determine whether the description and the actualities of the job mesh.

Clear Standards, Improved Quality Control

An important part of a successful, ongoing quality-control initiative is to have clear standards in place, against which you can compare your performance. Take yourself through a quality-control assessment by comparing your performance level as a postsecondary student with the performance standards for your state or institution of higher education. Educational standards for your school are likely posted on the school's Web site or within a student handbook. If you can't find standards specifically for your school, visit the Web site http://EdStandards.org (http://edstandards.org/Standards.html), which offers a state-by-state overview of educational standards for students at all educational levels. Print out the standards that best relate to you and your education. How are you doing on each item related to your course of study? Rate yourself in each category of assessment, using a 0 to 100% score. Average your various scores to arrive at an overall level of quality score.

MBO-approved Goals?

Take a moment and write down your goal or goals for the course you're currently taking. What sort of grade do you want to achieve? What do you hope to learn through this course? Are there any skills you plan to learn, develop, or refine? What about the people you're interacting with within the course—do you have any goals for these interactions? Write down your goal or goals and then consider the four critical characteristics for effective MBO objectives (section 7.5.3). Are your goals specific, time-defined, challenging, and measurable? Revise your goals so each is specific, time-defined, challenging, and measurable.

211

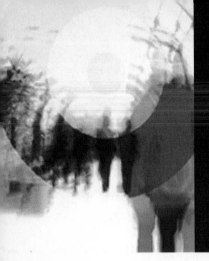

8

MAKING MAJOR CHOICES
Performing Strategic Analysis and Making Decisions

Starting Point

Go to www.wiley.com/college/Lombardi to assess your knowledge of the basics of analyzing and making decisions.
Determine where you need to concentrate your effort.

What You'll Learn in This Chapter

▲ Two responsibilities of strategic management
▲ Three levels of organizational strategy
▲ Essential values for making decisions
▲ The Portfolio Planning Approach to decision making
▲ Tools for preparing to make decisions
▲ Strategies for analyzing situations
▲ Three models for implementing decisions
▲ Ways to effectively communicate strategic decisions

After Studying This Chapter, You'll Be Able To

▲ Calculate the importance of competitive advantage in strategic decision making
▲ Examine typical levels, types, and steps of strategic decision making
▲ Apply common strategic decision-making tools and techniques
▲ Examine standardized procedures for formulating and implementing decisions
▲ Practice methods for communicating strategic decisions
▲ Distinguish methods of measuring the effectiveness of decisions

Goals and Outcomes

▲ Master the terminology and tools related to strategic decision making
▲ Describe the steps of strategic decision making
▲ Choose appropriate information-gathering tools for decision making
▲ Analyze situations as part of the decision-making process
▲ Compare methods for formulating and implementing strategic decisions
▲ Create plans and processes for strategic decision making
▲ Evaluate the appropriateness of strategic decisions

INTRODUCTION

The ability to analyze situations strategically and make timely decisions is a key managerial responsibility. Strategic decisions are formulated and implemented at various levels within organizations and for several common purposes. Good decisions are driven by values and utilize standardized approaches. To make strategic decisions, managers have a range of tools and techniques they can use to gather information, analyze the information, and finally implement their decisions. Throughout the decision-making process, communicating with others and evaluating outcomes are both critical to successfully making strong, strategic decisions.

8.1 Understanding Levels and Types of Strategy

In order to successfully make good decisions, managers need to understand the strategic demands and expectations that all modern businesses—including health care organizations—operate under.

An organization with **competitive advantage** operates with an attribute or combination of attributes that allows it to outperform its rivals. The goal for any organization, however, is not just to achieve competitive advantage but to make it sustainable, even as rivals attempt to duplicate and copy a success story. A **sustainable competitive advantage** is one that is difficult for competitors to imitate. Competitors have trouble catching up, let alone getting ahead.

A **strategy** is a comprehensive action plan that identifies long-term direction and guides resource utilization to accomplish an organization's mission and objectives with sustainable competitive advantage. It is a plan for using resources with consistent **strategic intent;** that is, with all organizational energies focused on a unifying and compelling target.[1]

To gain competitive advantage, an organization must deal with market and environmental forces better than its competitors.[2] The task of crafting strategies with this potential can be daunting.

While a discussion of strategy and competition may seem extreme or out-of-sync with the essential care-giving services and purposes of most health care organizations, the truth is that all organizations—including health care organizations—are competing for limited resources, patients, and money. For example:

▲ When a teaching hospital's public relations materials highlight the hospital's alliance with a research university and its ability to provide "state-of-the-art cancer care" to patients, the hospital is capitalizing on its competitive advantage.

▲ When a medical billing department partners with an outside collections service to begin offering three simple methods of low-term payment for its patients, the department is establishing a sustainable competitive advantage in the complex and often frustrating world of medical claims billing and collections.

▲ When a family planning clinic initiates a pilot program to facilitate adoption services (in addition to its already established birth-control and crisis-pregnancy services), the clinic is responding strategically to the needs of its patients.

8.1.1 The Strategic Management Process

The demands of intense competition call for strategies that are often bold and fast-moving. **Strategic management** is the process of formulating and implementing strategies that create competitive advantage and advance an organization's mission and objectives.

The essence of strategic management is to look ahead, understand the environment, and effectively position an organization for competitive success in changing times. Figure 8-1 describes two major responsibilities in the strategic management process.

The first responsibility is **strategy formulation**, which involves assessing existing strategies, organization, and environment to develop new strategies

Figure 8-1

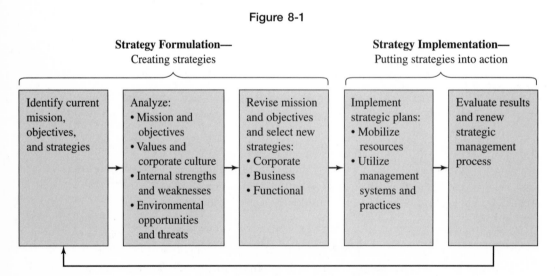

The responsibilities involved in the management process.

and strategic plans capable of delivering future competitive advantage. As management consultant Peter Drucker points out, this process asks five strategic questions:

1. What is our mission?
2. Who are our customers?
3. What do our customers value?
4. What have been our results?
5. What is our plan?[3]

The second responsibility is **strategy implementation.** After strategies are created, they must be acted upon successfully to achieve the desired results. As Drucker says, "The future will not just happen if one wishes hard enough. It requires decision—now. It imposes risk—now. It requires action—now. It demands allocation of resources and above all, of human resources—now. It requires *work*—now."[4] This work is the responsibility for actually putting strategies and strategic plans into action; it is the process of implementation. All this, in turn, requires a commitment to mastering the full range of strategic management tasks listed here.

▲ **Identify organizational mission and objectives.** *Ask:* What business are we in? Where do we want to be in the future?
▲ **Assess current performance in regards to mission and objectives.** *Ask:* How well are we currently doing?
▲ **Create strategic plans to accomplish purpose and objectives.** *Ask:* How can we get where we really want to be?
▲ **Implement the strategic plans.** *Ask:* Has everything been done that needs to be done?
▲ **Evaluate results; change strategic plans and/or implementation processes as necessary.** *Ask:* Are things working out as planned, and what can be improved upon?

For more information about the planning process, specifically mission statements, core values, and objectives, refer to section 6.4.

8.1.2 Levels of Strategy

Successful health care organizations formulate strategies at several specific levels.

At the level of **corporate strategy,** top management directs an organization as a whole toward sustainable competitive advantage. Corporate strategy describes the scope of operations by answering the strategic question, "In what industries, service sectors, and/or markets should we compete?"

In many of today's large-scale, diversified health care conglomerates such as university hospitals and multiclinic partnerships, corporate strategy identifies the different areas of business in which the larger organization intends to compete. Top-level managers and vice presidents typically make these high level corporate strategic decisions, determining resource allocation, new business acquisition and divestiture, and the overall mix of the organization's business portfolio. Increasingly, corporate strategies for large health care organizations include international ventures and strategic alliances.

At the level of **business strategy,** top- and mid-level management set the direction for a single business unit. Business strategy typically describes strategic intent with respect to a given market or major service/department, such as a hospital's surgery division or an inner-city's emphasis on diabetic services for lower-income patients. The selection of business strategy involves answering the strategic question, "How are we going to compete for customers within this industry, service sector, or market?" Typical business strategy decisions include choices about product/service mix, facility locations, new technologies, and the like.

At the level of **functional strategy,** middle- and low-level management guide the use of resources to implement business strategy. This level of strategy focuses on activities within a specific functional area of operations, such as marketing, patient care, finance, human resources, or research and development. The strategic question to be answered in selecting functional strategies is, "How can we best utilize resources to implement our business strategy?"

8.1.3 Types of Strategies

The types of strategies that health care organizations pursue can be classified in several general types.

Growth strategies pursue larger-size and expanded operations. Growth strategies are popular in part because growth is necessary for long-term survival in some sectors. There is a tendency to equate growth with effectiveness, but that is not necessarily true. Management must manage any growth in order to achieve the desired results. Some organizations grow through **concentration**— that is, by using existing strengths in new and productive ways and without taking the risks of great shifts in direction. Others grow through **diversification,** the acquisition of or investment in new businesses and services in previously unrelated areas.

Retrenchment strategies reduce the scale of operations in order to gain efficiency and improve performance. The decision to retrench can be difficult to make because some may (often incorrectly) perceive retrenchment as an admission of failure. But in today's era of challenging economic conditions and uncertainty, retrenchment strategies have gained renewed respect. Some common retrenchment strategies include

▲ **retrenchment by turnaround:** A strategy of "downsizing" to reduce costs and "restructuring" to improve operating efficiency;
▲ **retrenchment by divestiture:** Selling parts of the organization to refocus on core competencies, cut costs, and improve operating efficiency;
▲ **retrenchment by liquidation:** Closing operations through the complete sale of assets or the declaration of bankruptcy.

Stability strategies maintain the present course of action without major operating changes. Stability is sometimes pursued when an organization is doing well and the environment is not perceived to be changing. Stability strategies are also used when time is needed to consolidate organizational strengths after a period of growth or retrenchment. Of course, organizations can also pursue stability by default when decision makers are unwilling to make strategic changes.

Cooperation strategies are becoming increasingly popular, given the popularity of business networks and collaborative partnerships. **Strategic alliances**, in which two or more organizations join together in partnership to pursue an area of mutual interest, are becoming much more common in health care. One way to cooperate strategically is through **outsourcing alliances**, contracting to purchase important services from another organization. Many health care organizations today, for example, have begun outsourcing their IT functions to technical firms in the belief that these services are better provided by a specialist firm.

FOR EXAMPLE

Emergent Strategies

In the real world, strategy formulation is complex and demanding. Strategies are rarely developed at one point in time and then implemented step by step. Many strategies take shape, change, and develop over time as modest adjustments to past patterns. Such modern workplace realities have led management consultant Henry Mintzberg to identify what he calls emergent strategies,[5] which develop progressively over time as "streams" of decisions made by managers as they learn from and respond to work situations. **Emergent strategies** allow managers and organizations to become good at implementing and combining strategies, not just formulating and discarding strategies in rapid succession. For more real-world insight from Mintzberg, visit his Web site (www.henrymintzberg.com), which features free excerpts from his research, books, and presentations.

- Identify and define **competitive advantage, strategy,** and **strategic management process.**
- Compare competitive advantage and sustainable competitive advantage.
- Describe the two responsibilities of the strategic management process.
- List characteristics of strategies at corporate, business, and functional levels.
- Define various types of strategies, including growth, retrenchment, stability, and cooperation.
- Provide specific examples of growth, retrenchment, stability, and cooperation strategies.

8.2 Formulating Strategies and Making Decisions

When strategies are being developed, savvy health care organizations remember to focus on achieving sustainable competitive advantage. Major opportunities for competitive advantage include the following areas:[6]

- ▲ **Cost and quality:** Where strategy drives an emphasis on operating efficiency and/or product or service quality.
- ▲ **Knowledge and timing:** Where strategy drives an emphasis on learning, innovation and speed of delivery to market for new ideas.
- ▲ **Barriers to entry:** Where strategy drives an emphasis on creating a market stronghold that is protected from entry by others.
- ▲ **Financial resources:** Where strategy drives an emphasis on investments and/or loss sustainment that competitors can't match.

8.2.1 Appreciating What It Takes to Make Decisions

Managerial decisions have direct impact on the work lives and overall performance of other individuals. Given the limited resources in today's health care arena, managers also often make decisions that concern a number of areas: human resources, operational equipment, and financial expenditures, to name a few.

Every decision you make has consequence, not only on the work life of others, but also on the long-term progress of your department or team. Although at first this responsibility may seem overwhelming, it is something managers must confront on a daily basis.

Team members look to managers to direct their work activity, and the organization depends on managerial decisions to help effect positive action. Additionally, patients rely on managerial decisions for positive outcome with the health care they receive.

Five essential values drive the decision-making process for managers:

▲ **Accountability:** Managers must use all the tools available to them in accomplishing their set goals. In addition, they must be accountable for how those resources are used. In analyzing data and taking into account the potential ramifications of their decisions, managers assume accountability on several levels. They must be accountable not only for the decision made, but also for how the decision was determined, what data were analyzed, and which course of action was pursued in arriving at the final decision.

▲ **Adaptability:** To demonstrate the flexibility needed for managing health care delivery in a turbulent business climate, managers must embrace a certain degree of adaptability. *Adaptability* means being flexible in considering options, being able to deal with a wide range of people, and having a versatile business approach. Managers must take care, however, to avoid being too adaptable; that is, becoming wishy-washy or irresolute by constantly straying from an established course of action, or spending so much time considering options that the manager ultimately fails to arrive at a set course of action.

▲ **Dependability:** Staff depends on leaders to make timely decisions that, for the most part, are correct and specify a proper course of action. Constant reluctance to take stands or making decisions without communication or staff input does not promote the perception among staff and the organization that a manager is dependable.

▲ **Responsibility:** A strong manager embraces responsibility for making decisions, takes ownership for decisions, and views the management role as a commitment to organizational excellence. These attitudes mandate selfless participation in the decision-making process so as to consider at all times what is good for the organization and to consider both the positive and negative ramifications of a decision on staff and the entire organization. (All decision making must be done while keeping in mind the organization's objective of providing stellar health care service to all its patients.) Managers who shirk responsibility may be seen as being overly political, figureheads, or worse. Even when managers delegate a particular task, they ultimately must take responsibility for the outcome.

▲ **Visibility:** Visible leaders are present and on the scene. In conducting their activities, they are around to hear the cheers and the boos. Furthermore, a manager's visibility does not diminish in critical times or in situations that are out of the norm. At no time should a visible manager hear the question, "Who's in charge?"

FOR EXAMPLE

Adapting at Sloane-Kettering

Memorial Sloane-Kettering Cancer Center (www.mskcc.org) is known world-wide for its innovative research into the causes and treatment of cancer. In November 2004, the institution, frustrated by an ongoing shortage of exceptional cancer researchers, decided to respond creatively and flexibly to the situation and create its own innovative doctoral program. Sloane-Kettering's new Graduate School of Biomedical Sciences trains basic laboratory scientists to work in research areas directly applicable to human disease, particularly cancer. "Right now, there aren't enough basic scientists who understand the biological challenges faced by clinicians," MSKCC president Harold Varmus said. "The new program we've designed will provide unparalleled opportunities to gifted and creative students who are inspired to attack clinical problems through research." Beginning July 2006, 10 to 12 graduate students annually will enroll in the intensive program, which leads to the newly created degree of a PhD in cancer biology.

8.2.2 Utilizing the Portfolio Planning Approach

The **portfolio planning approach** is a basic method of formulating strategy and making decisions, in which managers allocate scarce organizational resources among competing opportunities. In the portfolio planning approach, *resources* include various products, services, business units, and departments or divisions.[7]

Figure 8-2 summarizes a portfolio planning approach developed by the Boston Consulting Group known as the BCG matrix. The matrix ties strategy formulation to an analysis of business opportunities according to market growth rate and market share.[8] The matrix shows the following four possibilities, with each linked to a possible strategic direction.

▲ **Stars** are high-market-share opportunities in high-growth markets. They produce large profits through substantial penetration of expanding markets. The preferred strategy for stars is *growth,* and further resource investments in them are recommended.

▲ **Question marks** are low-market-share businesses in high-growth markets. They do not produce much profit but compete in rapidly growing markets. They are the source of difficult strategic decisions. The preferred strategy is *growth,* but the risk exists that further investments may not result in improved market share. The most promising question marks should be targeted for growth; others are retrenchment candidates.

▲ **Cash cows** are high-market-share businesses in low-growth markets. They produce large profits and a strong cash flow. Because the markets

Figure 8-2

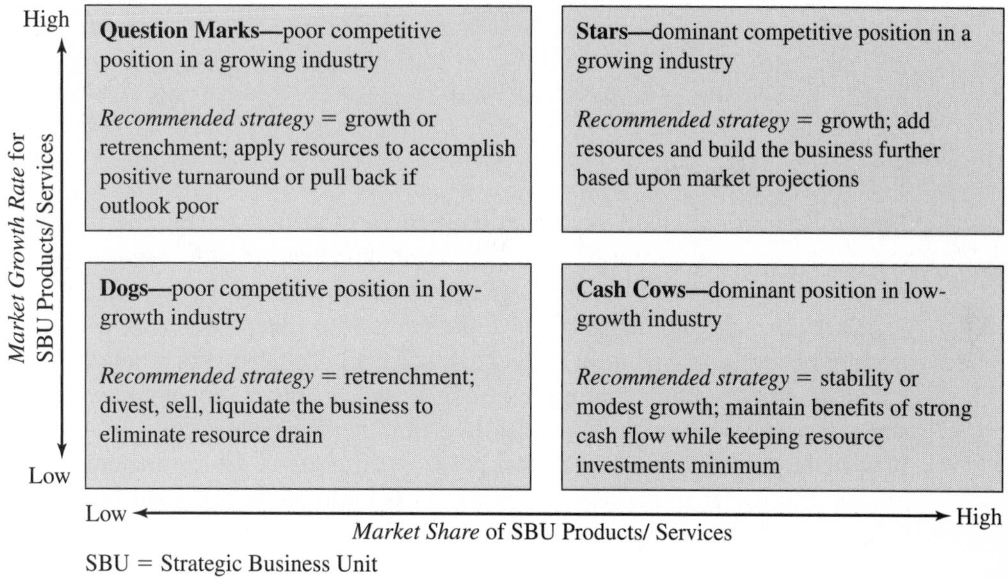

Market Growth Rate for SBU Products/Services

High

Question Marks—poor competitive position in a growing industry

Recommended strategy = growth or retrenchment; apply resources to accomplish positive turnaround or pull back if outlook poor

Stars—dominant competitive position in a growing industry

Recommended strategy = growth; add resources and build the business further based upon market projections

Dogs—poor competitive position in low-growth industry

Recommended strategy = retrenchment; divest, sell, liquidate the business to eliminate resource drain

Cash Cows—dominant position in low-growth industry

Recommended strategy = stability or modest growth; maintain benefits of strong cash flow while keeping resource investments minimum

Low

Low ← *Market Share* of SBU Products/Services → High

SBU = Strategic Business Unit

A portfolio model for corporate strategy formulation.

offer little growth opportunity, the preferred strategy is *stability* or *modest growth*. The choice of terms is very descriptive; "cows" should be "milked" to generate cash that can be used to support needed investments in stars and question marks.

▲ **Dogs** are low-market-share businesses in low-growth markets. They do not produce much profit, and they show little potential for future improvement. The preferred strategy for dogs is *retrenchment by divestiture*.

SELF-CHECK

- Identify and define **portfolio planning approach, opportunities, and resources.**
- List four business areas in which organizations can have competitive advantage.
- Discuss the five values that drive managerial decision making.
- Explain the purpose of the portfolio planning approach to strategic decision making.
- Describe the four possible outcomes of the portfolio planning approach.

8.3 Tools for Making Strategic Decisions

Managers can utilize numerous resources, strategies, and tools for data collection and analysis during the process of formulating strategic decisions. The following sections cover some of the most common and useful aids.

8.3.1 Collecting Data

Data collection and analysis should happen early in the strategic decision-making process. Managers must collect as much information as possible, and then make a timely decision based on the information at hand.

Often, health care managers have problems with this phase because they mistakenly believe that a magical answer can solve all problems. For example, if your organization cut your department's budget, as a manager, you may believe that some magical solution can help deal with limited financial resources and somehow make the department staff feel good about the cut. Unfortunately, no right answer exists toward addressing the dilemma imposed by a limited budget.

Managers can also make the mistake of believing that the more time that they spend collecting data, the more accurate their decision will be. Given the high visibility of a manager's position, too much time can be spent collecting information and becoming involved in a research process that instead of signaling a leader may demonstrate a manager who is afraid to make a decision. Not only is this perception extremely harmful to the manager's reputation, but also the manager who spends more time on research than action does not inspire confidence or generate positive results on a consistent basis.

Therefore, remember two guidelines when collecting data:

▲ **Try to obtain valid, realistic information.** Do not expect a one-size-fits-all solution from colleagues or other sources. By recognizing that each situation is unique, a manager brings his or her individual style and approach to problem resolution.

▲ **Recognize that the time frame for making a decision is as important as the decision itself.** After you have the information you need, rely on an intelligent gut feeling to arrive at an informed decision. Then initiate the action and begin implementation of your plan.

8.3.2 Studying Established Past Actions

Savvy managers utilize past action—including the actions of predecessors or peer managers—to help formulate new strategies. Assuming someone else's decision was correct, you can gain some insight into your problem and a potential solution.

Keep in mind, however, that what worked in the past may not necessarily suit current or future circumstances. Nonetheless, the overall dynamics of the situation may be similar and give you some clue for constructing your own plan of action.

For example, in examining how other managers at your health care organizations have responded to budget cuts, you can learn about potential reactions your staff may have toward working with reduced resources. By learning from others' mistakes as well as their positive contributions, you gain insight into what did not work and what did work. In a similar vein, you can ask colleagues for their ideas on what they would do or, better yet, what they did in the past to help staff deal with departmental budget cuts. In both cases, you can find valuable information that provides a strong general frame of reference for formulating your strategy.

8.3.3 Researching Formal References

Formal references are anything that can be construed as "book knowledge," including journals relevant to your technical area, management texts that offer pragmatic solutions, or your organization's manual of standard operating procedures. Standard operating procedures typically include specific protocols and policies that your organization has adopted or specific bylaws applicable to the situation that you are currently confronting.

8.3.4 Analyzing Hard Data

Hard data can include any information that may have been generated by a questionnaire, form, or survey. Measurable data, or quantitative information, can give you some outlook on the possible impact of your decision.

For example, a manager can gather hard data on departmental budget cuts by reviewing organizational history relative to adverse reaction to budget cuts

---

FOR EXAMPLE

Survey Data Points to Dramatic Increase in Peanut Allergies

According to research published in the December 2005 issue of *Journal of Allergy and Clinical Immunology* (JACI), peanut allergies in children have increased 100% from 1997 to 2002. Scott Sicherer, MD, and Hugh Sampson, MD, of Mount Sinai School of Medicine (www.mountsinaihospital.org) conducted 13,493 formal phone surveys and spend 2 years analyzing the hard data they collected. According to Sicherer and Sampson, their data shows that.4% of U.S. children were diagnosed with fatal peanut allergies in 1997, while.8% had been diagnosed in 2002. "This study confirms what we've been hearing from growing numbers of families, school administrators and other institutional leaders—food allergy is increasing," said Anne Muñoz-Furlong, founder and CEO of the Food Allergy & Anaphylaxis Network. Additional research, surveys, and analysis is planned to determine possible causes of the dramatic increase in peanut allergies.

and employee perceptions toward dealing with them. Whether a questionnaire is used or questions are asked informally in a meeting, a survey of staff attitudes to previous budget cuts generates data to assist you in making decisions. (Gathering hard data can also help strengthen the communication link between department colleagues and staff.)

8.3.5 Predicting Advantages and Potential Disadvantages

An important element of data collection is considering the advantages and disadvantages of your options. Who will benefit from your action? How might positive interpersonal effect best be achieved? Also consider when positive results may be realized, and set a time frame of realization of positive output.

Again using the budget-cut example, consider who would be involved with making the budget cuts, when some positive effects could be seen despite the cuts, and what the overall impact of the cuts might be. Set a projected implementation schedule and list the overall benefits, if any, that might emerge from the cuts.

At the same time, identify potential negative fallout, including adverse reactions and unfavorable perceptions that may arise. By anticipating negative fallout, you take the first step toward addressing problems and effecting positive action.

8.3.6 Following Your Instincts

The final element of data collection is trust in your instincts. Instinctual reaction gives credence to your insight into the problem at hand, the decision you have arrived at, and the action plan you implement. It also mandates a certain amount of introspection—that is, considering the impact a decision will have not only on staff but also on your own activities. Instinctual reaction also means trusting your intelligence and ability to consider the facts objectively, subjectively analyze data, and use common sense to arrive at a course of action.

SELF-CHECK

- Identify and define **hard data** and **formal references**.
- List and describe common tools for data collection and analysis.
- Discuss the process of data collection, including the two main guidelines for successful data collection.
- Compare the relative usefulness of studying past actions, reviewing formal references, analyzing hard data, making predictions, and following instincts as part of the decision-making process.

8.4 Analyzing Information

After collecting all significant data, you now must move to the action phase of the decision-making process. This phase entails reviewing all the information collected and setting a course of action and a specific plan for achieving the action. **Action analysis** allows managers to examine the viability of their plans and try to predict whether their decisions are sound and the courses of action will be effective.

Action analysis begins with a data review within the context of four essential factors: the environment, the various functions involved in the action plan, the business consequences of the action taken, and the historical precedent of the action. These four types of analysis allow you to examine every conceivable angle of a decision before taking action.

8.4.1 Environment Analysis

Environment analysis takes into account the theoretical and physical environment in which you operate and the action plan that will be undertaken. Figure 8-3 shows the sphere of influence surrounding a health care team, as well as interaction between critical groups (represented as arrows).

An environment analysis allows managers to look specifically at workplace dynamics while making decisions. The example in Figure 8-3 shows a rehabilitation unit at a metropolitan hospital. The model can assist managers in determining areas that may be most affected by budget cuts, identifying potential areas of concern, and arriving at some suggestions for undertaking the action.

Information that is helpful to consider while conducting an environment analysis include the department's size, the daily volume of patient services, and the revenue the department generates.

Less tangible environmental factors include the prevailing mood of the organization, employee morale in your department, and the administration's attitude toward your department. For example, a department that has direct patient contact traditionally has greater visibility within the organization and consequently gets quicker action and support for carrying out its actions. Hence, as a manager, you must consider your department's status as a factor in your decision-making process.

Finally, environment analysis must take place over a time continuum. Seek to determine what the past status of the department has been, what its present conditions and objectives are, and what its future objectives may be. This viewpoint can be expanded to include the entire organization. Past, present, and future objectives that might bear on the decision at hand should be factored into the decision-making equation.

Figure 8-3

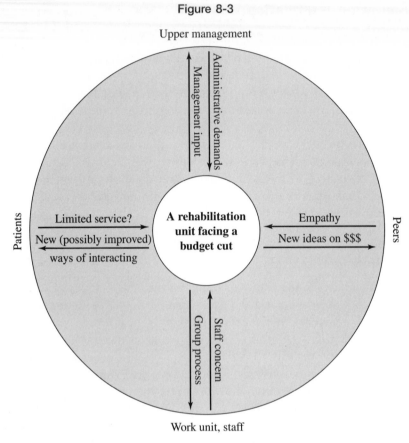

Sphere of influence for a health care team facing budget cuts.

8.4.2 Function (Role) Analysis

Function analysis basically asks, "Who can do what to make this happen?" In the following approach to function analysis, you evaluate every role affected by implementing and executing a strategic action plan.

1. **Consider function analysis on your immediate department.** Try to draw an accurate picture of how you can use various available staff resources, given the staff's roles and functions. Do you have enough staff to carry out the action? Is the range of staff talent sufficient (for example, in technical ability) and balanced in terms of individual contribution? Consider the performance levels of the various individuals in your department. If your action plan is to be a group process, be certain to include the stronger players on your action team. If significant individual action is required, again consider various individuals' roles, as well as their strengths and weaknesses, and then set your plan accordingly.

2. **Expand the function analysis to include related departments and colleagues.** For example, a decision you are about to implement may require the support and participation of other departments. You also may need the participation of specialists and other peers within the organization. Try to specify what roles or functions need to be assumed by these individuals and what is required from all participants in installing your plan.

3. **Consider what participation you need from your supervisor.** As your primary mentor, your supervisor is invaluable in guiding you as you implement and execute strategic designs. Also, you may require specific action from a supervisor (for example, influencing another individual within or outside the organization who can further empower your efforts). If you need political clout that only a supervisor can deliver, identify that role during function analysis and enlist participation as appropriate.

4. **Consider benefits to the overall organization.** Detail any specific advantages your organization may enjoy from your strategic decision. Brainstorm any contributions or roles the organization can assume in supporting your decision. Analyze any potential negative impact your decision may have on the organization.

8.4.3 Business Analysis

Before you can fully implement an action plan as a health care manager, you must analyze business-related dynamics.

First, consider the impact of your decision and its subsequent effect on patients. Specifically, what benefits will patients enjoy? What potential, short-term adverse outcomes may patients suffer as a result of your decision? (The qualifier *short-term* is key here: if any adverse impact falls to the patient, you have made a wrong decision.)

Two key quality-related themes underlie all aspects of business analysis:

▲ **Continuous quality improvement (CQI)** should drive all department activities. CQI dictates ongoing quality enhancement as the incentive that fuels everyday activities associated with optimum health care delivery.

▲ **Continuous business development (CBD)** connotes a building-block approach to all departmental activities in management efforts. Every effort undertaken by the department should be done to make the department a stronger, more progressive entity than it was prior to the effort.

Managers reinforce the dynamics of CQI and CBD asking the following questions:

▲ Will the decision mandate action that is quality conscious?
▲ Will the decision result in action that improves the quality of services?

▲ Will the decision initiate action that facilitates departmental mission of progressive development?

▲ What future departmental or organizational goals may evolve from this decision?

▲ What will be the ultimate benefit of this action to the patient and the organization?

Finally, in developing a business perspective through analysis, identify any potential negative impacts and business consequences. Specifically, what adverse effect may compromise appropriate use of resources (human, fiscal, and equipment, for example)? Could patients perceive that their welfare is not a top organizational priority? For example, does a construction project severely inconvenience patients? These questions all speak to business dynamics that managers must analyze throughout the decision-making process.

8.4.4 Historical Analysis

Historical analysis takes into account past precedents established in the organization. As a starting point, managers should consider precedents set by past action. What courses of action were taken that were similar in scope to the one you are contemplating?

Managers should review decisions from a political and psychological viewpoint in order to identify possible historical backers and detractors. Health care environments are not unlike other corporate cultures in that some individuals look with disdain on certain parts of their organizations. For example, in a metropolitan hospital, the human resource department may be discredited because, according to detractors, it never seems to fill open positions quickly enough. Hence, whenever the human resource department tries to enact a new program, the department experiences a certain resistance from individuals whose positions may be on the line. However, line personnel (such as medical support services) hold human resources in high regard because the department facilitates the training and education that are so vital to the workers' roles. Therefore, enlist the support of potential backers in your decision-making process; they can help sell your new plan.

Health care organizations are changing more dramatically and quickly than ever before. In light of ever-escalating competition and a variable fiscal climate, focusing on "how we've always done it before" can undercut a commitment to presenting new ideas openly and making decisions that explore new frontiers of organizational progress.

A commitment to *making* history is necessary in modern-day health care, where innovative problem-solving can mean the difference between success and failure.

8.4.5 Considering Relevance and Contribution to the Organization

After you make a strategic decision and plan a course of action, you should still take time to consider the ramifications of your decisions on the organization, from the perspective of what it can contribute to the organization's goals. By stressing the benefits of your action and gathering the appropriate operational and moral support, you can transform your decision from idea to action.

To crystallize these ramifications, ask yourself the following 10 questions:

1. How do the decision and action enhance the organization's commitment to patients?
2. How do the decision and action reflect the organization's stated values?
3. How do the decision and action contribute to attaining the organization's stated mission?
4. Who should support this decision?
5. Who in the organization will automatically support this decision?
6. How can nonsupporters be convinced of the decision's merits and positive contribution to the organization?
7. What are the overall benefits of the action to the organization?
8. How does the decision make the organization better in terms of effectiveness and efficiency?
9. How does my decision make my department a larger contributor to the organizational good?

FOR EXAMPLE

Business Analysis at Coastal Medical

Like many private practices throughout the United States, the Rhode Island physicians who make up Coastal Medical Inc. (www.coastaldocs.com) began combining office facilities and support staff in the mid-1990s to meet cost pressures from private insurers and Medicare. Through the process of business analysis, Coastal Medical was able to focus on creating a profitable, sustainable business while still providing outstanding patient care. From its analysis, Coastal Medical identified lab testing and X-rays as expensive services that the organization was paying larger outside facilities to conduct. Instead, Coastal Medical decided to set up its own in-house lab and is in the process of developing its own medical-imaging center. Now, Coastal Medical not only conducts and processes its own laboratory tests (which saves the group significant costs), but Coastal Medical also supplies laboratory services to physicians outside the group, generating considerable new profit.

10. What are two major benefits of this action that everyone in the organization can quickly recognize?

SELF-CHECK

- Identify and define **action analysis, environment analysis, function analysis, continuous quality improvement, continuous business development,** and **historical analysis.**
- Describe how spheres of influence impact environment analysis.
- Explain the four steps of the function analysis process.
- Discuss the relationship of continuous quality and continuous business development to business analysis.
- Compare environment, function, business, and historical analysis.

8.5 Models for Implementing Strategies and Decisions

Any strategy—no matter how well formulated—can achieve long-term success without proper implementation.

In order to successfully put strategies into action, the entire organization and all of its resources must be mobilized in support of them. Mobilizing the organization involves the complete management process—from planning and controlling through organizing and leading.

Common strategic planning pitfalls that hinder implementation include both failures of substance and failures of process.

▲ **Failures of substance** reflect inadequate attention to the major strategic planning elements—analysis of mission, values and objectives, organizational strengths and weaknesses, and environmental opportunities and threats.

▲ **Failures of process** reflect poor handling of the strategic planning process itself.

Strategies require supporting structures, well-designed tasks and workflows, and the right people. And strategies must be enthusiastically supported by leaders who can motivate everyone, build individual performance commitments, and utilize teams and teamwork to best advantage. Only with such total systems support can strategies be implemented well enough to actually achieve competitive advantage.

Numerous management consultants and authors have developed models that managers can follow to implement strategic decisions.

In addition to the three processes described here, SWOT analysis (see section 6.5) can also be a useful tool for making and implementing strategic decisions.

8.5.1 The Military Model

The military model involves the following five-part sequence:

1. **Define the objective.** Specify the need or needs and identify the desired outcomes. In defining the objective, identify the optimum outcome and the maximum result that can be achieved.
2. **Identify resources.** Identify all available resources, list their potential contribution to your action, and consider all related resources from other departments within the organization.
3. **Establish the plan.** Write down the specific action you require and establish a time sequence within which the action is needed.
4. **Lay out the course of action.** Set up an incremental plan and establish time checkpoints in which certain objectives should be achieved. For example, if you delegate a particular task to an individual as part of your decision-making and action-execution process, you establish not only a final objective but also interim checkpoints for that individual.
5. **Provide closure.** Closure is made up of those final benchmarks of success that indicate that the plan was successful and the objective reached (such as an accomplished objective or attained goal).

8.5.2 The Parliamentary Model

The parliamentary model is used in many legislative bodies and is similar to the military model in terms of outcomes. The eight-step process is as follows:

1. **Establish need.** Define the needed action and ultimate problem being addressed by the decision and the action taken.
2. **Define the optimum outcome.** What are the best possible results? How can maximum results be achieved by your decision?
3. **Conduct a stakeholder review.** Who is involved? Who has a stake in this action? Who needs to be in on the communication loop?
4. **List pros and cons.** Delineate the positives and negatives of the action taken.
5. **Make an option review.** Review all possible actions and alternative actions.
6. **Review potential consequences.** Consider all adverse reactions to your plan, as well as positive support that might be garnered.

FOR EXAMPLE

The QUICK Decision Model

In an effort to create an easy-to-remember model that utilizes the best military and parliamentary models (as well as several other less-used models), health care management consultant and author Donald N. Lombardi devised the QUICK decision model. As the name suggests, the method focuses on quickly making decisions and executing action. Each letter of the acronym QUICK stands for one of five particular activities that you should do in order to get things done effectively at work:

▲ Q = Question appropriate parties
▲ U = Understand your objective(s)
▲ I = Investigate all options
▲ C = Communicate clearly to all concerned parties
▲ K = Keep on top of things, monitoring and reporting progress

---

7. **Formulate a step-by-step plan.** Establish a plan and allow for a general preparation and time sequence as evidenced by the information collected in the data-gathering phase and confirmed by continuous contribution and communication with all parties involved.

8. **Analyze achievement.** After you reach the objective, analyze its results, considering the needed action and initial objective. This gives you a reliable measure of success and provides an educational and developmental opportunity for future decisions.

SELF-CHECK

- Identify and define **military model, parliamentary model,** and **QUICK decision model.**
- Discuss reasons that strategies sometimes fail.
- Compare failures of substance and failures of process.
- Sequence the five steps of the military model.
- Describe the process involved in the eight-step parliamentary model.

8.6 Completing Strategic Plan Execution

In the process of strategic analysis and decision making, much of your time as a manager is spend gathering information, evaluating options, formulating a plan, and executing that plan. However, the strategic decision making doesn't end after you execute a plan. Ongoing communication with everyone affected by the decision, as well as evaluation of all results are other important managerial responsibilities.

8.6.1 Communicating with Stakeholders

Regardless of which tools or models you employ as a health care manager, communication is a key element of any strategic decision. Savvy managers strive for maximum appropriate input from all parties involved in the decision-making process, during the initial data-collection process, and in later stages of executing a plan.

Communication must be comprehensive, open, and (when necessary) repetitive. You do not risk being redundant when you repeat the importance of the task and underscore the basic objective you are trying to achieve with your action. In addition to simply reviewing the goals and mission objective, review and present your expectations. Expectations make clear what specific level of achievement you want to accomplish toward your goal.

Make sure that you detail each aspect of the plan appropriately to key members of your staff and to other significant players in your action plan. Individuals should be apprised of their part in the planning and execution phase, and of the roles of others with whom they may interact.

Be certain to set your goals realistically, without expectation of a perfect model of excellence in all your endeavors. By setting unrealistic and unattainable expectations, you create false hope and will ultimately suffer the consequences of a disappointed staff and a disenchanted administration.

In particular, four communication keys are critical to executing action plans:

▲ **Clarity:** Be clear and comprehensive in all communication with your team.

▲ **Closure:** Bring all meetings and discussions to a positive end and leave no loose ends hanging.

▲ **Cohesion:** Make sure that your team works together as a focused unit by discussing their problems with each other in dedicated meetings. The key question to ask in eliciting this type of communication participation is, "What have we learned up to this point in the project?"

▲ **Command:** After you make a decision, take timely action. The speed with which you undertake a decision is vital, and although haste makes waste, you still must move quickly and positively toward your goal.

FOR EXAMPLE

Ongoing Communication at Saint Luke's Hospital

Introduced over the course of several years, the "Listening and Learning" process at Saint Luke's Hospital of Kansas City (www.saintlukeshealthsystem.org) is now core to the hospital's identity and success. Under the umbrella of its commitment to "Listening and Learning," Saint Luke's established the ongoing customer satisfaction research program to help the hospital gather patient-customer feedback, assess market demands, and measure customer satisfaction. By continually executing surveys, focus groups, and follow-up calls with patients, Saint Luke's better understands how its patients want to be treated and has gone on to set up a series of 12 customer contact requirements, which include expectations such as "Address patients/guests by last name unless otherwise told" and "Address all complaints within 24 hours or less." To further incorporate the principles into Saint Luke's everyday activities, employees now carry these requirements on a Very Important Principles Card, and permanent artwork with this theme is placed throughout the hospital.

Closely monitor progress throughout the project and get continuous feedback. Doing so gives a clear indication about who is in charge and allows you to command the freedom to give direction and provide advice as needed. As you take command of the action-execution phase, avoid guesswork and unfounded assumptions. Remember, data collection is a continuous process, and it becomes even more important after you undertake action. Remember also that being in command mandates a certain amount of participative management. Therefore, allow all staff members to become involved in the process, but without relinquishing your own authority.

The concept of command calls for a kind of balancing act. As you assume command of action execution and watch your decision turn into the reality of performance, you must delegate a certain amount of control to your staff and other participating parties. While delegating control, do not delegate command. Ultimately, you alone are accountable and responsible for the action taken.

8.6.2 Quantifying Outcomes

As you move closer to your goal, review progress periodically. Hold regular meetings with all significant players to discuss your progress and address any problems. Elicit the participation and suggestions of all players in resolving problems.

After you reach your goal and desired outcome, clearly and objectively quantify the gains your action has helped achieve.

Begin by comparing outcomes to initial decision-making criteria. Announce the benefits gained, both from a short-term and long-term perspective. Work with staff to review what was learned—individually and as a group—as a result of your action. Try to list at least three or four lessons learned in the process. If your goals were reached, a need was fulfilled, or action was taken that led to improved patient service, then you have made a significant contribution to the health care delivery process, which, after all, is your mission as a health care manager. Do not lose sight of this essential reward system as you go about daily activities.

Recognize that no matter how effective your action was or how accurate your decision might have been, any action-oriented process is, in a sense, a trial-and-error education even under the best of circumstances. The more decisions you make, the better your judgment will become and, ultimately, the better your management style and performance effectiveness will be.

Decision making and action execution mark the scope of a health care manager's responsibilities. By having the courage, foresight, and intelligence to make a decision, you are applying the basic building blocks used by effective health care leaders at the top levels of premier organizations.

SELF-CHECK

- Describe tools and techniques for enabling open communication during the strategic decision-making process.
- List the four communication traits essential to executing plans.
- Explain the importance of quantifying outcomes as part of the strategic decision-making process.
- Discuss ways to gather results information.

SUMMARY

Making major decisions requires managers to analyze situations, gather information, evaluate options, determine a course of action, and then follow through on a plan. Strategic decision making is the responsibility of managers at every level of an organization; each decision can generally be classified as a growth, retrenchment, stability, or cooperation strategy. Competitive advantage motivates managers to make major decisions, while approaches such as portfolio planning provide guidance. Managers use a variety of information-gathering tools to help identify options. Analysis can take various forms, but the purpose of analysis is to evaluate situations and plot a course of action. Models can guide managers through the execution phase of a decision. Open communication ensures stakeholders understand decisions, while quantifying outcomes measures the effectiveness of decisions.

KEY TERMS

Action analysis	The process of a manager examining the viability of a plan and predicting whether a decision is sound and the courses of action effective.
Business strategy	Top- and mid-level management set the direction for a single business unit.
Competitive advantage	An attribute or combination of attributes that allows an organization to outperform its rivals.
Concentration	Growth strategy that uses existing strengths in new and productive ways.
Continuous business development (CBD)	A building-block approach to all departmental activities in management efforts. Every effort undertaken by the department should be done to make the department a stronger, more progressive entity than it was prior to the effort.
Continuous quality improvement (CQI)	Ongoing quality enhancement as the incentive that fuels everyday activities associated with optimum health care delivery.
Corporate strategy	Top management directs an organization as a whole toward sustainable competitive advantage.
Diversification	Growth strategy that focuses on acquiring or investing in new businesses and services.
Emergent strategy	Strategy that develops progressively over time as managers learn from and respond to work situations.
Environment analysis	Analysis that takes into account the theoretical and physical environment in which you operate and in which the action plan will be undertaken.
Formal references	Information sources such as journals, management texts, or an organization's manual of standard operating procedures.

Functional strategy	Middle- and low-level management guide the use of resources to implement a specific business strategy.
Function analysis	Analysis in which you evaluate every role affected by implementing and executing a strategic action plan.
Growth strategy	Strategy that pursues larger-size and expanded operations.
Hard data	Any information that may have been generated by a test, questionnaire, form, or survey.
Historical analysis	Analysis that takes into account past precedents established in the organization.
Outsourcing alliance	Contracting to purchase important services from another organization.
Portfolio planning approach	A basic method of formulating strategy and making decisions, in which managers allocate scarce organizational resources among competing opportunities.
Retrenchment strategy	Strategy that reduces the scale of operations in order to gain efficiency and improve performance.
Stability strategy	Strategy that maintains a present course of action without major operating changes.
Strategic alliance	Two or more organizations join together in partnership to pursue an area of mutual interest.
Strategic intent	The focusing of all organizational energies on a unifying and compelling target.
Strategic management	The process of formulating and implementing strategies that create competitive advantage and advance an organization's mission and objectives.
Strategy	A comprehensive action plan that identifies long-term direction and guides resource utilization to accomplish an organization's mission and objectives with sustainable competitive advantage.
Strategy formulation	Assessing existing strategies, organizations, and environments to develop new strategies and strategic plans capable of delivering future competitive advantage.
Strategy implementation	Acting upon strategies successfully to achieve the desired results.
Sustainable competitive advantage	An attribute that is difficult for competitors to imitate.

ASSESS YOUR UNDERSTANDING

Go to www.wiley.com/college/Lombardi to evaluate your knowledge of the basics of analyzing and making decisions.
Measure your learning by comparing pretest and post-test results.

Summary Questions

1. A competitive advantage can be considered sustainable when it
   (a) consistently enables an organization to outperform competitors.
   (b) strategically eliminates the need for further research.
   (c) consciously forces an organization to analyze its processes.
   (d) None of the above
2. The two main responsibilities of the strategic management process are
   (a) strategic formulation and strategic integration.
   (b) strategic initiatives and group motivation.
   (c) strategic formulation and strategic implementation.
   (d) competitive advantage and strategic alliance.
3. At the level of business strategy, top management directs an entire organization toward sustainable competitive advantage. True or false?
4. When an organization follows a growth strategy, it pursues larger-size and expanded operations, often through the process of concentration or diversification. True or false?
5. An organization has the opportunity to create competitive advantage in all the following, except
   (a) knowledge and timing.
   (b) cost and quality.
   (c) financial resources.
   (d) schedules and budget.
6. In the strategic decision-making process, managers are accountable for any decisions made as well as for how the decision was determined. True or false?
7. In the portfolio planning approach to decision making, cash cows produce large profits and strong cash flow. The preferred strategy for cash cows is a growth strategy. True or false?
8. Data collection should happen continually throughout the decision-making process. True or false?
9. Which of the following information-gathering tools is most appropriate in an organization with a history of good leadership?
   (a) Analyzing hard data
   (b) Studying established past actions

    (c) Following your instincts

    (d) Collecting data

10. Hard data can be collected from

    (a) surveys.

    (b) tests.

    (c) questionnaires.

    (d) all the above.

11. Continuous quality improvement (CQI) means quality is always more important than speed or cost-effectiveness to responsible health care organizations. True or false?

12. Which type of action analysis strives to evaluate every role affected by implementing and executing a strategic action plan?

    (a) Environment analysis

    (b) Business analysis

    (c) Function analysis

    (d) Historical analysis

13. When using function analysis to help make a decision, you should start by considering the benefits to the overall organization, then move to benefits for your supervisor, related departments, and finally to your immediate department. True or false?

14. Strategic plans can fail for a variety of reasons. In a failure of process,

    (a) the execution process has unexpected errors.

    (b) the planning process was poorly handled.

    (c) the research process was poorly designed.

    (d) None of the above

15. The appropriate sequence of the military model is

    (a) identify resources, establish the plan, define the plan, lay out the course of action, provide closure.

    (b) define the objective, establish the plan, lay out the course of action, identify resources, provide closure.

    (c) define the objective, lay out the course of action, establish the plan, identify resources, provide closure.

    (d) define the objective, identify resources, establish the plan, lay out the course of action, provide closure.

16. During the strategic decision-making process, communication can be repetitive in order to communicate the importance of the task at hand. True or false?

17. You can delegate some control during the execution phase of a decision, but you must retain

    (a) command.

    (b) counsel.

(c) critical judgment.

(d) collective bargaining.

18. An activity that helps quantify the outcomes of a strategic decision is
    (a) reviewing with staff what has been learned from the decision.
    (b) announcing short- and long-term benefits realized because of the decision.
    (c) writing a summary report about the impact of the decision.
    (d) all the above.

Review Questions

1. The process of strategic implementation has five main steps. What are these steps?

2. Business strategies set the direction for a single business unit. What levels of management typically devise business strategies?

3. Strategically speaking, middle and lower management are typically responsible for the use of resources to best implement a business strategy. What is this level of strategy?

4. Retrenchment strategies reduce the scale of operations in order to gain efficiency and improve performance. What are the three most common types of retrenchment strategies?

5. How does a strategic alliance differ from an outsourcing alliance?

6. Which essential value for decision making is a manager demonstrating when she is around to accept praise as well as complaints and criticism?

7. Business opportunities that offer high market share in high-growth markets are known are considered *stars*. What is the preferred strategy for responding to stars?

8. The portfolio planning approach compares business opportunities on what two factors?

9. To effectively collect data as part of the strategic decision-making process, managers need to keep two guidelines in mind. One guide is to obtain valid, realistic information. What is the other guideline?

10. When a manager reviews department manuals and searches for a process that his staff can utilize to solve a current problem, the manager is using what information-gathering tool?

11. What sort of strategy is an urban hospital utilizing when it decides to build a state-of-the-art pediatric AIDS unit in response to recent rises in infant AIDS cases?

12. The third shift manager in an intensive care unit can probably make the greatest impact on what level of strategy for her suburban hospital?

13. What are the four types of analysis that make up process of action analysis?

14. During environment analysis, managers look specifically at workplace dynamics while making decisions. In particular, what sort of factors should managers pay attention to?

15. When a manager asks how instituting a new billing procedure will affect patients, positively and negatively, in the short term and long term, what form of action analysis is the manager engaging in?

16. In the parliamentary model, what is the equivalent of the final military model step of providing closure?

17. Plans usually fail because of substance or process. What are some aspects that can constitute a failure or substance?

18. Communication is especially critical during the execution phase of a strategic decision. What are the four communication traits to keep in mind during execution?

19. When is it appropriate for plan-related communication to become repetitive?

Applying This Chapter

1. A county hospital serving primarily rural patient-customers is concerned about losing market share to several new franchised walk-in clinics that have opened in the area in the last year. How might the hospital establish sustainable competitive advantage?

2. A mammography clinic wants to grow its business and effectively treat 35% more patients in the next year. In assessing ways to reach this goal, the clinic is considering offering a state-of-the-art digital scanning technique to its patients. The technique is new and will probably become an industry standard in 5 years. However, the clinic is known primarily for offering affordable mammograms to inner-city women. Based on the portfolio model, which opportunity has the clinic identified?

3. You're the manager of a nursing staff at a large urban hospital. Your supervisors would like your input on a major report they're preparing. You've been asked to present recommendations of the ways in which nursing staffs are and should be scheduled for work. What information-gathering tools should you consider utilizing as you prepare your recommendations for your supervisors?

4. What "sphere of influence" groups should the manager of a medical laboratory facility consider engaging as her department undergoes the process of construction and improvements that will close or limit laboratory function over the next fiscal year?

5. You manage the clerical and support staff in a small-town emergency room. In addition the daily challenges and rapid changes associated with

emergency-room work, your hospital is undergoing construction and management reorganization in an effort to become the leading facility in the tri-country region. Which model—military, parliamentary, or QUICK—would you choose as you make strategic decisions for your department in the next year?

6. As the manager of a student health center at small private school, you and your staff have been charged with developing and introducing a plan for improving student health during winter months, when flu-infection rates typically rise to dangerously high levels. Who are the stakeholders that you and your team need to connect with in order to create an effective winter-health plan? How might you interact with these stakeholders?

YOU TRY IT

Levels of Strategy at SSM Health Care

Successful health care strategy involves planning at corporate, business, and functional strategic levels. Take a look at the strategic plans of your current employer or of a health care organization you're interested in working for. If you don't have or can't locate a strategic plan, review the Recognized Best Practices for SSM Health Care (search for "best practices" at www.ssmhc.com). Identify at least one corporate, business, and functional strategic plan for the organization.

Your Essential Values

The five essential values for making strategic decisions (section 8.2.1) apply to more than just business decisions. These five values can be essential to success in your career and your education—even your personal life. For example, consider how the five values might come into play in a job interview situation. If an interviewer asked you for a specific example of time in your educational or work life when you exhibited outstanding accountability, what would you say? What about adaptability, dependability, responsibility, or visibility? Look over your resume (or start drafting one if you don't have one yet) and consider experiences that highlight each of the five values. Can you include some (or perhaps all) the descriptive words *accountable*, *adaptable*, *dependable*, *responsible*, and *visible* into your resume?

Formal and Informal References

Formal references (books, journals, management texts, written documents, and so on) as well as informal references (insights, experiences, relationships, and so on) are important sources of data that can help you make strategic decisions more quickly and effectively. As the manager of an inner-city infant vaccination program (with nurse-practitioners, social workers, and administrative assistants on your staff), what are some formal and informal references you can capitalize on to increase the number of participants in your programs by 25% over the next year?

Considering Ramifications

Strategic decisions almost always produce both positive and negative ramifications. Of course, you can't avoid ramifications altogether, but you can work to minimize negative ramifications and maximize positive ramifications. Consider the difficult situation of a manager who chose to respond to budgetary pressures by slightly reducing each employee's wage, rather than eliminating one or more workers' positions. Run through the 10 questions in section 8.4.5. How might this manager answer these 10 questions?

Following the Military Model

Look back on a recent strategic decision your school or employer made. A strategic decision could be to reorganize a department; to reposition the organization to appeal to a different audience; or to invest money in a new program, equipment, or building. (If your school or workplace hasn't made recent strategic decisions, check out press releases associated with the new Brain Institute at Providence Health System at www.providence.org/brain.) In what ways was the military model followed? How did the organization define its objectives? How did the organization identify resources and establish its plan? Was a course of action clearly laid out? What about closure?

Your Stakeholders

Every decision, large or small, has stakeholders—individuals and groups that are affected by the decision and often play some role in making the decision. Who in your career or education are your key stakeholders? Create a list of all the people who would be impacted if you make a significant change in your course of study or your work situation. Add to this list people who may influence your educational or career decisions; you may want to include instructors, professors, outstanding professionals, friends, co-workers and more here. Now, review your list of stakeholders and rank each person based on how important he or she is in your decision-making process. Rewrite your list and keep a copy in a notebook, electronic organizer, wallet, or purse. The next time you're unsure of how to proceed on a decision, pull out your list and consider how you can involve your stakeholders in your decision-making process.

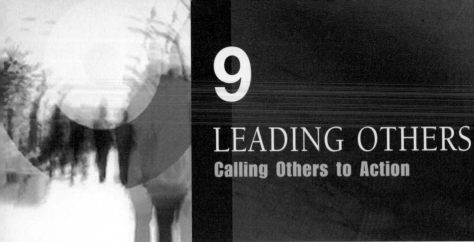

9
LEADING OTHERS
Calling Others to Action

Starting Point

Go to www.wiley.com/college/Lombardi to assess your knowledge of the basics of leadership.
Determine where you need to concentrate your effort.

What You'll Learn in This Chapter

▲ Common definitions of leadership and five models of leadership
▲ Relationship between vision and leadership
▲ Three types of position power and two types of personal power
▲ Techniques for developing leadership skills
▲ Transformational leadership characteristics
▲ The role of morals and ethics in leadership

After Studying This Chapter, You'll Be Able To

▲ Demonstrate characteristics of strong leadership
▲ Distinguish ways to establish, share, and maintain vision
▲ Compare position power and personal power
▲ Examine appropriate ways to empower others while leading
▲ Differentiate between leadership models and types
▲ Employ the continuous leadership development process
▲ Interpret possible roles of gender, morals, and ethics in strong leadership

Goals and Outcomes

▲ Master the terminology and tools related to leadership
▲ Describe characteristics of strong leadership
▲ Compare leadership models
▲ Employ traditional leadership development models
▲ Choose appropriate leadership styles and techniques
▲ Model strong leadership characteristics within work teams
▲ Perform leadership duties and responsibilities within a team setting
▲ Evaluate leadership styles and effectiveness

INTRODUCTION

Leadership is the catalyst of action in any group. Although various definitions of leadership exist, one of a leader's central responsibilities is establishing and sharing his or her vision. Leaders have various types of power and must use this power wisely. Additionally, a leader can empower others. Leadership models are useful tools for describing different styles of leading others. In general, leaders are made not born—managers can and should work to develop leadership skills over the course of their careers. Superior leadership requires a manager to also be aware of the moral and ethical implications of their activities as leader.

9.1 Defining Leadership

What is great leadership? Perhaps at its most simple, great leaders are individuals who are able to bring out the best in other people.

In the words of management consultant Tom Peters, "Leaders get their kicks from orchestrating the work of others—not from doing it themselves."[1] He goes on to say that the leader is "rarely—possibly never?—the best performer." They don't have to be; they thrive through and by the successes of others.

Leadership—the process of inspiring others to work hard to accomplish important tasks—is one of the most popular management topics.[2]

As Figure 9-1 shows, leadership is also critical to the management process. Planning sets the direction and objectives; organizing brings the resources together to turn plans into action; leading builds the commitments and enthusiasm needed for people to apply their talents fully to help accomplish plans; and controlling makes sure things turn out right.

Figure 9-1

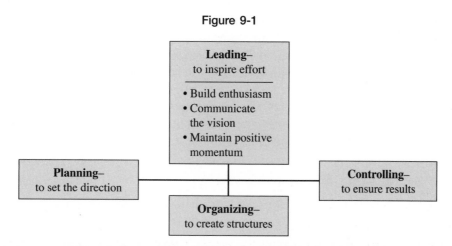

Leading viewed in relationship to the other management functions.

9.1.1 Understanding Leadership and Vision

"Great leaders," it is said, "get extraordinary things done in organizations by inspiring and motivating others toward a common purpose."[3] More and more frequently, great leadership is associated with *vision*. This term is generally used to describe someone who has a clear sense of the future and an understanding of the actions needed to get there successfully. But there is more. Leading requires turning vision into results. Five core principles for meeting the challenges of visionary leadership are:[4]

- ▲ **challenge the process:** Be a pioneer—encourage innovation and support people who have ideas;
- ▲ **be enthusiastic:** Inspire others through personal enthusiasm to share in a common vision;
- ▲ **help others to act:** Be a team player and support the efforts and talents of others;
- ▲ **set the example:** Provide a consistent role model of how others can and should act;
- ▲ **celebrate achievements:** Bring emotion into the workplace and rally "hearts" as well as "minds."

9.1.2 Maintaining a Clear Vision for Leadership

A strong leader must maintain a clear vision of what he or she wants to accomplish with a work group. The adage "If you can dream it, if you can conceive it, then you can achieve it," captures the essence of visionary leadership.

Leaders who do not have a vision are not true leaders. People need to share a vision to get meaning from and excited about their daily responsibilities and individual work. A tremendous motivator for health care professionals—one that unfortunately is often overlooked—is the feeling that one is making a contribution to "the big picture." Health care professionals like to know that their efforts contribute to a greater, larger good. If a leader fails to provide a **vision**—a goal that provides patients with solid health care, for example—the work group has nothing to get excited about and little inspiration during difficult professional times. To work through adversity—and everyone experiences adversity at some time in his or her work life—you must have a sense of moving toward accomplishment of an important, even if difficult, goal.

9.1.3 Establishing and Sharing Vision

To establish a vision, managers consider what they want to see happen within their work groups. To begin the process, list five or six major goals you want your work group to accomplish in the next year. Base these goals on interaction and communication with peers and supervisors, as well as your entire frame of reference.

Write these goals on an index card or a word-processing file; keep the list easily accessible in your briefcase, PDA, or computer. Every few weeks, review this list. Make sure that you present the elements of your vision to staff members on a regular basis, beginning with the start of your management activities. Staff should feel that the vision is achievable, viable, and important to their professional aspirations.

A shared vision is a terrific motivator. Individuals who feel that the vision represents something that can provide them with a great deal of satisfaction and opportunity for career growth are more likely dedicated to helping make the vision a reality.

The vision does not necessarily have to be measured quantitatively, as long as its content and achievement are positive and worthy of team effort. For example, a vision statement for a director of rehabilitation services at a small community hospital may include the following:

> *Make every patient feel as though he or she is the most important person in the building.*
>
> *Provide the opportunity for the entire staff to grow and develop every day.*
>
> *Provide the best rehabilitation services possible at all times.*
>
> *Support each other fully and give each other the benefit of the staff's talents and personal attributes.*
>
> *Be totally uncompromising in pursuing the goal of making patients feel as though the organization does everything possible to assist them in enhancing their life and health.*

Savvy managers involve their work group in creating and defining vision statements. For example, after establishing the basic framework of your vision, involve your team in the vision process simply by asking them to list criteria that ascertains whether the department is maintaining its vision.

FOR EXAMPLE

Visionary Leadership at Dosher Memorial Hospital

Although small in size and remotely located, Dosher Memorial Hospital (www.dosher.org) is still a health care and community leader in Southport, North Carolina, a small historic town about a mile from Cape Fear. Through its comprehensive vision statement (visit www.dosher.org/vision.htm), the 100-bed hospital clearly articulates its vision to both employees and patients. For example, the hospital realizes that due to its size, it cannot offer every type of medical service. Therefore, the hospital pursues a policy of "network development with other providers to establish a continuum of quality yet efficient healthcare."

SELF-CHECK

- Identify and define **vision, leadership,** and **visionary leadership.**
- Describe how leading fits with other responsibilities of the management process.
- Explain the role of vision in effective leadership.
- List the five core principles for meeting challenges of visionary leadership.
- Discuss ways a manager can share vision with teams or departments.

9.2 Leadership and Power

Leadership involves influencing the behavior of other people. **Power,** in this sense, is the ability to get someone else to do something you want done. Power is also the ability to make things happen for the good of the group or organization as a whole.[5] This positive aspect of power is the foundation of effective leadership.[6]

Figure 9-2 divides possible sources of power into those that trace to one's position in an organization and those that come from personal qualities.[7]

9.2.1 Position Power

A manager's official status, or position, in the organization's hierarchy of authority provides access to **position power.** Position power includes the power of rewards, punishments, and legitimacy.

Reward power is the ability to influence through rewards. It is the capability to offer something of value—a positive outcome—as a means of influencing

Figure 9-2

Sources of power...

Power of the POSITION: based on things managers can offer to others.		**Power of the PERSON:** based on the ways managers are viewed by others.	
Rewards:	"If you do what I ask, I'll give you a reward."	**Expertise:**	as a source of special knowledge and information.
Coercion:	"If you *don't* do what I ask, I'll punish you."	**Reference:**	as a person with whom others like to identify.
Legitimacy:	"Because I am the boss; you *must* do as I ask."		

Sources of position power and personal power used by leaders.

the behavior of other people. This involves the control of rewards or resources such as pay raises, bonuses, promotions, special assignments, and verbal or written compliments. To mobilize reward power, a manager says, in effect, "If you do what I ask, I'll give you a reward."

Coercive power is the ability to influence through punishment. It is the capacity to punish or withhold positive outcomes as a way to influence the behavior of other people. A manager may attempt to coerce someone by threatening him or her with verbal reprimands, pay penalties, and even termination. To mobilize coercive power, a manager says, in effect, "If you don't do what I want, I'll punish you."

Legitimate power is the ability to influence through formal authority—the right by virtue of one's organizational position or status to exercise control over people in subordinate positions. It is the capacity to influence the behavior of other people by virtue of the rights of office. To mobilize legitimate power, a manager says, in effect, "I am the boss and therefore you are supposed to do as I ask."

9.2.2 Personal Power

Power can also derive from a manager's or leader's unique personal qualities. Two bases of **personal power** are expert power and referent power.

Expert power is the ability to influence through special expertise. It is the capacity to influence the behavior of other people because of one's knowledge, understanding, and skills. Expertise derives from the possession of technical know-how or information pertinent to the issue at hand.[8]

Expert power is developed by acquiring relevant skills or competencies or by gaining a central position in relevant information networks. It is maintained by protecting one's credibility and not overstepping the boundaries of true understanding. When a manager uses expert power, the implied message is, "You should do what I want because of my special expertise or information."

Referent power is the ability to influence through identification. It is the capacity to influence the behavior of other people because they admire you and want to identify positively with you. Reference is a power derived from charisma or interpersonal attractiveness. It is developed and maintained through good interpersonal relations that encourage the admiration and respect of others. When a manager uses referent power, the implied message is, "You should do what I want in order to maintain a positive self-defined relationship with me."

9.2.3 Using Power Wisely

Good leaders appreciate the ramifications of power and know how to use it effectively. Most organizations give health care managers a significant scope of authority in formatting policy, executing decisions, and establishing plans for progressive performance. With this trust comes power.

On the management power continuum, two extremes are possible: At one end is the manager who is reluctant to use power; at the other is the autocrat. A reluctant manager does not want to exert authority over staff activities, holds back from making decisions, or perhaps tries to be one of the group. In a sense, the reluctant manager does not want to accept the responsibilities of management and would rather maintain a low profile by being part of the work group. This stance causes problems because these managers cannot garner the respect necessary to have their plans and initiatives followed and carried through. Furthermore, they are in effect abandoning their responsibility to the organization and belying the organization's trust.

Successful health care leadership includes the proper use of power by exerting appropriate pressure when necessary to help realize the department's vision. The following four basic strategies suggest ways to properly utilize your power base:

▲ **Let people know you are in charge.** From your first day as manager, emphasize in appropriate words that you are indeed the manager and will make decisions. Of course, new managers need to take time to learn about their department and get to know each staff member, but you can still emphasize your intent to take appropriate action when necessary in the interest of achieving top performance.

▲ **Let people know where you stand.** From the outset, communicate feedback to all members of your staff. Let them know when they are doing a good job in moving toward top performance and, conversely, when their performance is less than satisfactory. In this way you communicate to your staff that you are interested in their activities *and* are setting high standards for performance.

▲ **Be forceful when necessary.** Someone in the department—usually a poor performer—is sure to challenge your authority early on. When this happens, meet with the person privately in your office and tactfully provide specific evidence of their poor performance and contrast it to the high performance standards you have delineated. You must take an immediate stand with subversive or poor performers. (See section 5.5.6 for more information about dealing with problem employees.)

▲ **Be action-oriented.** From the first day, never hesitate to make decisions (after you gather enough information) or to take appropriate action to enhance departmental performance. New health care managers often take too much time to make decisions or fail to empower staff with the resources necessary to take action. Procrastination causes departmental stagnation and can cripple performance. (Sections 6.3, 8.2, and 8.3 offer decision-making strategies.)

FOR EXAMPLE

Position Power at National Health Information Network

In May 2004, President George W. Bush created the position of national coordinator for Health Information Technology within the Health & Human Services Department (www.hhs.gov) in an effort to promote a National Health Information Network. The department's goal of giving every American an electronic record of their health care by 2014 is aggressive, but the National Coordinator position has been given with considerable position power, including a close relationship with the White House and a substantial PR and marketing budget. To learn more about the national coordinator position and the U.S. Department of Health Information Technology, visit www.hhs.gov/healthit.

SELF-CHECK

- Identify and define **power, personal power, and position power.**
- Compare position power and personal power.
- Describe and contrast the three types of position power: reward power, coercive power, and legitimate power.
- Describe and contrast the two types of personal power: expert power and referent power.
- Discuss four strategies for using power wisely.

9.3 Leadership and Empowerment

Health care management today is rich with the processes of **empowerment,** the process through which managers enable and help others to gain power and achieve influence within the organization. Effective leaders know that when people feel powerful, they are more willing to make the decisions and take the actions needed to get their jobs done.[9]

Savvy managers realize that power in organizations is not a "zerosum" quantity—that is, in order for someone to gain power, it isn't necessary for someone else to give it up. Indeed, to master the complexity and pace of challenges

FOR EXAMPLE

Open Doors at Baptist Hospital

In the mid-1990s, low satisfaction surveys from patients, families, and staff led Baptist Hospital Inc. (www.ebaptisthealthcare.org) of Florida to radically restructure nearly every aspect of its business, including leadership policies. One of the hospital's first restructuring actions (based on feedback from listening events and surveys) was to create a flat, fluid, and open leadership system designed to facilitate easier communication. Under the new system, staff is not just encouraged, they are expected, to contact anyone in the organization, including the hospital's president, at any time to discuss work issues and improvement opportunities. To symbolize management's commitment to "open-door" communication policies, a large glass window that faces into a busy area of the hospital was installed in the president's office. Additionally, senior leaders are charged with creating a "no secrets" environment by facilitating short informational meetings during which management and employees gather together and review the hospital's daily staff newsletter.

faced in today's environments, an organization's success may well depend on how much power can be mobilized throughout an organization's workforce.

Managers have numerous ways of empowering others:[10]

▲ Get others involved in selecting their work assignments and the methods for accomplishing tasks.

▲ Create an environment of cooperation, information sharing, discussion, and shared ownership of goals.

▲ Encourage others to take initiative, make decisions, and use their knowledge.

▲ When problems arise, find out what others think and let them help design the solutions.

▲ Stay out of the way; give others the freedom to put their ideas and solutions into practice.

Leadership through empowerment is helping others use their knowledge and judgment to make a real difference in daily workplace affairs. This occurs as people work in responsible jobs, as they participate in cross-functional task forces and teams, and as they function in work environments that respect them as capable and creative human beings.

SELF-CHECK

- Identify and define **empowerment** and **leadership through empowerment.**
- Explain how empowering others is a form of leadership.
- Describe methods for empowering others.

9.4 Exploring Leadership Models

For centuries, people have recognized that some persons perform very well as leaders, whereas others do not. The questions still debated are, Why? and What determines leadership success?

Several models for leadership have emerged over the years. Five of the most common models for leadership include leading based on

▲ behaviors;

▲ contingencies;

▲ situation;

▲ paths and goals;

▲ participation.

9.4.1 Leadership Based on Behaviors

The behavioral theories of leadership sought to determine which **leadership style**—the recurring pattern of behaviors exhibited by a leader—worked best.[13] Given a preferred style, the goal was to be able to train leaders to become skilled at using a certain style to best advantage.

Most research in the leader behavior tradition has focused on the degree to which a leader's style displays concern for the task to be accomplished and/or concern for the people doing the work. The behavioral characteristics of each dimension are quite clear:

▲ **A leader high in concern for task plans** defines work to be done, assigns task responsibilities, sets clear work standards, urges task completion, and monitors performance results.

▲ **A leader high in concern for people** acts warm and supportive toward followers, develops social rapport with them, respects their feelings, is sensitive to their needs, and shows trust in them.

FOR EXAMPLE

Common Leadership Traits?

An early tradition in leadership research involved a search for **universal traits** that separate effective and ineffective leaders. The results of many years of research on leadership traits can be summarized as follows:[11] Physical traits such as a person's height, weight, and physique make no difference in determining leadership success. On the other hand, followers do appear to admire certain things about leaders. One study of more than 3,400 managers, for example, found the most respected leaders were described as honest, competent, forward-looking, inspiring, and credible. Such positive feelings may enhance a leader's effectiveness, particularly with respect to creating vision and a sense of empowerment. Among the personal traits now considered most important as personal foundations for leadership success are drive, desire to lead, motivation, honesty, integrity, self-confidence, intelligence, knowledge, and flexibility.[12]

The results of leader behavior research at first suggested that followers of people-oriented leaders would be more productive and satisfied than those working for more task-oriented leaders. Later results, however, suggested that truly effective leaders were high in both concern for people and concern for task.[14]

As shown in Figure 9-3, the preferred style of leadership involves sharing decisions with subordinates, encouraging participation, and supporting the teamwork needed for high levels of task accomplishment.

Figure 9-3

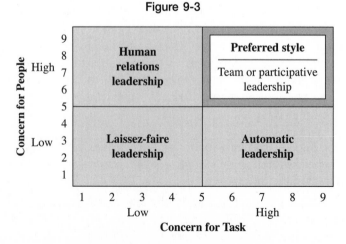

Implications of leader behavior research.

9.4.2 Leadership Based on Contingencies

Instead of searching for the one best style, **contingency leadership theory** (developed by Fred Fiedler) suggests that leadership success depends on a match between leadership style and situational demands.[15] The theory suggests that leadership style is part of one's personality and is therefore relatively enduring and difficult to change. Rather than trying to train leaders to adopt new styles, the theory recommends matching leaders' existing styles with situations for which they are the best fit.

According to the theory, people's leadership styles tend to be either *task motivated* or *relationship motivated*. Extensive research suggests that neither style is effective all the time. Instead, each works best when used in the right situation.

To diagnose leadership, you must understand and evaluate three contingency variables:

▲ The quality of *leader-member relations* (good or poor) measures the degree to which the group supports the leader.

▲ The degree of *task structure* (high or low) measures the extent to which task goals, procedures, and guidelines are clearly spelled out.

▲ The amount of *position power* (strong or weak) measures the degree to which the position gives the leader power to reward and punish subordinates.

Figure 9-4 shows eight possible combinations that range from the most favorable situation for a leader (good leader-member relations, high task structure,

Figure 9-4

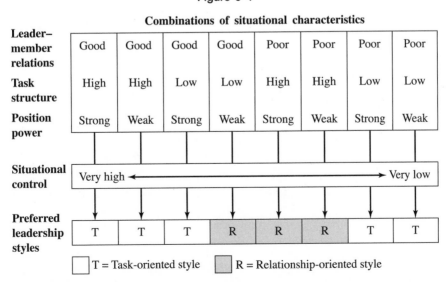

Combinations of situational characteristics

Matching leadership style and situations based on contingency leadership theory.

strong position power) to the least favorable situation (poor leader-member relations, low task structure, weak position power).

Two significant implications of Figure 9-4 and the contingency theory are

▲ a task-oriented leader is more successful in either very favorable (high-control) or very unfavorable (low-control) situations;

▲ a relationship-oriented leader is more successful in situations of moderate control.

9.4.3 Leadership Based on Situation

Hersey-Blanchard's **situational leadership model** suggests that successful leaders adjust their styles depending on the readiness of followers to perform in a given situation.[16] Readiness, in this sense, is based on how able, willing, and confident followers are to perform required tasks.

As Figure 9-5 shows, the possible leadership styles that result from different combinations of task-oriented and relationship-oriented behaviors are as follows:

▲ **Delegating:** Allowing the group to make and take responsibility for task decisions; a low-task, low-relationship style.

▲ **Participating:** Emphasizing shared ideas and participative decisions on task directions; a low-task, high-relationship style.

▲ **Selling:** Explaining task directions in a supportive and persuasive way; a high-task, high-relationship style.

▲ **Telling:** Giving specific task directions and closely supervising work; a high-task, low-relationship style.

Figure 9-5

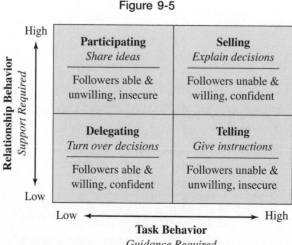

Leadership implications of the situational leadership model.

Anyone using the situational model must be able to implement the alternative leadership styles as needed. For example, a delegating style works best in high-readiness situations of able, willing, and confident followers; the telling style works best at the other extreme of low readiness. In between, the participating style is recommended for low to moderate readiness and the selling style for moderate to high readiness.

Hersey and Blanchard further believe that leadership styles can and should be adjusted as followers in a given situation change over time. The model also implies that if the correct styles are used in lower readiness situations, followers can grow in ability, willingness, and confidence. Not only is this a positive result in itself, but it also allows the leader to become less directive.

9.4.4 Leadership Based on Paths and Goals

The **path-goal theory,** as advanced by Robert House,[17] suggests that an effective leader is one who clarifies paths through which followers can achieve both task-related and personal goals. A good leader helps people progress along these paths, removes any barriers, and provides appropriate rewards for task accomplishment. Four leadership styles exemplify a path-goal model of leadership:

▲ **Directive leadership:** Letting subordinates know what is expected; giving directions on what to do and how; scheduling work to be done; maintaining definite standards of performance; clarifying the leader's role in the group.

▲ **Supportive leadership:** Doing things to make work more pleasant; treating group members as equals; being friendly and approachable; showing concern for the well-being of subordinates.

▲ **Achievement-oriented leadership:** Setting challenging goals; expecting the highest levels of performance; emphasizing continuous improvement in performance; displaying confidence in meeting high standards.

▲ **Participative leadership:** Involving subordinates in decision making; consulting with subordinates; asking for suggestions from subordinates; using these suggestions when making a decision.

The path-goal leadership theory advises a manager always to use leadership styles that complement the needs of situations. This means that the leader "adds value" by contributing things that are missing from the situation or that need strengthening. She or he specifically avoids redundant behaviors. The important contingencies for making good path-goal leadership choices include the work environment (tasks, authority, and group) and subordinate personal characteristics (ability, experience, and locus of control). For example,

▲ when job assignments are unclear, an effective manager provides directive leadership to clarify task objectives and expected rewards;

▲ when worker self-confidence is low, the effective manager provides supportive leadership to clarify individual abilities and offers needed task assistance;

▲ when performance incentives are poor, the effective manager provides participative leadership to identify individual needs and appropriate rewards;

▲ when task challenge is insufficient, the effective manager provides achievement oriented leadership to raise performance aspirations.

Path-goal theory has led some to identify substitutes for leadership.[18] **Substitutes for leadership** are aspects of the work setting and the people involved that can reduce the need for a leader's personal involvement. In effect, these substitutes make outside leadership unnecessary because leadership is already built into the situation. Possible substitutes for leadership include staff characteristics such as ability, experience, and independence; task characteristics such as routineness and availability of feedback; and organizational characteristics such as clarity of plans and formalization of rules and procedures.

9.4.5 Leadership Based on Participation

The Vroom-Jago **leader-participation model** is designed to help a leader choose the method of decision making that best fits the nature of the problem being faced. In this approach, an effective leader is someone able to consistently choose and implement from the following alternatives the most appropriate decision models:[19]

▲ **Authority decisions** are made by the leader and then communicated to the group. Participation is minimized. No input is asked of group members other than to provide specific information on request.

▲ **Consultative decisions** are made by the leader after asking group members for information, advice, or opinions. In some cases, group members are consulted individually; in others, the consultation occurs during a meeting of the group as a whole.

▲ **Group decisions** require all members to participate in making a decision and working together to achieve a consensus regarding the preferred course of action. This approach to decision making is a form of empowerment, and it is successful to the extent that each member is ultimately able to accept the logic and feasibility of the final group decision.[20]

For a manager who wants to be successful at leading through participation, the challenge in effectively managing the decision process is twofold. First, the

Figure 9-6

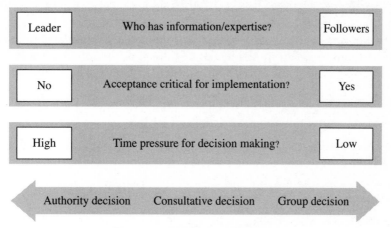

Leader	Who has information/expertise?	Followers
No	Acceptance critical for implementation?	Yes
High	Time pressure for decision making?	Low

Authority decision   Consultative decision   Group decision

Recommended Decision Methods

Implications of participatory styles of leadership.

leader must know when each decision method is the preferred approach. Second, the leader must be able to properly implement decision-making methods when needed.

No decision-making method is considered universally superior to any others. Rather, leadership success results when the decision method used correctly matches the characteristics of the problem to be solved.

Figure 9-6 shows when to choose among authority, consultative, and group decisions.

Using participative decision-making methods offers important benefits to the leader.[21] Participative decisions help improve decision quality by bringing more information to bear on the problem. They help improve decision acceptance as participants gain understanding and become committed to the process. And they contribute to the development of leadership potential in others through the experience of active participation in the problem-solving process.

However, a cost must also be considered: The greater the participation, the more time required for the decision process. Leaders do not always have sufficient time available; some problems must be resolved immediately. In such cases, the authority decision may be the only option. The more authority-oriented decisions work best when leaders personally have the expertise needed to solve the problem, they are confident and capable of acting alone, others are likely to accept the decision they make, and little or no time is available for discussion.

SELF-CHECK

- Identify and define **leadership style, contingency leadership theory, situational leadership model, path-goal theory, substitutes for leadership, leader-participation model,** and **strategic management process.**

- Contrast the characteristics and relative strengths of the five leadership models.

- Explain the importance of tasks and people in behavioral leadership models.

- Discuss task motivation and relationship motivation in contingency leadership theory.

- Define the role of readiness in the situational leadership model.

- Define the four path-goal leadership styles.

- Compare decision models in leader-participation theory, including authority decisions, consultative decisions, and group decisions.

9.5 Developing Leadership Skills

A magic formula for great leadership does not exist. Often, the circumstances and types of individuals in your department have much to do with the type of leadership style that's most effective.

However, a second part of the equation—your own preferences, personality, and predilections—is equally important. Personal characteristics dictate the type of leadership style you use, as they define what you feel comfortable with and find to be effective in daily activities. Accordingly, first examine the influences that played most prominently in developing your leadership style. Then ascertain which ones were most influential in the development of your innate leadership identity.

In addition to the leadership models covered in section 9.4, the best health care managers continuously seek new applications of leadership, learn about the latest insights into leadership styles, and attempt to upgrade their leadership effectiveness.

9.5.1 Continuous Leadership Development

To ensure that your leadership style develops progressively and your effectiveness grows over time, remember the following strategies:

▲ **Get as diverse and as much feedback as possible on leadership effectiveness.** Influences on your leadership style can be numerous and diverse; have family, peers, and trusted subordinates give you feedback on your leadership effectiveness. Get suggestions from all these individuals and try to incorporate any good ideas into your future efforts.

▲ **Give clear direction at all times to all staff members.** Try to specify exactly what is expected and provide as much insight as appropriate on why something should be done. Sharing this information with employees can build trust and allow you to have two-way communication, which is important for a successful leader. Use appropriate follow-up methods to ensure that progress is being made and provide as much additional instruction as possible as employees strive to achieve their goals. Doing so enhances communication and trust, two commodities that are always helpful.

▲ **Give staff an appropriate amount of freedom.** Assume that staff members know what they are doing until they prove otherwise. Providing too much direction or constraining performance can create the perception that you are unnecessarily overbearing or not trusting of your staff. Closely monitor performance, provide inspiration, and measure goal attainment of all staff members.

▲ **Balance positive and negative information realistically.** You must occasionally give your staff bad news. Provide this information on a timely basis, try to identify an upside (if possible), and deal with problems realistically. On these occasions, verbally stress your confidence that the group can handle adversity and rebound from negative circumstances. Strong leaders participate in adversity as much as in prosperity.

▲ **Try to keep perspectives on all issues.** The true measure of leaders, in the opinion of many, is their reaction to things that are above and beyond the call of duty or beyond the norm. Try to maintain a balanced view of things, and exhibit the courage and strength necessary to handle tough situations.

▲ **Learn from every situation.** Health care offers learning opportunities every day. Collect as much information as possible, process that information, and incorporate it into your leadership efforts. Remember that one of the best ways to learn things is to ask appropriate questions. These may be questions that you ask yourself about what you have learned from a situation or questions you ask your peers and your supervisor about their insights and experiences. The more you learn, the greater your frame of reference becomes and the better leader you become.

▲ **In all cases, be yourself.** Whatever makes sense to you should inspire the judgments you make. Whatever you are comfortable communicating or exhibiting in your words and actions should rule the way you communicate ideas, thoughts, and objectives. Your actions and words are being closely examined by your staff because they provide the impetus and inspiration for staff's activities. Therefore, in the long run, whatever is most natural and comfortable is likely the most progressive precedent to set.

▲ **Pace your activities both inside and outside the workplace.** Do not try to accomplish everything at once, and make time to enjoy your responsibilities rather than unnecessarily allowing them to be burdensome. Strike a balance between the things that you like to do and the things that you have to do.

▲ **Trust your instincts.** Your instincts and intelligence are what got you the management job to begin with. As a leader, your good intentions, frame of reference, and basic values are the greatest strengths you have to offer those who want you to succeed.

Perhaps the most important point to remember is that the health care organization wants you to succeed, your staff wants you to succeed (if for no other reason than it makes their lives easier), and of course you want to succeed. This innate desire, coupled with all the factors discussed throughout this chapter, can allow you to become a strong, positive leader.

9.5.2 Becoming a Transformational Leader

The term **transformational leadership** is often used to describe someone who uses charisma and related qualities to raise aspirations and shift people and organizational systems into new high-performance patterns. This contrasts with **transactional leadership** in which a leader adjusts tasks, rewards, and structures to help followers meet their needs while working to accomplish organizational objectives.[22]

Transactional leadership meets only part of an organization's requirements in today's dynamic environment. A manager must also lead in an inspirational way and with a compelling personality. The transformational leader provides a strong aura of vision and contagious enthusiasm that substantially raises the confidence, aspirations, and commitments of followers. The transformational leader arouses followers to be more highly dedicated, more satisfied with their work, and more willing to put forth extra effort to achieve success in challenging times.

The special qualities that are often characteristic of transformational leaders include

▲ **vision:** Having ideas and a clear sense of direction; communicating them to others; developing excitement about accomplishing shared dreams;

▲ **charisma:** Arousing others' enthusiasm, faith, loyalty, pride, and trust in themselves through the power of personal reference and appeals to emotion;

▲ **symbolism:** Identifying leadership heroes, offering special rewards, and holding spontaneous and planned ceremonies to celebrate excellence and high achievement;

▲ **empowerment:** Helping others develop, removing performance obstacles, sharing responsibilities, and delegating truly challenging work;

▲ **intellectual stimulation:** Gaining the involvement of others by creating awareness of problems and stirring their imagination to create high-quality solutions;

▲ **integrity:** Being honest and credible, acting consistently out of personal conviction, and by following through on commitments.[23]

9.5.3 Embracing Emotional Intelligence

Over the last decade, the concept of **emotional intelligence**—the ability to understand emotions in one's self and others and the ability to use that understanding to guide behavior—has caught the attention of leadership scholars and consultants.[24]

Emotional intelligence is now recognized as an important contributor to leadership success. Research indicates that emotional intelligence may even be more important than technical and cognitive skills in creating performance excellence. Emotional intelligence becomes increasingly important as you move into higher levels of management responsibility. Technical or knowledge-based skills and cognitive or analytical skills are "threshold capabilities" for leadership.[25] They are baseline or entry-level requirements for performing in a leadership capacity. The achievement of true excellence in leadership, however, depends on the presence of emotional intelligence.

In this sense, emotional intelligence is not an option or a "nice to have" leadership component; it is a necessity. Someone low in emotional intelligence, for example, may fail to spot signs of excessive stress or burnout in members of a work team. Without this awareness and the ability to act on it, the team leader may push too hard to meet performance expectations and find members responding with anger, job avoidance, and/or poor performance. By contrast, a leader high in emotional intelligence has the interpersonal insight and sensitivity to recognize that emotions are running high. He or she also has the confidence and expertise to take actions that help team members balance work demands and find relief from stressful conditions.

One of the important implications of research on emotional intelligence is the notion managers can make the improvement of emotional intelligence an important component in any leadership development agenda. For example, the following five components can be enhanced in the modern health care workplace:

▲ **Self-awareness:** The ability to understand one's moods, emotions, drives, and how they affect others.

▲ **Self-regulation:** The ability to think before acting and to control disruptive impulses or moods.

▲ **Motivation:** The ability to work for more than money or status, and to work with perseverance and high energy.

▲ **Empathy:** The ability to understand emotions of others and deal with them according to their emotional states.

▲ **Social skill:** The ability to manage relationships, build interpersonal networks, and establish social rapport.

By consciously and persistently seeking to acquire and develop these skills, anyone can improve upon his or her leadership effectiveness.

9.5.4 Gender and Leadership

One leadership theme of continuing interest is the question of whether gender influences leadership styles or effectiveness. Overall, evidence clearly supports the belief that both women and men can be effective leaders.[26]

However, men and women do tend to exhibit somewhat different styles.[27] Research regarding gender differences in respect to the leaderparticipation model discussed in section 9.4.5[28] indicates that female managers are significantly more participative than their male counterparts. Although followers in these research studies value participation by all leaders, they tended to value participation by female leaders more highly than by men.

Women may tend toward a style sometimes referred to as **interactive leadership**.[29] This style focuses on the building of consensus and good interpersonal relations through communication and involvement. Interactive leaders display behaviors typically considered democratic and participative—such as showing respect for others, caring for others, and sharing power and information with others. This interactive style also has qualities in common with transformational leadership discussed earlier in this section.[30]

Men, by contrast, may tend to utilize transactional leadership, relying more on directive and assertive behaviors and using authority in a traditional "com-

---

FOR EXAMPLE

Advice on Leadership Skills from the Academy of Achievement

Established in 1961, the not-for-profit Academy of Achievement (www. achievement.org) has sponsored awards for leaders "who represent the pinnacle of achievement in their respective fields." Each year, new inductees participate in public forums in which high school and college students can ask questions about each leader's style, skills, accomplishments, and personal development. More than 30 leaders have been honored in the areas of science and medicine, including Jonas Salk, David Ho, and Andrew Weil. Transcripts and audio recordings of the forums are free and downloadable from the Academy's Web site, along with detailed biographies and profiles.

mand and control" sense. Given the emphasis on shared power, communication, cooperation, and participation in health care organizations today, these results are provocative.

Gender issues aside, interactive leadership styles seem to be an excellent fit with the demands of a diverse and evolving health care workplace. Regardless of whether the relevant behaviors are displayed by women or men, future leadership success rests more often on one's capacity to lead through positive relationships and empowerment than through aloofness and formal authority.

SELF-CHECK

- Identify and define **transformational leadership, transactional leadership, emotional intelligence,** and **interactive leadership.**
- Describe strategies for continuous leadership development.
- Compare transformational leadership with transactional leadership.
- List six characteristics of transformational leaders.
- Explain the importance of emotional intelligence in today's health care workplace.
- List five common components of emotional intelligence.
- Discuss the role of gender in leadership.
- Contrast interactive leadership with transactional leadership.

9.6 Moral and Ethical Leadership

Regardless of the leadership model a health care manager or a health care organization ascribes to, **integrity**—a leader's honesty, credibility, and consistency in putting his or her values into action—is a critical management trait.

As section 2.3 explains, health care leaders have an undeniable responsibility to set high ethical standards to guide the behavior of followers. For managers, the ethical aspects of leadership are important and everyday responsibilities. They are central to the notion of **moral leadership**—that is, leadership that by actions and personal example sets high ethical standards for others to follow. Most health care organizations and professional groups have codes of ethics that offer managers guidance for appropriate behavior.

Concerned about what he perceives as a lack of momentum in organizational life, author and consultant John W. Gardner suggests that managers have a moral obligation to supply the necessary spark to awaken the potential of each individual, to urge each person "to take the initiative in performing leader-like acts."[31] Gardner points out that high expectations tend to generate high performance. Gardner's premise is that people with a sense of ownership of their jobs naturally outperform those who feel they are outsiders. Moral leaders instill ownership by truly respecting others and helping them to do their best. By doing so, they build organizations that consistently perform to society's expectations.[32] Moral leadership, therefore, must be clearly and strongly anchored in a true commitment to people.

9.6.1 Forging a Value-Driven Orientation

Leaders incorporate certain values and ethical principles into the work environment at the outset. Many health care teams fail because they lack a proper ethical orientation. Volumes of books and a score of management development programs focus on medical ethics, but this concept of **value-driven leadership** is relatively new to—though gaining wide acceptance in—modern health care leadership. Many strong health care organizations have very sound value-driven leadership at all organizational levels and enjoy a solid record of health care provisions and organizational growth.

The lack of value-driven leadership in a health care environment presents a number of problems. First, animosity can invade a work group in which ethical values are not an important or integral part of the everyday work process. The major catalyst in establishing a value-driven environment is the leader. If the leader fails to demonstrate value-driven action—actions that demonstrate decency and compassion, for instance—these qualities may not be valued and demonstrated by subordinates, and eventually this can have a detrimental effect on the department's performance.

9.6.2 Identifying Appropriate Values

As a health care manager, you need to determine which values are important for a health care department to maintain and enhance. A logical starting point is to examine the larger organization's values as they are expressed in the mission statement or in other organizational literature.

In general, the following value-based elements should be part of any value-driven health care leadership strategy:

▲ **Care** mandates the provision of health services to patients with the added "human touch" that all staff members should demonstrate when dealing with each patient.

▲ **Concern** should be shown by the staff not only to patients, but also to each other. Staff should be concerned about the welfare and development of fellow employees, helping each other through crises, as well as sharing the joy of daily victories.

▲ **Compassion** is a cornerstone of successful health care organizations and must be present at all levels of a facility—including your department.

FOR EXAMPLE

"Good Old-Fashioned" Leadership

Noted management scholar and consultant Peter Drucker (www.peter-drucker.com) takes a practical approach to workplace leadership by focusing on what he calls the "good old-fashioned" view of the leadership as hard work. Specifically, the work of a leader is threefold: First, good leaders define and establish a sense of mission by setting clear goals, priorities, and standards. Second, good leaders accept their roles as *responsibility* rather than *rank*; hence, good leaders aren't afraid to develop strong and capable subordinates. Third, great leaders understand the importance of earning and keeping the trust of others. The followers trust good leaders and believe their leaders mean what they say and act in ways consistent with what is said. "Effective leadership . . . is not based on being clever," says Drucker, "it is based primarily on being consistent."

Sensitivity and perceptiveness should be demonstrated by all team members toward the professional needs and desires of fellow team members and certainly toward the patient.

▲ **Community,** the sense that "we are in this together," should be promoted throughout the work group.

Initially, you may simply want to list the preceding four value-based elements on a chalkboard or flip chart and encourage discussion among team members about the importance of each one. Discussion may center on the definition of each element, the importance that you as leader place on each one, and how team members perceive them to help contribute to success of the larger health care organization.

You may want to enhance the list with your own short list of five or six additional value-based elements, perhaps including allegiance, dignity, optimization of resources, quality, societal awareness, and commitment (just to mention a few).

SELF-CHECK

- Identify and define **integrity, moral leadership,** and **value-driven leadership.**
- Discuss the place of morals, ethics, and values in leadership today.
- List the four common values in today's health care organizations.

SUMMARY

In addition to planning, organizing, and controlling, health care managers must devote time to leading their staffs, teams, and departments. Leadership can be defined in numerous ways, but establishing and sharing vision is a key trait of any successful leader. Leaders are aware of their power, in all its many forms, and use these powers appropriately. Managers who empower their teams can improve the effectiveness of individuals as well as entire departments. Models are useful tools for identifying proven methods of leadership success. Developing leadership skills can and should be a continuous process for managers. In health care workplaces, in particular, managers must also consider aspects of moral and value-driven leadership.

KEY TERMS

Authority decision	Decision made by the leader and then communicated to the group.
Coercive power	The ability to influence through punishment, a type of position power.
Consultative decision	Decision made by the leader after asking group members for information, advice, or opinions.
Contingency leadership theory	Leadership theory in which a leader's success depends on a match between leadership style and situational demands.
Emotional intelligence	The ability to understand emotions in one's self and others and then use this understanding to guide behavior.
Empowerment	The process through which managers enable and help others to gain power and achieve influence within the organization.
Expert power	The ability to influence through special expertise; a type of personal power.
Group decision	All members to participate in making a decision and working together to achieve a consensus regarding the preferred course of action.
Integrity	Honesty, credibility, and consistency in putting one's values into action.
Interactive leadership	A leader focuses on building consensus and good interpersonal relations through communication and involvement.

Leader-participation model	Leadership model in a leader chooses the method of decision making that best fits the nature of the problem being faced.
Leadership	The process of inspiring others to work hard to accomplish important tasks.
Leadership style	The recurring pattern of behaviors exhibited by a leader.
Leadership through empowerment	Helping others use their knowledge and judgment to make a real difference in daily workplace affairs.
Legitimate power	The ability to influence through formal authority, a type of position power.
Moral leadership	Leadership that by actions and personal example sets high ethical standards for others to follow.
Path-goal theory	Leadership theory that suggests an effective leader is one who clarifies paths through which followers can achieve both task-related and personal goals.
Personal power	Power derived from a leader's unique personal qualities.
Position power	Power from a manager's official status in the organization's hierarchy of authority.
Power	The ability to get someone else to do something you want done; the ability to make things happen for the good of the group or organization as a whole.
Referent power	The ability to influence the behaviors of other people because they admire you and want to identify positively with you; a type of personal power.
Reward power	The ability to influence through rewards; a type of position power.
Situational leadership model	Successful leaders adjust their styles depending on the readiness of followers to perform in a given situation.
Substitutes for leadership	Aspects of a work setting and the people involved that can reduce the need for a leader's personal involvement.
Transactional leadership	A leader adjusts tasks, rewards, and structures to help followers meet their needs while working to accomplish organizational objectives.

Transformational leadership	A leader uses charisma and related qualities to raise aspirations and shift people and organizational systems into new high-performance patterns.
Value-driven leadership	Leaders incorporate certain values and ethical principles into the work environment.
Vision	An overarching goal that manager/leader has for his or her department or team.

ASSESS YOUR UNDERSTANDING

Go to www.wiley.com/college/Lombardi to evaluate your knowledge of the basics of leadership.

Measure your learning by comparing pretest and post-test results.

Summary Questions

1. Managers who lead with vision
   (a) celebrate differences.
   (b) challenge processes.
   (c) help others do their jobs.
   (d) set budgets and schedules.
2. A manager without vision can still be a leader. True or false?
3. To establish a vision, a manager can
   (a) present your departmental goals to your staff on a regular basis.
   (b) list five major goals you want the department to accomplish in the next year.
   (c) base goals on your interaction and communication with peers and supervisors.
   (d) All of the above
4. The two main types of power are position power and personal power. Position power is derived from staff respect for a leader's accomplishments, while personal power is derived from the leader's status. True or false?
5. When a manager offers staff gift certificates for taking on additional shift work, what type of power is he or she exercising?
   (a) Expert power
   (b) Coercive power
   (c) Reward power
   (d) Legitimate power
6. Letting your staff know where you stand on issues and being action-oriented are two appropriate manners of utilizing managerial power. True or false?
7. Power is essentially a "zero-sum" proposition: If someone gains power, someone else must lose power. True or false?
8. Leadership through empowerment happens when
   (a) staff has opportunities to participate in cross-functional teams.
   (b) managers trust staff enough to eliminate status reports.

(c) staff can provide critical feedback to management.

(d) managers require two signatures for a purchase request.

9. Emotional intelligence, although a natural skill for some managers, can be learned or enhanced in managers who have limited relational or social-interaction skills. True or false?

10. Leader behavior research shows that task-oriented leaders generally outperform people-oriented leaders. True or false?

11. In contingency leadership theory, the degree of task structure measures the extent to which

(a) schedules and budgets are determined by upper management.

(b) task goals, procedures, and guidelines are clearly spelled out.

(c) job descriptions are made available to all employees.

(d) None of the above

12. In the situational leadership model, delegating works best in

(a) high-readiness situations of confident followers.

(b) low-readiness situations of confident followers.

(c) high-readiness situations of reliant followers.

(d) low-readiness situations of reliant followers.

13. Leading through participation offers the benefit of

(a) improving decision quality.

(b) bringing more information to bear on the problem.

(c) developing leadership potential in others.

(d) all of the above.

14. Which of the following is NOT an appropriate strategy for continuous leadership development?

(a) Give staff an appropriate level of freedom

(b) Learn from every situation

(c) Refer to organizational procedures to solve problems

(d) Balance positive and negative information realistically

15. Transactional leaders adjust tasks and rewards to help staff meet their needs while accomplishing organizational objectives; transformational leaders use personal quality to raise staff aspirations and encourage high-performance patterns from people and organizations. True or false?

16. Emotional intelligence includes five main components:

(a) Self-awareness, self-regulation, motivation, empathy, and social skills

(b) Self-direction, self-sacrifice, empowerment, sympathy, and analytical skills

(c) Self-regulation, self-analysis, intuition, integrity, and interpersonal skills

(d) Self-motivation, self-starting, honesty, empathy, and problem-solving skills

17. In moral leadership, a leader's actions and personal examples
    (a) override the policies and procedures in company manuals.
    (b) set high ethical standards for others to follow.
    (c) are more important than the staff's actions and examples.
    (d) are open to critical feedback from the team.

18. Although value-driven health care leadership differs, most approaches include care, concern, compassion, and
    (a) charisma.
    (b) continuity.
    (c) civility.
    (d) community.

Review Questions

1. A manager's vision does not have to be measurable in a quantitative sense. What characteristics does the vision need to have?

2. A leader with vision has a clear sense of the future, as well as what other characteristics?

3. If you tell a staff member that he must work 4 hours of overtime this week because you're the manager and you set the schedule, you are exercising what type of power?

4. What sort of power is the shift manager at a nursing care facility using when he tries to persuade his staff to alter a procedure based on his 10 years of hands-on elderly care?

5. Some managers are reluctant to utilize power, while others focus solely on maintaining and using their power. Why is either extreme undesirable?

6. What is a manager doing when she takes time to find out what her staff thinks may be causing an accounting problem for the department, rather than assuming she already knows the answer?

7. Based on the contingency leadership model, a relationship-oriented manager is likely to be more successful in what types of management situations?

8. Based on the situational leadership model, what leadership style best describes a manager who hosts bimonthly brainstorming sessions to problem-solve issues facing his department?

9. In path-goal theory, substitutes for leadership are aspects of the work setting and people involved that can reduce the need for the leader's personal involvement. What are some common substitutes?

10. To respond to recent budget cuts, a shift manager asks individual team members for opinions on how to deal with the situation. The manager then presents her plan for saving money within the department based on this feedback. Within the leader-participation model, which type of decision does this represent?

11. Participative decision making offers many benefits; however, what is the drawback of this model of decision making?

12. A manager decides to look at every situation she encounters during her day as an opportunity to collect new information and reevaluate her leadership style. Which strategy for continuous leadership development is the manager utilizing?

13. Being honest and credible, acting consistently out of personal conviction, and following through on commitments are all examples of which aspect of transformational leadership?

14. Moral leaders instill their teams with a sense of ownership of their jobs. How do moral leaders go about doing this?

15. Where should a leader look first when determining appropriate values to include in a value-driven leadership approach?

16. What four values are an appropriate part of most any value-driven leadership approach in today's health care workplace?

Applying This Chapter

1. The new shift manager at large nursing care facility presents her vision for her team as follows: Each patient is a "unit of care," which includes the patient, as well as the patient's families. Staff must do everything possible to satisfy medical and housing needs of this unit of care and avoid legal action. Is this an appropriate vision for leading a team or department?

2. How might the office manager of a multidoctor family medicine practice utilize reward power and coercive power to improve the efficiency of a new billing/claims representative in his department?

3. The team you manage at a student health center at a small liberal arts college looks to you to make all treatment decisions, solve day-to-day problems, sign off on all paperwork, and set their daily schedule and priorities. What are some things you can do as a manager to empower your staff?

4. For a nursing team leader to effectively utilize contingency leadership, what three variables must the leader understand and evaluate on an ongoing basis?

5. Jan has managed the record-keeping staff in an inner-city clinic for 5 years. Although her department generally runs smoothly, she has been challenged to think strategically about the hospital's record-keeping policies and improve the effectiveness and performance of her department. Jan decides to focus first on her style of leadership, which has been very by-the-book since she became a manager. What skills and abilities should Jan develop if she wants to grow from being a transactional leader to a transformational leader?

Building a Leadership Matrix

Many health care managers look to history books to help define the characteristics of great leadership. Create your own leadership matrix to help identify leadership examples that you consider important and meaningful. Along one side of a piece of paper, list figures from U.S. and world history (as well as current figures) who impress you because of their notable actions and achievements. In a second column, list next to each leader the characteristic (or two characteristics) that you believe the individual represents. After identifying 10 or so leaders, share your list with someone else and add to your list as you learn about additional impressive individuals. Consider reading online and print biographies about individuals who most intrigue you, noting inspirational quotes or anecdotes along the way. Some noteworthy individuals (along with outstanding characteristics they exemplify) can include Abraham Lincoln (honesty, integrity); Franklin D. Roosevelt (courage to implement innovative programs); Mother Theresa (compassion, human spirit); Benjamin Franklin (imagination, innovation); John F. Kennedy (charisma, vision); Dr. Martin Luther King Jr. (recognized that little things launch big things); Winston Churchill (ability to get the job done); Mohandas Gandhi (regard for others interests and needs); Eleanor Roosevelt (compassionate communication).

How You Use Power

Consider a recent event in which you used power to make a decision or get something done. The event doesn't have to be major; it could be that you made the decision of which movie to see or that you changed someone's mind while shopping. Maybe you assigned a task to someone in a study group or in a workplace setting. Maybe you disciplined a young child or successfully debated a topic with a parent or elder. Whatever the case, which of the two main types of power did you use: personal or position? Did you use both types of power? If you used personal power, was it reward, coercive, or legitimate? If you used position power, was it expert or referent?

Using Nominal Group Process

Developed in the 1970s, nominal group process is a popular approach for leading and empowering groups. During nominal group process, the goal is to select one solution based on group consensus (rather than total agreement). Research suggests that in many situations, nominal process produces better results than unstructured group interactions. To facilitate nominal process on group decision (perhaps determining the topic for a group project/presentation, or selecting a movie for you and your friends to see), guide your group through the following series of specific interactive steps. First, have everyone generate ideas individually and silently. Share ideas in round-robin fashion, encouraging feedback from the group only after *all* ideas have been presented. Ask each group member to establish their final recommendation and record this decision. Finally, mathematically combine all recommendations and produce a ranked list of final ideas.

Role Model Roundup

Role models are sources of inspiration for your leadership style. The ways in which your role models approach their responsibilities and conduct their activities shows you how you might lead and what choices you might make as a leader. Consider the success stories behind one of your role models—perhaps a family member, a favorite teacher, a youth group leader, a successful co-worker, or an inspiring religious or community leader. On three index cards, list the role model's name and position or title. On each card, list a brief "success story" associated with the role model. (For example, "hired an entirely new nursing staff in one month's time" or "empowers staff to present one new idea at each monthly staff meeting" are briefly stated success stories.) Read over the three success stories and consider the challenges or negative aspects the role model may have encountered prior to the success story; list one or two challenges on each card. Finally, read through the cards one last time. This time consider why the role model may have been successful (despite the challenges); list one or two reasons for success on each card. Clip the three cards together and keep them in your purse, briefcase, or backpack. During free moments over the next month, take out the cards, shuffle through the success stories, and the lesson each story offers to you and your career as a health care manager.

Your Continuous Leadership Development

Leaders aren't born, they're made. Developing leadership skills is a daily activity that you can engage in today, even if you're not yet working in your chosen career field. Review the nine strategies for continuous leadership development in section 9.5.1 and select one aspect that you can begin working on in little ways *today*. For example, if you choose to develop your ability to "balance positive and negative information realisti-

cally," how might this play out in your daily life? How might you interact differently with your friends, family, partner or spouse, and classmates? How might you act/react differently to horrible news story or a day when nothing seems to be going your way?

Your Health Care Values

Value-driven leadership continues to be an important topic in today's health care workplace. If you apply for or work as a manager within an organization, you will, most likely, be asked to discuss some of your values as they relate to patient care and your leadership style. Although every manager's values are different, the four basic values outlined in section 9.6.2—care, concern, compassion, and community—are all strong values for today's health care manager. Review these four values and formulate a specific example of a time each value played a significant role in your education, work life, or personal life. Consider incorporating an outstanding example of one or more of these values into your resume or cover letter.

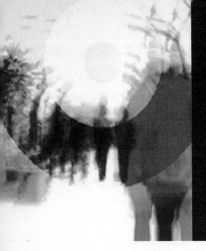

10

MOTIVATING OTHERS
Encouraging Great Results and Outstanding Contributions

Starting Point

Go to www.wiley.com/college/Lombardi to assess your knowledge of the basics of motivating to meet needs.
Determine where you need to concentrate your effort.

What You'll Learn in This Chapter

▲ Three theories of needs-based motivation
▲ Maslow's five levels of need
▲ Three theories of process-based motivation
▲ Strategies for successful goal setting
▲ Fours ways to reinforce behaviors
▲ Nontraditional work arrangements for today's workplace

After Studying This Chapter, You'll Be Able To

▲ Differentiate between internal and external motivators
▲ Interpret Maslow's hierarchy of needs
▲ Apply tools and techniques for motivating others
▲ Use common behavior-reinforcement techniques
▲ Examine the role of job design in motivation
▲ Compare various job design alternatives in today's workplace

Goals and Outcomes

▲ Master the terminology and tools related to motivation
▲ Describe motivational techniques that involve needs, processes, and goal
▲ Compare motivational theories and approaches
▲ Choose appropriate alternative job designs and work arrangements
▲ Use needs, processes, and goals to motivate others
▲ Choose appropriate methods of behavior reinforcement
▲ Propose motivation strategies for a team or department
▲ Formulate alternative job designs
▲ Evaluate motivation techniques and strategies

INTRODUCTION

Managers know that "productivity through people" is an important ingredient for long-term success in today's demanding, people-intensive health care workplace. Managers have a variety of techniques and tools to motivate others. Unfulfilled needs can motivate workers to avoid poor conditions and strive for better work experiences. The various process theories of motivation all suggest ways to get employees to choose to work harder for more positive outcomes. Managers can utilize external factors—especially positive reinforcement and punishment—to influence how staff works. By designing appropriate, compelling jobs, managers can encourage employees to motivate themselves. In today's rapidly changing health care workplace, job design and alternative work arrangements are major methods of encouraging outstanding worker performance.

10.1 Motivation Based on Human Needs

The term **motivation** is used in management theory to describe forces within individuals that account for the level, direction, and persistence of effort they expend at work. Simply put, a highly motivated person works hard at a job; an unmotivated person does not.

Health care managers who lead teams and staff through motivation create conditions under which other people feel continually inspired to work hard and perform to the best of their abilities.

By understanding what motivates people, health care managers can appreciate where team members are coming from; they can also better direct the energies of team members to achieve truly great things for their organizations. The following sections explore a variety of ways that people find motivation in the modern workplace.

Needs are unfulfilled physiological or psychological desires of an individual. Some theories of motivation use individual needs to explain the behaviors and attitudes of people at work. Although each of the theories in this section focuses on a slightly different set of needs, all the theories agree that needs cause tensions that influence attitudes and behavior.

Good managers and leaders establish conditions in which people can satisfy important needs through their work. They also take action to eliminate things that can block the satisfaction of important needs.

10.1.1 Hierarchy of Needs

Abraham Maslow's theory of human needs provides an important foundation for management thinking. Maslow views people as seeking the satisfaction of the five levels of needs, as Figure 10-1 shows. Lower-level needs include physiological, safety, and social concerns, while higher-level needs include esteem and self-actualization concerns.[1]

Figure 10-1

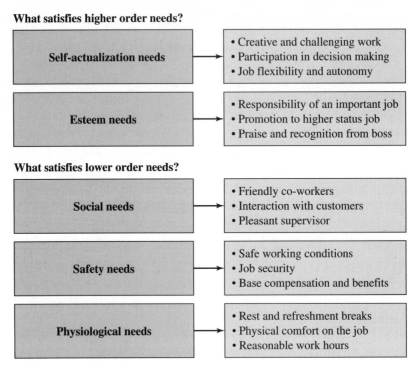

What satisfies higher order needs?

| **Self-actualization needs** | → | • Creative and challenging work
• Participation in decision making
• Job flexibility and autonomy |

| **Esteem needs** | → | • Responsibility of an important job
• Promotion to higher status job
• Praise and recognition from boss |

What satisfies lower order needs?

| **Social needs** | → | • Friendly co-workers
• Interaction with customers
• Pleasant supervisor |

| **Safety needs** | → | • Safe working conditions
• Job security
• Base compensation and benefits |

| **Physiological needs** | → | • Rest and refreshment breaks
• Physical comfort on the job
• Reasonable work hours |

Work motivation and Maslow's hierarchy of needs.

Two principles are central to Maslow's theory:

▲ The **deficit principle** holds that a satisfied need is not a motivator of behavior. People are expected to act in ways that satisfy deprived needs—that is, needs for which a "deficit" exists.

▲ The **progression principle** holds that a need at one level does not become activated until the next lower level need is already satisfied. People are expected to advance step by step up the hierarchy in their search for need satisfactions. At the level of self-actualization, the more these needs are satisfied, the stronger they are supposed to grow. According to Maslow, a person should continue to be motivated by opportunities for self-fulfillment as long as the other needs remain satisfied.

Maslow's theory advises managers to recognize that blocked or deprived needs may negatively influence work attitudes and behaviors. By the same token, providing opportunities for need satisfaction may have positive motivational consequences. Figure 10-1 gives some examples of how managers can use Maslow's ideas to better meet the needs of people at work.

10.1.2 Two-Factor Theory

Frederick Herzberg's **two-factor theory** offers another framework for understanding motivation in the workplace.[2]

The theory was developed from a pattern identified in the responses of almost 4,000 people to questions about work. When questioned about what "turned them on," respondents tended to identify things relating to the nature of the job itself. Herzberg calls these **satisfier factors.** When questioned about what "turned them off," they tended to identify things relating more to the work setting. Herzberg calls these **hygiene factors.**

As shown in Figure 10-2, the two-factor theory associates hygiene factors, or sources of job dissatisfaction, with aspects of job context. That is, "dissatisfiers" are considered more likely to be a part of the work setting than of the nature of the work itself. The hygiene factors include such things as

▲ working conditions;

▲ interpersonal relations;

▲ organizational policies and administration;

▲ technical quality of supervision;

▲ base wage or salary.

Herzberg's two-factor theory argues that improving the hygiene factors, such as by adding piped-in music or implementing a no-smoking policy, can make people less dissatisfied with these aspects of their work. But these changes do not in themselves contribute to increases in satisfaction.

To really improve motivation, Herzberg advises managers to give proper attention to the satisfier factors. As part of job content, the satisfier factors deal

Figure 10-2

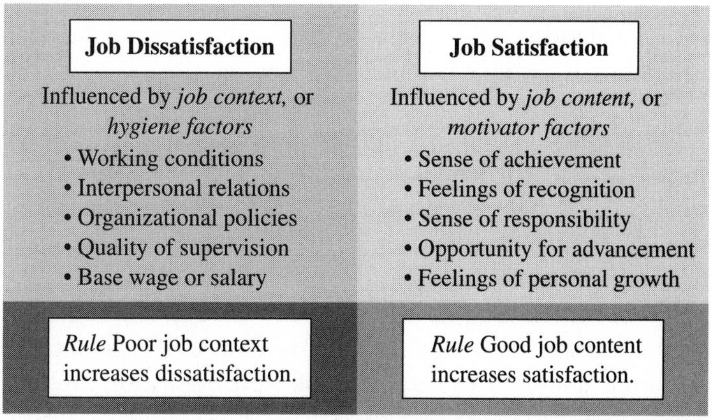

Job Dissatisfaction	Job Satisfaction
Influenced by *job context,* or *hygiene factors*	Influenced by *job content,* or *motivator factors*
• Working conditions	• Sense of achievement
• Interpersonal relations	• Feelings of recognition
• Organizational policies	• Sense of responsibility
• Quality of supervision	• Opportunity for advancement
• Base wage or salary	• Feelings of personal growth
Rule Poor job context increases dissatisfaction.	*Rule* Good job content increases satisfaction.

Two-factor theory in the workplace.

with what people actually do in their work. By making improvements in what people are asked to do in their jobs, Herzberg suggests that job satisfaction and performance can be raised. Important satisfier factors include

▲ a sense of achievement;
▲ feelings of recognition;
▲ a sense of responsibility;
▲ opportunity for advancement;
▲ feelings of personal growth.

Scholars have criticized Herzberg's theory as being methodbound and difficult to replicate.[3] Yet, the two-factor theory remains a useful reminder that there are two important aspects of all jobs:

▲ **Job content:** What people do in terms of job tasks.
▲ **Job context:** The work setting in which they do it.

Furthermore, Herzberg's advice to managers is still timely: (1) Always correct poor context to eliminate actual or potential sources of job dissatisfaction; and (2) be sure to build satisfier factors into job content to maximize opportunities for job satisfaction.

10.1.3 Acquired Needs Theory

David McClelland offers another motivation theory based on individual needs.[4]

▲ **Need for achievement** is the desire to do something better or more efficiently, to solve problems, or to master complex tasks.
▲ **Need for power** is the desire to control other people, to influence their behavior, or to be responsible for them.
▲ **Need for affiliation** is the desire to establish and maintain friendly and warm relations with other people.

According to McClelland, people acquire or develop these needs over time as a result of individual life experiences. In addition, each need carries a distinct set of work preferences. Managers are encouraged to recognize the strength of each need in themselves and in other people. Attempts can then be made to create work environments responsive to them.

People high in the need for achievement, for example, like to put their competencies to work, they take moderate risks in competitive situations, and they are willing to work alone. As a result, the work preferences of high-need achievers include individual responsibility for results, achievable but challenging goals, and feedback on performance.

FOR EXAMPLE

Complex Needs in Today's Health Care Organization

Researcher Milton Hammerly sees needs driving not only health care employees and managers, but also patients, insurance agents, and independent providers. In reports he's written for *American Journal Medical Quality*, Hammerly focuses on the complexity theory of needs, in which Maslow's hierarchy of needs drives the behavior of everyone involved in providing health care. Hammerly recommends that health care organizations must of course satisfy lower-order needs (survival), but that they must also provide opportunities for everyone to satisfy higher-order needs (actualization). Employers aware of actualization needs can maintain a stronger workforce for longer periods of time. Patients who work toward actualization needs (perhaps through more active collaboration with their caregivers) can experience more than mere survival—they can experience truly improved health and wellness.

SELF-CHECK

- Identify and define **motivation, needs, two-factor theory, and acquired needs theory.**
- Compare the three main theories of motivation based on need.
- Describe Maslow's hierarchy of needs, including the deficit principle and progression principle.
- Contrast elements of the two-factor theory: satisfier factors and hygiene factors.
- Compare the three types of needs that make up acquired needs theory.

10.2 Motivation Based on Process

Although the details vary, each of the need theories described in section 10.1 can help managers understand individual differences and deal positively with workforce diversity.

The following **process theories** can add further to this understanding. The equity, expectancy, and goal-setting theories each offer advice and insight on how people actually make choices to work hard or not, based on their individual preferences, the available rewards, and possible work outcomes.

10.2.1 Equity Theory

The **equity theory** of motivation is known best through the work of J. Stacy Adams.[5] The essence of the theory is that perceived inequity is a motivating state—that is, when people believe that they have been inequitably treated in comparison to others, they will try to eliminate the discomfort and restore a sense of equity to the situation.

Equity comparison typically occurs whenever managers allocate extrinsic rewards, especially monetary incentives or pay increases. Inequities occur whenever people feel that the rewards received for their work are unfair given the rewards other people appear to be getting. A worker may compare his or her situation to other co-workers in the group, to workers elsewhere in the organization, and even to people employed by other organizations.

Adams predicts that people will deal with perceived inequity by changing

▲ their work inputs by putting less effort into their jobs;
▲ the rewards received by asking for better treatment;
▲ the comparison points by finding ways to make things seem better;
▲ the situation by transferring or quitting the job.

Much of Adams's research has been laboratory based and focuses on **perceived negative inequity,** a condition that most managers would want to avoid. People who feel underpaid and perceive negative inequity, for example, tend to reduce their work efforts to compensate for missing rewards. These workers are less motivated to work hard in the future.

People who feel overpaid and perceive positive inequity, by contrast, have been found to increase the quantity or quality of their work. However, many questions involving this particular issue remain to be answered.

Informed managers anticipate perceived negative inequities whenever especially visible rewards—such as pay or promotions—are allocated. Instead of letting equity concerns get out of hand, they carefully communicate the intended value of rewards being given, clarify the performance appraisals upon which they are based, and suggest appropriate comparison points.

10.2.2 Expectancy Theory

Victor Vroom's **expectancy theory** of motivation asks a central question: What determines the willingness of an individual to work hard at tasks important to the organization?[6]

Expectancy theory suggests that "people *will* do what they *can* do when they *want* to do it." More specifically, Vroom suggests that the motivation to work depends on the relationships among the following three factors:

▲ **Expectancy:** A person's belief that working hard will result in a desired level of task performance being achieved.

▲ **Instrumentality:** A person's belief that successful performance will be followed by rewards and other potential outcomes.

▲ **Valence:** The value a person assigns to the possible rewards and other work-related outcomes.

Expectancy theory suggests that motivation (M), expectancy (E), instrumentality (I), and valence (V) are related to one another in a multiplication-based equation:

$$M = E \times I \times V$$

In other words, motivation is determined by expectancy times instrumentality times valence. The multiplier effect has important managerial implications. Mathematically speaking, a zero at any location on the right side of the equation (for E, I, or V) results in zero motivation.

For example, a typical assumption is that people will be motivated to work hard to earn a promotion. But is this necessarily true? If expectancy is low, motivation will suffer. The person may feel that he or she cannot achieve the performance level necessary to get promoted. So why try? If instrumentality is low, motivation will suffer. The person may lack confidence that a high level of task performance will result in being promoted. So why try? If valence is low, motivation will suffer. The person may place little value on receiving a promotion. It simply isn't much of a reward. So, once again, why try?

As Figure 10-3 shows, the management implications of expectancy theory include being willing to work with each individual and try to maximize his or her expectancies, instrumentalities, and valences in ways that support organizational objectives. Stated a bit differently, a manager can apply expectancy theory by clearly linking effort and performance, linking performance to work outcomes, and choosing work outcomes valued by the individual.

10.2.3 Goal-Setting Theory

Task goals, in the form of clear and desirable performance targets, are the basis of Edwin Locke's **goal-setting theory.**[7] The theory's basic premise is that task goals can be highly motivating—if they are properly set and if they are well managed. Specifically, goals

▲ give direction to people in their work;

▲ clarify the performance expectations between a supervisor and subordinate, between co-workers, and across subunits in an organization;

▲ establish a frame of reference for task feedback;

▲ provide a foundation for behavioral self-management.

According to Locke, goal setting can enhance individual work performance and job satisfaction. To achieve these benefits, however, managers and team leaders must work together to set the right goals in the right ways. The degree to which

Figure 10-3

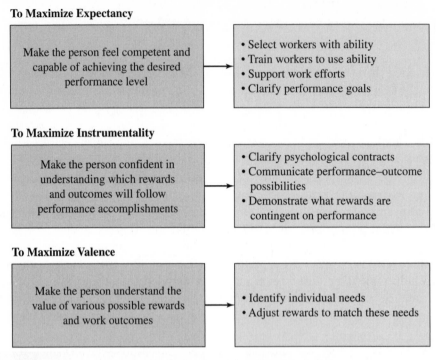

To Maximize Expectancy

Make the person feel competent and capable of achieving the desired performance level

→
- Select workers with ability
- Train workers to use ability
- Support work efforts
- Clarify performance goals

To Maximize Instrumentality

Make the person confident in understanding which rewards and outcomes will follow performance accomplishments

→
- Clarify psychological contracts
- Communicate performance–outcome possibilities
- Demonstrate what rewards are contingent on performance

To Maximize Valence

Make the person understand the value of various possible rewards and work outcomes

→
- Identify individual needs
- Adjust rewards to match these needs

Managerial implications of expectancy theory.

people are involved in setting performance goals can influence their satisfaction and performance. Research indicates that a positive impact is most likely to occur when the participation (1) allows for increased understanding of specific and difficult goals and (2) provides for greater acceptance and commitment to them.

Some additional tips for successful goal-setting include the following:

▲ **Set specific goals:** Specifically worded goals ("To complete three preoperative consultations every hour," for example) lead to higher performance than more generally stated ones ("Do your best").

▲ **Set challenging goals:** As long as goals are viewed as realistic and attainable, more difficult goals lead to higher performance than do easy goals.

▲ **Build goal acceptance and commitment:** People work harder for goals that they accept and believe in; they tend to resist goals forced on them.

▲ **Clarify goal priorities:** Make sure that expectations are clear as to which goals should be accomplished first and why.

▲ **Reward goal accomplishment:** Don't let positive accomplishments pass unnoticed; reward people for doing what they set out to do.

FOR EXAMPLE

Setting Goals and Priorities

Vision 2010, the aggressive 5-year growth plan for Harrison Hospital in Kitsap County, Washington (www.harrisonhospital.org), relies heavily on Locke's goal-setting theories of motivation. After extensive research and information gathering—including a survey of more than 2,500 employees and patients—Vision 2010's 13-member team of hospital leaders presented a detailed plan with long- and short-term goals, complete with specific "milestone" checkpoints and public accountability measures (www.harrisonhospital.org/main/vision.html). Additionally, the plan sets employees' priorities by focusing on nine areas for improvement: market position, expanded services, customer service, clinical excellence, physician and hospital alignment, employee engagement, financial performance, information systems, and location and function of facilities.

The concept of management by objectives (see section 7.5.1) is a good illustration of such a participative approach to goal setting.

SELF-CHECK

- Identify and define **process theories, equity theory, perceived negative inequity, expectancy theory,** and **goal-setting theory.**
- Describe how inequity can motivate according to equity theory.
- Compare the effects of perceived negative inequity and perceived positive inequity.
- Discuss the relationship between the three expectancy theory factors of expectancy, instrumentality, and valence.
- Explain the importance of goals in the workplace.
- Suggest strategies setting effective goals.

10.3 Motivating through External Forces

The theories described in section 10.2 rely on cognitive explanations of behavior. They explain why people do things in terms of satisfying needs, resolving felt inequities, or pursuing positive expectancies and task goals.

By contrast, **reinforcement theory** explains human behavior as a result of one's environment. Instead of looking within the individual to explain motivation and behavior, reinforcement theory focuses on the external environment and the consequences it holds for individuals.

The basic premises reinforcement theory is based on what E. L. Thorndike called the **law of effect:** Behavior that results in a pleasant outcome is likely to be repeated; behavior that results in an unpleasant outcome is not likely to be repeated.[8]

10.3.1 Reinforcing Behaviors

Psychologist B. F. Skinner popularized the concept of **operant conditioning,** or learning by reinforcement. In management, reinforcement systematically reinforces desirable work behavior and discourages undesirable work behavior.

Four strategies of reinforcement are used in operant conditioning:

▲ **Positive reinforcement** strengthens or increases the frequency of desirable behavior by making a pleasant consequence contingent on its occurrence. *Example:* A manager nods to express approval to someone who makes a useful comment during a staff meeting. Section 10.3.2 deals with positive reinforcement in greater detail.

▲ **Negative reinforcement** increases the frequency of or strengthens desirable behavior by making the avoidance of an unpleasant consequence contingent upon its occurrence. *Example:* A manager who has been nagging a worker every day about tardiness does not nag when the worker comes to work on time one day.

▲ **Punishment** decreases the frequency of or eliminates an undesirable behavior by making an unpleasant consequence contingent on its occurrence. *Example:* A manager issues a written reprimand to an employee who reports late for work one day.

▲ **Extinction** decreases the frequency of or eliminates an undesirable behavior by making the removal of a pleasant consequence contingent on its occurrence. *Example:* A manager observes that a disruptive employee is receiving social approval from co-workers; the manager counsels co-workers to stop giving this approval.

For example, Figure 10-4 shows how a manager can apply all four reinforcement strategies to influence continuous improvement among employees. Note, too, that the strategies of both positive and negative reinforcement strengthen desirable behavior when it occurs. The punishment and extinction strategies weaken or eliminate undesirable behaviors.

10.3.2 Utilizing Positive Reinforcement

Among the reinforcement strategies, positive reinforcement deserves special attention. Positive reinforcement can be a valuable motivational tool.

Figure 10-4

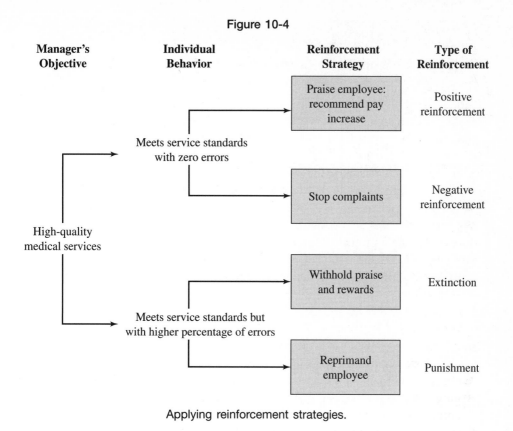

Applying reinforcement strategies.

When using positive reinforcement in the workplace, managers need to always be mindful of two important laws:

▲ **The law of contingent reinforcement:** For a reward to have maximum reinforcing value, it must be delivered only if the desirable behavior is exhibited. For example, an insurance call center manager should reward her staff for their prompt attention to calls only after the center fully meets its goal of answering every call within 60 seconds.

▲ **The law of immediate reinforcement:** The more immediate the delivery of a reward after the occurrence of a desirable behavior, the greater the reinforcing value of the reward. For example, a manager should complement a perpetually late staffer for arriving on time to work as early in the day as possible.

The following are additional tips for effectively using positive reinforcement:

▲ Clearly identify desired work behaviors.
▲ Maintain a diverse inventory of rewards.

FOR EXAMPLE

Employee Recognition Programs

Over the last decade, many health care organizations have developed and enhanced employee recognition programs in an effort to encourage high levels of performance from all workers. Many recognition programs now salute contributions beyond (and in addition to) traditional "employee of the month" type recognition and anniversary of service awards. Overlake Hospital in Bellevue, Washington (www.overlakehospital.org), has five employee recognition programs to better identify and celebrate outstanding effort within the organization. For example, the hospital's Bravo program enables employees to recognize co-workers for "going above and beyond the call of duty" on a single project or task. After completing a simple application form, Bravo awards can be issued at any time in any public forum (like a weekly team meeting). Bravo award items have included complementary movie tickets, small gift certificates, and celebratory "cookie cards."

▲ Inform everyone what must be done to get rewards.

▲ Recognize individual differences when allocating rewards.

The timing of positive reinforcement can also make a difference in its impact.

▲ A **continuous reinforcement schedule** administers a reward each time a desired behavior occurs.

▲ An **intermittent reinforcement schedule** rewards behavior only periodically.

In general, a continuous reinforcement elicits a desired behavior more quickly than an intermittent reinforcement. By contrast, behavior acquired under an intermittent schedule is often more permanent than behavior acquired under a continuous schedule.

Managers can mobilize the power of positive reinforcement through the process of **shaping,** which is the creation of a new behavior by the positive reinforcement of successive approximations to it.

One way to succeed with a shaping strategy is to give reinforcement on a continuous basis until the desired behavior is achieved. Then use an intermittent schedule to maintain the behavior at the new level.

10.3.3 Using Punishment

As a reinforcement strategy, punishment attempts to eliminate undesirable behavior by making an unpleasant consequence contingent with its occurrence. To punish an employee, for example, a manager may deny the individual a valued reward, such as verbal praise or merit pay, or the manager may administer an unpleasant outcome, such as a verbal reprimand or pay reduction. Like positive reinforcement, punishment can be done poorly or it can be done well.

Unfortunately, punishing is often done poorly. To effectively use punishment,

▲ tell the person what specifically he or she is doing wrong;

▲ tell the person what specifically he or she is doing right;

▲ make sure the punishment matches the behavior;

▲ administer any punishment in private;

▲ follow the laws of immediate and contingent reinforcement;

▲ combine punishment with positive reinforcement for maximum effectiveness.

SELF-CHECK

- Identify and define **reinforcement theory, operant conditioning, and shaping.**
- Compare the four operant conditioning techniques: **positive reinforcement, negative reinforcement, punishment, and extinction.**
- Explain how law of effect impacts all reinforcement theories.
- Describe strategies for effectively using positive reinforcement.
- Contrast characteristics and effectiveness of continuous and intermittent reinforcement schedules.
- List strategies for effectively utilizing punishing in the workplace.

10.4 Motivating through Job Design

The process of **job design** is one of creating or defining jobs by assigning specific work tasks to individuals and groups.

Done appropriately, job design can contribute to the accomplishment of two major goals—job performance and job satisfaction. One without the other is simply insufficient to meet the high standards expected of today's health care workplace.

10.4.1 Defining and Designing Good Jobs

Job performance is the quantity and quality of tasks accomplished by an individual or group at work. Performance, as is commonly said, is the "bottom line" for people at work. It is a cornerstone of productivity, and it should contribute to the accomplishment of organizational objectives.

Indeed, more and more health care organizations now consider a value-added aspect when evaluating the worthwhileness of jobs and/or jobholders. The performance of every job should add value to the organization's production of useful goods and/or services.

In addition to its performance potential, any job should also provide opportunities for job satisfaction. This indicator of quality of work life is defined as the degree to which a person feels positively or negatively about various aspects of a job.[9]

An important goal in job design is to always create jobs rich with potential satisfaction. This means managers must consider such things as pay, tasks, supervision, co-workers, work setting, and advancement opportunities. Employers can address all these facets of job satisfaction in the attempt to improve attitudes and raise the quality of work life.

10.4.2 Exploring Job Design Alternatives

Job design in many ways is an exercise in "fit." A good job provides a fit between the needs and capabilities of workers and tasks so that both job performance and satisfaction are high.

To tailor job design to better fit workers unique abilities and situations, managers can utilize several common job design alternatives, including job simplification, job enlargement and rotation, and job enrichment.

▲ **Job simplification** involves streamlining work procedures so that people work in well-defined and highly specialized tasks.

Simplified jobs are narrow in job scope, with a limited number and variety of different tasks a person performs. The logic is straightforward: Because some jobs don't require complex skills, workers can be easier and quicker to train, less difficult to supervise, and easy to replace if they leave. Furthermore, because tasks are precisely and narrowly defined, workers can become good at doing the same tasks over and over again.

However, there are some downsides to highly simplified jobs. Productivity can suffer as unhappy workers drive up costs through absenteeism and turnover and through poor performance caused by boredom and alienation. The most extreme form of job simplification is automation, or the total mechanization of a job.

The process of job simplification dates back to industrial assembly lines, in which each worker did a specific, simple task to help create a complex product, like an automobile. Today, however, job simplification is less common, particularly in complex health care workplaces. In fact, many health care jobs are becoming more complex (see section 10.5). Still, some entry-level positions (particularly clerical and technical positions within large health care organizations) can still be focused and simplified.

One way to move beyond job simplification is to expand job scope by increasing the number and variety of tasks involved in a job.

▲ **Job rotation** increases task variety by periodically shifting workers between jobs involving different task assignments.

Job rotation in health care settings can include clinical, office, and laboratory settings with a series of functional job stations that workers are assigned to and shuffled on an hourly or daily basis.

▲ **Job enlargement** increases task variety by combining two or more tasks that were previously assigned to separate workers. The process often involves combining tasks done immediately before or after the work performed in the original job.

Frederick Herzberg (see section 10.1.2) questions the value of the job rotation and job enlargement. "Why," he asks, "should a worker become motivated when one or more meaningless tasks are added to previously existing ones or when work assignments are rotated among equally meaningless tasks?" By contrast, he says, "If you want people to do a good job, give them a good job to do."[10]

▲ **Job enrichment** that builds more opportunities for satisfaction into a job by expanding not just job scope but also job depth—that is, the extent to which task planning and evaluating duties are performed by the individual worker rather than the supervisor.

10.4.3 Relying on the Core Job Characteristics

Job rotation, enlargement, and enrichment may not be adequate tools for designing truly satisfying jobs in today's demanding health care workplace.

The **core characteristics model** developed by Richard Hackman and his associates offers a way for health care managers to create jobs, enriched or otherwise, that best fit the needs of people and organizations.[11]

The model, shown in Figure 10-5, identifies five core job characteristics:

▲ **Skill variety:** The degree to which a job requires a variety of different activities to carry out the work and involves the use of a number of different skills and talents of the individual.

▲ **Task identity:** The degree to which the job requires completion of a "whole" and identifiable piece of work—that is, one that involves doing a job from beginning to end with a visible outcome.

▲ **Task significance:** The degree to which the job has a substantial impact on the lives or work of other people elsewhere in the organization or in the external environment.

Figure 10-5

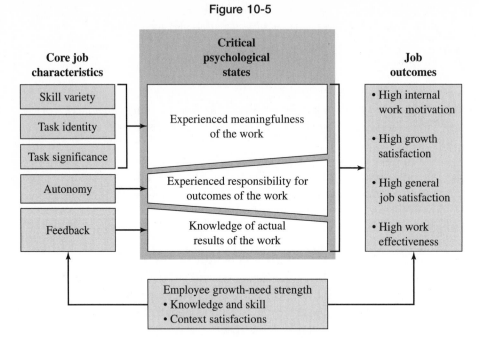

Core job characteristics and job design.

- ▲ **Autonomy:** The degree to which the job gives the individual substantial freedom, independence, and discretion in scheduling the work and in determining the procedures to be used in carrying it out.
- ▲ **Feedback from the job itself:** The degree to which carrying out the work activities required by the job results in the individual obtaining direct and clear information on the results of his or her performance.

A job that is high in the core characteristics is considered enriched; the lower a job scores on the core characteristics, the less enriched it is. However, these core characteristics do not affect all people in the same way. Generally speaking, people who respond most favorably to enriched jobs have strong higher-order needs and appropriate job knowledge and skills. They are typically satisfied with their job context.

When job enrichment is a good job design choice, you have four main ways of improving the core characteristics:

- ▲ **Form natural units of work.** Make sure that the tasks people perform are logically related to one another and provide a clear and meaningful task identity.
- ▲ **Combine tasks.** Expand job responsibilities by pulling together into one larger job a number of smaller tasks previously done by others.

> ### FOR EXAMPLE
>
> #### Nursing: A Wealth of Alternative Designs
>
> Even though there are currently more than 2.5 million nurses in the United States, most regions of the country are experiencing a nursing crisis. (According to the U.S. Bureau of Labor Statistics, job options for registered nurses will grow faster than the average for all occupations through 2008.) To respond to shortages, hospitals and other health care providers are developing a range of job designs to attract and retain quality nursing staffs. Established in 2001, CampusRN.com (www.campusrn.com) not only lists thousands of entry-level nursing opportunities around the country, the site reports on hiring and job-design trends—including flexible schedule, traveling nurses, independent contracting, and more—on its Nurse Corner area (www.campusrn.com/students/nurses_corner.asp).

▲ **Open feedback channels.** Provide opportunities for people to receive performance feedback as they work and to learn how performance changes over time.

▲ **Practice vertical loading.** Give people more control over their work by increasing their authority to perform the planning and controlling previously done by supervisors.

SELF-CHECK

- Identify and define **job design, job performance, job simplification, job rotation, job enlargement, job enrichment,** and **core characteristics model.**
- Explain how job design can affect employee motivation.
- Identify work situations where job simplification, rotation, enlargement, and enrichment are each appropriate job designs.
- List the five job characteristics that make up core characteristics model.

10.5 Exploring Alternative Work Arrangements

Not only is the content of jobs changing for individuals and groups in today's health care workplace, but the context is changing too. Work/life balance is increasingly at issue for a diverse workforce, and the increasing technology-based work environment is bringing new employment opportunities.[12]

Among the more significant developments is the emergence of a number of alternative ways for people to schedule their time to balance work and personal/family needs.[13] The following sections cover some of the most popular and effective new developments in the way jobs are structured today.

10.5.1 Compressed Workweek

A **compressed workweek** is any work schedule that allows a full-time job to be completed in less than the standard 5 days of 8-hour shifts. In health care, a very common form is the "4/40" or the "3/12" that is, accomplishing 40 hours of work in four 10-hour days or three 12-hour days.

One advantage of these compressed schedules is that the employee receives 3 or 4 consecutive days off from work each week. This benefits the individual through more leisure time and lower commuting costs. The organization may also benefit through lower absenteeism and improved performance. Potential disadvantages include increased fatigue and family adjustment problems for the individual, as well as increased scheduling problems, possible patient complaints, and possible union objections.

10.5.2 Flexible Working Hours

The term **flexible working hours,** also called *flexitime* or *flextime,* describes any work schedule that gives employees some choice in the pattern of their daily work hours. Some employees may choose to come in earlier and leave earlier, while still completing an 8-hour day; others may choose to start later in the morning and leave later. In between these extremes are opportunities to attend to personal affairs, such as dental appointments, home emergencies, visits to children's schools, and so on.

Flexible working hours are a challenging fit with the shift-driven schedules of clinical or medical positions at many health care facilities. However, for health care departments with less interaction with patients (accounting, administrative, laboratory), flexible working hours are becoming more common.

However, despite the challenges of incorporating flexible working hours in health care settings, the advantages are especially important to members of a diverse workforce. Flexibility is important to many dual-career couples who face the complications of managing careers and other responsibilities, including parenting. Single parents with young children and employees with elder-care responsibilities also find it very attractive to have the option of adjusting work schedules to allow for other obligations to be met. The added discretion flextime provides may also encourage workers to have more positive attitudes toward the organization.

10.5.3 Job Sharing

Another important development for today's workforce is **job sharing,** whereby one full-time job is split between two or more people.

Job sharing often involves each person working one-half day, but it can also be done on weekly or monthly sharing arrangements. When it is feasible for jobs to be split and shared, organizations can benefit by employing talented people who would otherwise be unable to work. For example, a qualified specialist who is also a parent may be unable to stay away from home for a full workday but may be able to work a half day. Job sharing allows two such people to be employed as one. Although adjustment problems and benefit-costs concerns are challenging, a job-sharing arrangement can be good for all concerned.

10.5.4 Telecommuting

Telecommuting, sometimes called *flexiplace* or *cyber-commuting,* is a work arrangement that allows at least a portion of scheduled work hours to be completed outside of the office, facilitated by various forms of electronic communication and computer-mediated linkages to clients, patients, and a central office.

Telecommuting frees the jobholder from the normal constraints of commuting, fixed hours, and special work attire. The new vocabulary of telecommuting practices includes *hoteling*—where telecommuters come to the central office and use temporary office facilities, and virtual offices that include everything from an office at home to mobile workspace in automobiles.

Traditional health care workers who have little direct interaction with patients are the most appropriate candidates for telecommuting work arrangements. Additionally, as online and phone-based health care services—everything from Dial-a-Nurse to medical-claims consulting to phone-based psychological counseling—become increasingly common, health care workers can look for health care careers that are not bound to a specific geographic location.

Telecommuting options offer both advantages and disadvantages from a job design and management perspective. On the positive side are the freedom to be your own boss and the benefit of having more time for yourself. On the negative side are the possibilities of working too much, difficulty separating work and personal life, feelings of isolation, and loss of visibility for promotion. Managers, in turn, may be required to change their routines and procedures to accommodate the challenges of supervising people from a distance.

10.5.5 Independent Contracting and Part-Time Work

Among the developments in more flexible work arrangements is a growing use of **independent contracting,** where specific health care-related tasks or projects are assigned to outsiders rather than full-time workers. Cleaning, case management, administrative work, specialized technical work, and dozens of other activities make up the services health care organizations provide and are frequently completed by independent health care contractors.

When the project is completed, the contractor moves on to another assignment elsewhere. This benefits the organization by allowing for the hiring of special talents and expertise "as needed" and without the need to engage in a long-term employment relationship. For the independent contractors, it can allow flexibility and variety in their jobs while providing opportunities for personal choice in work-life balance.

Independent contractors are examples of the growing number of American workers who work on a part-time basis. In fact, employers are increasingly relying on contingency workers, or **permatemps**, who supplement the full-time workforce, often on a long-term basis. Because part-time or contingency workers can be easily hired, contracted with, and/or terminated in response to changing needs, many employers like the flexibility they offer in controlling labor costs and dealing with cyclical demand.[14] On the other hand, some worry that temporary workers lack the commitment of permanent workers and may lower productivity.

Perhaps the most controversial issue of the part-time work trend relates to the different treatment part-timers may receive from employers. They may be paid less than their full-time counterparts, and they often fail to receive important benefits, such as health care, life insurance, pension plans, and paid vacations. The social and economic implications of the growing role of part-time and contingent employment is an area that managers at all levels need to be mindful of and monitor carefully over the next decade as U.S. health care demands continue to grow and change.[15]

FOR EXAMPLE

Family-Friendly Health Care Organizations

Working Mother magazine (www.workingmorther.com) annually evaluates thousands of U.S. workplaces—including hundreds of health care organizations—using a rigorous application with more than 500 questions that focus on job design and worker motivation. Although the target audience for *Working Mother's* research is female workers with children, all health care professionals looking for dynamic organizations with flexible hours, enriching work environments, and motivating advancement opportunities can benefit from reviewing the magazine's 100 Best Places to Work list. For example, in 2004, the magazine identified Children's Memorial Hospital (www.childrensmemorial.org) in Chicago, Illinois, as an outstanding health care organization. In addition to family-friendly scheduling options (job sharing, flextime, and so on), Children's Memorial also offers a wide range of innovative childcare-specific services, including 80 hours of free in-home childcare, backup care, discounts at area centers, summer programs, and flexible spending accounts.

SELF-CHECK

- Identify and define **compressed workweek, flexible working hours, job sharing, telecommuting,** and **independent contracting.**
- Describe appropriate situations for various alternative work arrangements being used in today's health care workplace.
- List advantages and disadvantages of various alternative work arrangements.
- Compare various forms of telecommuting.
- Discuss the pros and cons of today's growing reliance on independent contractors and part-time employees.

SUMMARY

Motivating others not only makes for a more pleasant workplace and happier workers, doing so also benefits an organization's bottom line because of lower turnover rates and less need to dismiss workers. According the hierarchy of needs, the two-factor theory, and acquired needs theory, human needs can motivate people's actions and attitudes. People's choices to work hard are the basis of various process theories of motivation, which include equity theory, expectancy theory, and goal-setting theory. Managers can set up external forces—particularly positive reinforcement and punishment—to influence and motivate workers. Designing jobs that are appropriate for individual's skills and career goals is a popular, relatively inexpensive way to motivate employees. Job design in today's dynamic health care organizations requires managers to consider several alternative work arrangements such as telecommuting and job sharing.

KEY TERMS

Compressed workweek	Any work schedule that allows a full-time job to be completed in less than the standard 5 days of 8-hour shifts.
Continuous reinforcement schedule	Rewarding behavior each time a desired behavior occurs.
Core characteristics model	Richard Hackman's motivation theory with five core job characteristics, skill variety, task identity, task, significance, autonomy, and feedback from the job itself.

Deficit principle

In Maslow's needs theories, only an unsatisfied need—one for which a deficit exists—can be a motivator of behavior.

Equity theory

Motivation theory in which people who believe that they have been inequitably treated in comparison to others will try to eliminate the discomfort and restore a sense of equity to the situation.

Expectancy

In expectancy theory, a person's belief that working hard will result in a desired level of task performance being achieved.

Expectancy theory

Victor Vroom's motivation theory based on an individual's willingness to work hard at tasks important to the organization.

Extinction

In operant conditioning, anything that decreases the frequency of or eliminates an undesirable behavior by making the removal of a pleasant consequence contingent on its occurrence.

Flexible working hours

Any work schedule that gives employees some choice in the pattern of their daily work hours, also called *flexitime* or *flextime*.

Goal-setting theory

Edwin Locke's theory that clear, desirable performance targets (goals) can motivate.

Hygiene factors

In two-factor theory, things relating more to the work setting.

Independent contracting

Specific health care-related tasks or projects are assigned to outsiders rather than full-time workers.

Instrumentality

In expectancy theory, a person's belief that successful performance will be followed by rewards and other potential outcomes.

Intermittent reinforcement schedule

Rewarding behavior only periodically.

Job design

The process of creating or defining jobs by assigning specific work tasks to individuals and groups.

Job enlargement

The process of increasing task variety by combining two or more tasks that were previously assigned to separate workers.

Job enrichment

The process of building more opportunities for satisfaction into a job by expanding not just job scope but also job depth.

Job performance	The quantity and quality of tasks accomplished by an individual or group at work.
Job rotation	The process of increasing task variety by periodically shifting workers between jobs involving different task assignments.
Job sharing	One full-time job is split between two or more people.
Job simplification	The process of streamlining work procedures so that people work in well-defined and highly specialized tasks.
Law of contingent reinforcement	In operant conditioning, for a reward to have maximum reinforcing value, it must be delivered only if the desirable behavior is exhibited.
Law of effect	In behavior reinforcement theory, behavior that results in a pleasant outcome is likely to be repeated; behavior that results in an unpleasant outcome is not likely to be repeated.
Law of immediate reinforcement	In operant conditioning, the more immediate the delivery of a reward after the occurrence of a desirable behavior, the greater the reinforcing value of the reward.
Motivation	Forces within individuals that account for the level, direction, and persistence of effort they expend at work.
Need for achievement	In acquired needs theory, the desire to do something better or more efficiently, to solve problems, or to master complex tasks.
Need for affiliation	In acquired needs theory, the desire to establish and maintain friendly and warm relations with other people.
Need for power	In acquired needs theory, the desire to control other people, to influence their behavior, or to be responsible for them.
Needs	Unfulfilled physiological or psychological desires of an individual.
Negative reinforcement	In operant conditioning, anything that increases the frequency of or strengthens desirable behavior by making the avoidance of an unpleasant consequence contingent upon its occurrence.
Operant conditioning	B. F. Skinner's concept of learning by reinforcement.

Perceived negative inequity   In equity theory, a condition people who perceive negative inequity tend to reduce their work efforts to compensate for missing rewards.

Permatemps   Long-term temporary workers who supplement the full-time workforce.

Positive reinforcement   In operant conditioning, anything that strengthens or increases the frequency of desirable behavior by making a pleasant consequence contingent on its occurrence.

Process theory   Motivational theory focuses on how people actually make choices to work hard or not, based on their individual preferences, the available rewards, and possible work outcomes.

Progression principle   In Maslow's hierarchy of needs, a need at one level does not become activated until the next lower level need is already satisfied.

Punishment   In operant conditioning, anything that decreases the frequency of or eliminates an undesirable behavior by making an unpleasant consequence contingent on its occurrence.

Reinforcement theory   Motivational theory that explains human behavior as a result of one's external environment.

Satisfier factors   In two-factor theory, things relating to the nature of a job itself.

Shaping   The process of creating a new behavior by the positive reinforcement of successive approximations to it.

Telecommuting   A work arrangement that allows at least a portion of scheduled work hours to be completed outside of the office, facilitated by various forms of electronic communication and computer-mediated linkages to clients, patients, and a central office; sometimes called *flexiplace* or *cyber-commuting*.

Two-factor theory   Frederick Herzberg's motivation theory that focuses on the nature of the job itself and the work setting.

Valence   In expectancy theory, the value a person assigns to the possible rewards and other work-related outcomes.

ASSESS YOUR UNDERSTANDING

Go to www.wiley.com/college/Lombardi to evaluate your knowledge of the basics of motivating to meet needs.
Measure your learning by comparing pretest and post-test results.

Summary Questions

1. Which of the following statements about motivation is true?
   (a) Managers who lead through motivation create conditions under which others feel inspired to work hard.
   (b) Managers who understand what motivates people can appreciate where staff are coming from.
   (c) Managers can better direct the energies of staff when they understand motivation.
   (d) All of the above

2. All the needs-based theories on motivation contend that needs cause
   (a) perceptions that inspire attitudes and beliefs.
   (b) tensions that influence attitudes and behaviors.
   (c) desires that encourage action.
   (d) passions that inspire loyalty.

3. In Maslow's hierarchy of needs, the deficit principle states that a need at one level does not become activated until the next lower need is already satisfied. True or false?

4. In two-factor theory of motivation, a satisfier factor would be
   (a) the sense of achievement you get from doing your job.
   (b) the salary and bonus you receive.
   (c) the relationship you have with your boss.
   (d) the length of your lunch break.

5. The process theories of motivation all focus on an employee's choice to work hard (or not) based on
   (a) individual responsibilities, implied rewards, and desired job promotion.
   (b) individual rewards, available options, and potential job growth.
   (c) individual preferences, available rewards, and possible work outcomes.
   (d) none of these.

6. In expectancy theory, the free motivating factors (expectancy, instrumentality, and valence) have a multiplier effect, which means a zero for any factor results in zero motivation. True or false?

7. Goals are useful in the workplace because they clarify hiring strategies and establish a frame of reference for worker retention. True or false?

8. Punishment can be an effective management tool. True or false?

9. In operant conditioning, anything that decreases the frequency of or eliminates an undesirable behavior by making an unpleasant consequence contingent on its occurrence is

    (a) punishment.

    (b) extinction.

    (c) negative reinforcement.

    (d) positive reinforcement.

10. In order for positive reinforcement to be effective, rewards can be given when a desirable behavior is partially exhibited. True or false?

11. Job simplification allows work tasks to be narrowly defined and makes training easier. True or false?

12. Which of the following situations is an example of job rotation?

    (a) Workers moving among various job stations during the workday

    (b) Flexible scheduling that enables each work to set their workday

    (c) Two part-time workers sharing one full-time position

    (d) An interdepartmental team that meets weekly to discuss differing work experiences

13. In the core characteristics model of job design, the degree to which a job has substantial impact on the lives of others in the organization or the external environment is known as

    (a) task identity.

    (b) autonomy.

    (c) skill variety.

    (d) task significance.

14. Job enrichment can be accomplished through vertical loading, which gives managers greater opportunity to assign a diversity of tasks to staff. True or false?

15. Flexible schedule is becoming a more common work choice in health care departments with

    (a) less interaction with patients.

    (b) more interaction with patients.

    (c) more union membership.

    (d) less union membership.

16. An alternative work arrangement in which a portion of scheduled work hours are completed outside the office is know as

    (a) job sharing.

    (b) flextime scheduling.

(c) independent contracting.

(d) telecommuting.

17. Long-term temporary workers are sometimes paid less than their full-time counterparts, and they often do not receive health care benefits. True or false?

Review Questions

1. Based on two-factor theory, which type of factors must a manager address in order to improve motivation?

2. According to acquired needs theory, a shift nurse who has a strong desire to influence others and take responsibility for situations and projects has a high level of which type of need?

3. Place Maslow's five levels of need in order, from low-level needs to high-level needs: esteem, safety, physiological, self-actualization, and social.

4. A medical billing center manager implements a policy in which employees can come to work 2 hours early on Fridays and then leave 2 hours earlier at the end of the day. Based on Herzberg's two-factor theory, which factor is the manager focusing on?

5. Which need in Maslow's hierarchy of needs is a manager addressing when he makes an effort to celebrate each staff member's birthday?

6. If a worker perceives an inequity in the workplace, he may become so uncomfortable with the situation that he will attempt to restore equality. What are two examples of actions that can deal with perceived inequity?

7. Setting goals can be effective motivation. What should manager and employee do in order to make goal setting effective?

8. When a manager makes a special effort to provide positive feedback every day on appropriate patient charting, the manager is relying on which law or positive reinforcement?

9. What are the benefits of using a continuous reinforcement schedule or an intermittent reinforcement schedule?

10. Punishment can be done poorly or well. What are two strategies to effective deliver punishment?

11. The third-shift manager at a 24-hour convenience clinic decides to save her organization's money by eliminating one front desk person during her shift and having nurses take on additional admission tasks. What job design alternative is the manager utilizing?

12. The core characteristics model of job design focuses on five key job characteristics. Which characteristic pays attention to an employee's freedom and independence?

13. Simplified jobs make training easier and allow for less managerial supervision. However, these jobs also have some downsides. What is a downside of a simplified job?

14. Compressed workweeks are becoming a popular scheduling choice in many health care organizations. What are some disadvantages of this type of work arrangement?

15. Telecommuting has advantages and disadvantages for today's health care organizations. What are some pros and cons of this type of alternative work arrangement?

Applying This Chapter

1. Lisa, an LPN on your team, is an average worker, but you sense she has greater potential. Lisa has been on-staff for about 3 months and largely keeps to herself. She doesn't seem particularly proud of the work she does, but she is satisfied with her salary and benefits. How might you use Maslow's progression principle to identify ways to motivate Lisa to achieve a higher level of work?

2. Byron has worked in the intact desk at an emergency room for 5 years. He has never received a promotion, although he has received annual cost-of-living raises. Overall, his work attitude is "Why try? I get paid the same amount no matter how many patients I interact with." Using Vroom's expectancy theory (and the equation $M = E \times I \times V$), what might be affecting Byron's performance?

3. How might the manager of the pediatric unit at a research hospital utilize shaping to positively reinforce the training and skill development of a new nursing intern?

4. The manager of a student health clinic is asked to work more job rotations into the job designs of his staff. What are some things the manager should consider?

5. To give your staff of eight full-time nurses greater flexibility and opportunity to spend more time at home with their young families, you decide to utilize job sharing. What are some possible job-sharing arrangements you might consider trying?

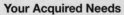
Your Acquired Needs

Part of what makes McClelland's acquired needs theory so powerful is that the work environments and job responsibilities can—and in fact, should—be tailored to meet workers' specific needs. Consider the three types of needs described in section 10.1.3. Of achievement, power, or affiliation, which is the strongest need you have? What type of position would be most likely to satisfy your greatest need?

Do Your Job Goals Motivate You?

According to the goal-setting theory of motivation, appropriately formulated and presented goals can lead workers to deliver outstanding performance on a daily basis. Evaluate the job-related goals of your current health care position based on the five-point criteria suggested by the goal-setting theory. Are your job-related goals specifically worded, challenging, built on employee acceptance and buy-in, prioritized in terms of relative importance, and linked to clear rewards? (If you don't have job-related goals for a current position, review the goals of the Pharmacy Residency program at Mercy and Unity Hospitals of Minnesota at www.mercy-unity.com/ahs/mercyunity.nsf/page/PharmGenMedRotation.)

Four Ways to Reinforce

As the shift manager of the critical care nursing staff at a small community hospital, your greatest managerial challenge centers around two highly experienced nurses who have frequently been passed over for promotions due to lack of interpersonal skills. These senior nurses frequently disregard new procedures you've been trying to implement; they also undermine your authority by engaging in overly critical conversations with newer staff members. How can you utilize the four types of behavior modification—positive reinforcement, negative reinforcement, punishment, and extinction—to attempt to modify the nurses' behaviors?

Alternative Designs

As the leader of a group of four students assigned to create a group presentation about current health care employment trends, discuss the pros and cons of dividing up work for the presentation based on the job design alternatives discussed in this chapter, specifically, job simplification, job rotation, job enlargement, and job enrichment.

Which Alternatives Suit You?

In today's dynamic workplace, even entry-level health care workers are given opportunity to work under the alternative work arrangements described in section 10.5. Nine-to-five, Monday through Friday jobs are rare in health care, so before you assume that you'll have a "regular" job, take time to consider each of the alternatives that section 10.5 discusses. Considering these alternative arrangements can open up a world of additional job opportunities. How would a compressed workweek fit with your lifestyle and commitments? How might you utilize flexible working hours or telecommuting, if either option were available to you? Does independent contracting have any appeal to you?

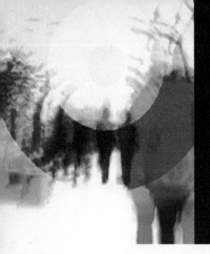

11

CHANGE OF LEADERSHIP IN THE WORKPLACE
Guiding Others through Challenging Times

Starting Point

Go to www.wiley.com/college/Lombardi to assess your knowledge of the basics of leadership transfer.
Determine where you need to concentrate your effort.

What You'll Learn in This Chapter

▲ The characteristics of positive change leadership
▲ Phases of planned change
▲ Commonly used change strategies
▲ Reasons for resisting change
▲ Reasons why people and groups resist change
▲ Various forms of stress

After Studying This Chapter, You'll Be Able To

▲ Analyze reasons for change
▲ Examine common change goals
▲ Apply strategies for effective change leadership
▲ Demonstrate responses to change-resistant individuals and groups
▲ Practice healthy responses to stress

Goals and Outcomes

▲ Master the terminology and tools related to change leadership
▲ Compare change leadership strategies
▲ Choose appropriate change leadership strategies
▲ Respond effectively to change resistance
▲ Select and practice effective stress management techniques
▲ Evaluate stress management techniques

INTRODUCTION

Health care organizations must be prepared not only to change, but to change continuously and in the face of ever-present uncertainties. Health care managers are in a powerful position to help lead a positive response to change. In particular, the planned change process offers managers multiple opportunities to inspire effective responses to change. Change strategies—including force-coercion, rational persuasion, and shared power strategies—are all ways to introduce and encourage change. Some individuals and groups may resist change, but effective managers can respond to concerns and utilize interventions to further enhance the change process. An effective managerial response to change includes an understanding of the role stress plays in a staff's work experience.

11.1 Understanding Change Leadership

The world of health care is undergoing significant transformation. Various regulatory changes and changes in the patient base, how health care services are delivered, and the financial structures that support the health care industry are only a few of the innovations that managers must address. Although change is not necessarily negative, many new managers may perceive it in a negative light because it confronts them with the unknown, requires them to change daily routines and readjust work goals.

In addition to public scrutiny, patient expectation, and patient demand, two additional external dynamics in the current health care environment affect managers and their staffs.

▲ **Shrinking financial resources.** The cliché of "having to do more with less" continues to apply throughout the health care industry. As a manager, become familiar with the fiscal resources available in your organization and balance those against departmental needs.

▲ **Government intervention.** With the advent of federal government intervention in health care, along with state and local regulatory agencies, managers must be keenly aware of regulatory compliance requirements and policy administration. Make a concerted effort to understand all regulatory issues and government intervention activities as they affect your organization and, what is more important, share pertinent information with your manager and your staff about the extent that legislative and regulatory compliance affects your department.

11.1.1 Responding Positively to Change

Organizations and their managers must continually innovate and adapt to new situations if they are to survive and prosper over the long run. A **change leader**

Figure 11-1

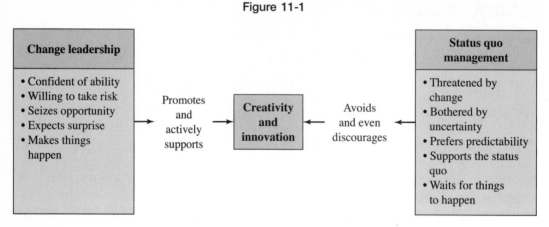

Change leadership versus status-quo management.

is a person or group who takes leadership responsibility for changing the existing pattern of behavior of another person or social system. A key part of every manager's job is to lead change in the work setting. This requires being alert to situations or to people needing change, being open to good ideas, and being able to support the implementation of new ideas in actual practice.

Figure 11-1 contrasts a change leader with a status-quo manager. A change leader is forward-looking, proactive, and embraces new ideas. A status-quo manager is backward-looking, reactive, and comfortable with habit. Obviously, the new workplace demands change leadership.

As sections 4.1 and 4.2 discuss, everyone in a team has the potential to lead by serving group needs for task and maintenance activities. A similar notion applies when leading change in an organization—the responsibilities for change leadership are ideally distributed and shared from top to bottom.

In **top-down change**, strategic and comprehensive changes are initiated with the goal of comprehensive impact on the organization and its performance capabilities. But change that is driven from the top runs the risk of being perceived as insensitive to the needs of lower-level personnel. It can easily fail if implementation suffers from excessive resistance and insufficient commitments to change. The success of top-down change is usually determined by the willingness of middle- and lower-level workers to actively support top-management initiatives.

Bottom-up change is also important. Here, the initiatives for change come from people throughout an organization and are supported by the efforts of middle- and lower-level managers acting as change agents. Bottom-up change is essential to organizational innovation and is very useful in terms of adapting operations and technologies to the changing requirements of work. Managers make bottom-up change possible by empowering staff and actively being involved in challenges staff faces.

11.1.2 Identifying Forces and Targets for Change

Planned change occurs as a result of the specific efforts of a change leader. Planned change is a direct response to someone perceiving a **performance gap**, or a discrepancy between the desired and actual state of affairs. Performance gaps may represent problems to be resolved or opportunities to be explored. Performance gaps and the impetus for change can arise from a variety of external forces, including market competition, economic conditions, government laws and regulations, technological developments, and social forces.[1]

As a health care organization's general and specific environments develop and change over time, the organization must adapt as well. Any change in one part of the organization as a complex system—perhaps a change initiated in response to one or more of the external forces just identified—can create the need for change in another part of the system.

Internal or organizational targets for change are highly interrelated and can include[2]

- ▲ **tasks:** The nature of work as represented by organizational mission, objectives, and strategy and the job designs for individuals and groups;
- ▲ **people:** The attitudes and competencies of the employees and the human resource systems that support them;
- ▲ **culture:** The value system for the organization as a whole and the norms guiding individual and group behavior;
- ▲ **technology:** The operations and information technology used to support job designs, arrange workflows, and integrate people and machines in systems;
- ▲ **structure:** The configuration of the organization as a complex system, including its design features and lines of authority and communications.

11.1.3 Identifying Goals and Processes for Organizational Development

In the world of management consulting, **organization development**, or OD, is a comprehensive approach to planned organizational change that involves applying behavioral science in a systematic and long-range effort to improve organizational effectiveness.[3]

Organization development helps organizations cope with environmental and other pressures for change, while also improving their internal problem-solving capabilities. Organization development, in this sense, brings the quest for continuous improvement to the planned change process.

In organization development, two types of goals are pursued simultaneously:

- ▲ **Outcome goals** focus on task accomplishments.
- ▲ **Process goals** focus on the way people work together.

Figure 11-2

Organization Development Process

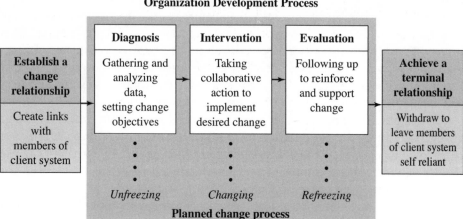

Organization development and the planned change process.

The inclusion of process goals strongly differentiates OD from more general attempts at planned change in organizations. Think of OD as "planned change plus," with the *plus* meaning that change is accomplished in such a way that organization members develop a capacity for continued self-renewal—that is, OD tries to achieve change while helping people become more active and self-reliant, so they can continue changing in the future.

Another aspect that makes OD unique is its commitment to strong humanistic values and established principles of behavioral science. OD is committed to improving organizations through freedom of choice, shared power, and self-reliance—and by capitalizing on what is known about human behavior in organizations.

Figure 11-2 presents a general model of OD and shows its relationship to Lewin's three phases of planned change (see section 11.2).

A traditional OD process consists of the following steps:

1. **Establish a change relationship.** An outside consultant or facilitator connects with members of an organization or team for the purpose of facilitating change.
2. **Diagnosis.** The consultant, manager, and team members gather and analyze data to assess the situation and set appropriate change objectives. This phase of the OD process can help with unfreezing as well as pinpointing appropriate directions for action.
3. **Intervention.** The consultant and/or manager actively intervene, pursuing change objectives through a variety of specific interventions, a number of which section 11.5 discusses.

> ## FOR EXAMPLE
>
> ### A Change Management Leader at Clarian Health
>
> In 2002, Clarian Health Partners (www.clarian.org) of Indianapolis upgraded its organization-wide software suite. The upgrade promised to help Clarian Health better manage hospital data, streamline business processes, and reduce costs. Because previous upgrades had met with resistance, Clarian Health appointed a well-respected peer to serve as the project's Change Management Leader. This individual's sole responsibility for several months prior to and after the software change was to champion the project, emphasize positive aspects, recognize team members for their contributions and achievements, and recruit others to serve as "Change Agents." Through a series of presentations hosted by the Change Management Leader at Clarian's 20-plus locations, more than 900 employees were introduced to the new software in a positive manner.

4. **Evaluation.** The consultant and/or manager examine the process to determine if things are proceeding as desired and if further action is needed.
5. **Achieve a terminal relationship.** Eventually, the consultant or facilitator leaves the client able to function on its own.

If OD has been done well, the system and its members should be better prepared to manage their ongoing need for self-renewal and development.

SELF-CHECK

- Identify and define **change leader, planned change, performance gap,** and **organizational development.**
- Describe two major external dynamics that impact change.
- Compare characteristics of top-down change and bottom-up change.
- List common targets for change.
- Compare characteristics of outcome goals and process goals.
- Discuss five steps in the organizational development process (OD) for planned change.

11.2 Leading during Planned Change

Change is much more likely to be successful when people are ready for it. In particular, planned change has little chance for long-term success unless people are open to doing things differently. Managers can give the process of planned change shape and structure by breaking the process into distinct phases and utilizing various proactive strategies during each phase of the change process.

11.2.1 The Phases of Planned Change

Psychologist Kurt Lewin recommends that managers view any planned change effort as a three-phase process, as shown in Figure 11-3.[4]

Figure 11-3

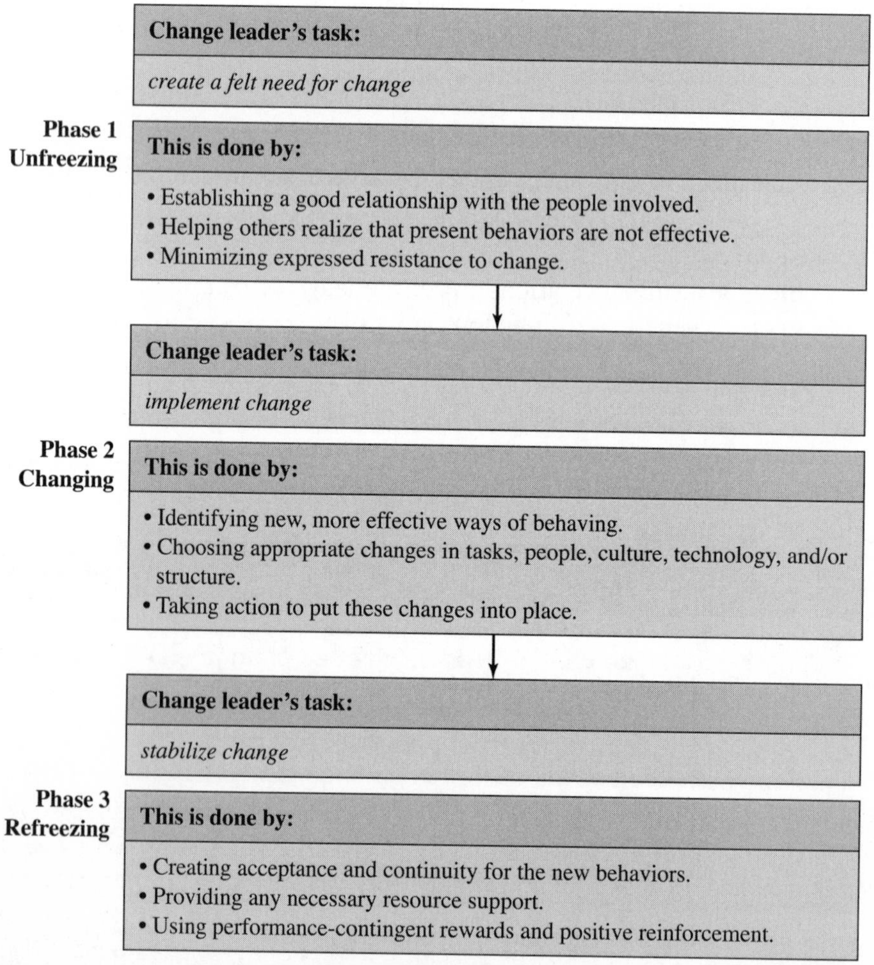

Phase 1 Unfreezing

Change leader's task:

create a felt need for change

This is done by:

• Establishing a good relationship with the people involved.
• Helping others realize that present behaviors are not effective.
• Minimizing expressed resistance to change.

Phase 2 Changing

Change leader's task:

implement change

This is done by:

• Identifying new, more effective ways of behaving.
• Choosing appropriate changes in tasks, people, culture, technology, and/or structure.
• Taking action to put these changes into place.

Phase 3 Refreezing

Change leader's task:

stabilize change

This is done by:

• Creating acceptance and continuity for the new behaviors.
• Providing any necessary resource support.
• Using performance-contingent rewards and positive reinforcement.

Three phases of planned organizational change.

According to Lewin, the planned change process can be described as a process of unfreezing, changing, and refreezing:

▲ During the **unfreezing stage**, the need for change is recognized and a situation is prepared for change. Several factors can facilitate unfreezing: environmental pressures for change, declining performance, the recognition of problems or opportunities, and the observation of behavioral models that display alternative approaches. When handled well, conflict can actually be an important unfreezing force in organizations. Conflict can help people break old habits and recognize alternative ways of thinking about or doing things.

▲ In the **changing stage**, something new takes place in a system, and change is actually implemented. This is the point at which managers initiate changes in such organizational targets as tasks, people, culture, technology, and structure. Ideally, any change is done in response to a good diagnosis of a problem and a careful examination of alternatives. However, many managers enter the changing phase prematurely, quickly changing things and creating resistance to change. When managers implement change before people feel a need for it, there is an increased likelihood of failure.

▲ During the **refreezing stage**, a manager is concerned about stabilizing the change and creating the conditions for its long-term continuity. Refreezing is accomplished by appropriate rewards for performance, positive reinforcement, and providing necessary resource support. Managers must also evaluate results carefully, provide feedback to the people involved, and make any required modifications in the original change. When refreezing is done poorly, changes are forgotten or abandoned over time. When refreezing is done well, change can be more long lasting.

The first two phases of the planned change process can be considered the *proactive phases* of change. During these phases, leaders can make plans and motivate staff participation in making the change happen.

Many health care leaders make the fundamental mistake of entering the change process without proper planning and without enlisting staff support. A more progressive approach is to set a course for change and enter a process of garnering staff support by proactively defining the benefits of the imminent change.

11.2.2 Focusing on Benefits

Early on, managers need to completely delineate the benefits of the proposed project or new process leading to change. Managers can hold a discussion with staff and encourage active participation. Along the way, managers identify benefits, both apparent and underlying, and relate them to the change process. Benefits may include more expedient patient service, improved operational flow, or obvious cost savings.

FOR EXAMPLE

Three-Phase Leadership Rollout at Lenior Memorial

In 2002, Lenoir Memorial Hospital (www.lenoirmemorial.org) determined that in order to meet its mission of becoming the "provider of choice in eastern North Carolina," the organization needed to introduce a new leadership model and provide dynamic ongoing leadership training to its employees. Over the next 2 years, new leadership training was developed and delivered to more than 65 executives, directors, managers, and supervisors in three distinct phases. During Phase 1, a select group of directors mapped out the process and debated specific environmental challenges. Phase 2 featured a series of "leadership development intensives," off-site exercises aimed at fostering collaboration and decision making between managers and within work teams. In Phase 3, an outside consulting firm evaluated individual and organizational performance and changes; the consultants also provided recommendations for further leadership training.

During this discussion, managers and the group try to identify less apparent benefits, including

- ▲ time saved by implementing new processes;
- ▲ energy saved by more efficient processes;
- ▲ a competitive edge that the organization may gain;
- ▲ a safer working environment;
- ▲ reduced boredom;
- ▲ increases in organizational progress (which helps ensure organizational stability and individual job security);
- ▲ elimination of hurdles or headaches associated with outmoded or cumbersome processes.

By brainstorming the preceding (and other) nonapparent benefits with the group, a savvy manager can add reality and truth to the change management discussion.

11.2.3 Planning in Detail

Another early objective in the planned change process is to delineate a plan for change. Managers can construct a plan of action by answering the following questions:

- ▲ **Why** must the change plan take place? Use the benefits identified by the group as the major catalysts for change.

▲ **When** will the major events in the change plan occur? Include a time sequence of the start, midpoint, and finished product.

▲ **How** will the plan take shape? Visualize the steps needed to implement the change.

▲ **Who** will make the plan happen? Include an appropriate discussion of group and individual responsibilities.

Managers need to also discuss the meaning of any plan. First, the leader and the group discuss what the change dynamic means in the near-term in terms of potential implementation problems, variations in daily routines, and any other pertinent topics. Second, the long-term meaning of the change is discussed fully, replete with a reiteration of benefits, relevance to the big picture of the organization and its relationship with its patient constituency, and other positive probabilities.

Too often, change management discussions focus only on short-term pain and not on long-term gain. Both components must be considered and especially examined sequentially, so that all members of the group recognize that the initial discomfort can ultimately lead to a better way of doing things.

11.2.4 Dealing with Nonplayers

During the proactive phase of a planned change, managers also need to properly manage **nonplayers**, those team members who do not agree with the change and even work against it. Typically, nonplayers use an assortment of verbal contentious challenges to derail the change process.

Fortunately, proactive managers can respond to common nonplayer complaints effectively, for example:

Nonplayer ploy: *"That will never work!"*

Manager response: *"Well, then tell us specifically what will work."*

Nonplayer ploy: *"I have got a problem with this."*

Manager response: *"Redefining problems is useless. Give us a solution that might be useful to achieve our goals."*

Nonplayer ploy: *"We tried that before, but it did not work."*

Manager response: *"We are dealing with the present. How can this work now?"*

Nonplayer ploy: *"With all this change, maybe I should find another job."*

Manager response: *"I will accept your resignation immediately because change will be constant for years to come in health care."*

As these responses indicate, managers can use three principles in managing the nonplayer's resistance.

▲ **Issue a direct, tactful challenge to the complaining nonplayer.** Do not allow the nonplayer to complain or cast dispersions on group plans without contributing a better idea. The only individual more detrimental to a health care organization than a nonplayer in this regard is a manager who allows negativity to become acceptable behavior without holding the nonplayer accountable for constructive contribution, not just destructive criticism.

▲ **Use plural pronouns, such as *we* and *us*.** Doing so encourages the group to recognize that the nonplayer is questioning the entire group's capability, not just yours. This encourages other team members to become accountable for group direction and goal formation and enlists their participation in countering ill-conceived negativity.

▲ **Use bottom-line vernacular.** Use words such as *useless* and *immediately,* so that the nonplayers are clear in their understanding that game playing, dissention, and group denigration are intolerable when striving for group achievement.

A final component of the proactive stage is your display of natural emotions. Don't be a Pollyanna or Jack Armstrong-esque with an unwarranted positive outlook in the change process; show honest emotion. The group usually recognizes that a manager is in the same boat as they are and will continue to "row" accordingly.

SELF-CHECK

- Identify and define the phases of planned change: **unfreezing, changing,** and **refreezing.**
- Describe activities for each of the three phases of planned change.
- Discuss the importance of focusing on benefits and planning in detail during the planned change process.
- Compare nonplayers and active team members.
- List strategies to effectively respond to nonplayer complaints.

11.3 Exploring Change Strategies

Change leaders use various approaches when trying to get others to adopt a desired change. Three common change strategies—force-coercion, rational persuasion, and shared power—are graphically depicted in Figure 11-4.

Figure 11-4

Change Strategy	Power Bases	Managerial Behavior	Likely Results
Force-Coercion Using position power to create change by decree and formal authority	Legitimacy Rewards Punishments	*Direct forcing* and unilateral action *Political maneuvering* and indirect action	Temporary Fast compliance
Rational Persuasion Creating change through rational persuasion and empirical argument	Expertise	*Informational efforts* using credible knowledge, demonstrated facts, and logical argument	
Shared Power Developing support for change through personal values and commitments	Reference	*Participative efforts* to share power and involve others in planning and implementing change	Slow Longer term internalization

Change strategies and their managerial implications.

11.3.1 Force-Coercion

A **force-coercion strategy** uses the power of legitimacy, rewards, and punishments as the primary inducements to change. As Figure 11-4 shows, the likely outcomes of force-coercion are immediate compliance but little commitment.

Managers can pursue force-coercion in at least two ways, both of which can be commonly observed in health care organizations:

▲ In a **direct forcing strategy**, a manager takes direct and unilateral action to "command" that change take place. Direct forcing requires someone to exercise formal authority or legitimate power (see section 9.2), offer special rewards, and/or threaten punishment.

▲ In **political maneuvering**, a manager works indirectly to gain special advantage over other people and thereby make them change. Political maneuvering involves bargaining, obtaining control of important resources, or granting small favors.

In both versions, the force-coercion strategy produces limited results. Although managers can implement this strategy rather quickly, most people respond to this strategy out of fear of punishment or hope for a reward, resulting in only temporary compliance with the manager's desires. The new behavior continues only so long as the opportunity for rewards and punishments is present. For this reason, force-coercion is most useful during the unfreezing phase of change as a device that helps people break old patterns of behavior and gain initial impetus to try new ones.

A manager who seeks to create change through force-coercion believes that people who run things are basically motivated by self-interest and by what the situation offers in terms of potential personal gains or losses. The manager capitalizes on formal authority, rewards, and punishments. Additionally, a manager relying on force-coercion strategies exploits weaknesses and works extensively to build political alliances within the organization.[5]

11.3.2 Rational Persuasion

A **rational persuasion strategy** attempts to bring about change through persuasion backed by special knowledge, data, and rational argument. The likely outcome is eventual compliance with reasonable commitment. Rational persuasion is an informational strategy that assumes that rational people are guided by facts, reason, and self-interest when deciding whether to support a change.

A manager using rational persuasion must convince others that the cost-benefit value of a planned change is high and that it will leave them better off than before. Convincing others depends to a large extent on the presence of expert power (see section 9.2), which can come directly from the manager or can be obtained from consultants and other outside experts. When successful, a rational persuasion strategy is especially helpful during the unfreezing and refreezing phase of change. Although slower than force-coercion, rational persuasion tends to result in longer lasting and more internalized change.

A manager utilizing rational persuasion believes that people are inherently rational and are guided by reason in their actions and decision making. After the manager demonstrates that a specific course of action is in someone's self-interest, he or she assumes that reason and rationality will cause the person to adopt it. Thus, the manager uses information and facts to communicate the essential desirability of change. If the logic is sound, the manager is confident that others will adopt and support the proposed change.

11.3.3 Shared Power Strategies

A **shared power strategy** engages people in a collaborative process of identifying values, assumptions, and goals from which support for change will naturally emerge. The process is slow, but it is likely to yield high commitment. This approach is based on empowerment and is highly participative in nature. Shared power strategies rely on involving others in examining personal needs and values, group norms, and operating goals as they relate to the issues at hand. Power is shared by the manager and other people as they work together to develop a new consensus to support needed change.

Managers using shared power as an approach to planned change need reference power (see section 9.2) and related skills to work effectively with other people in group situations. They must be comfortable allowing others to participate

FOR EXAMPLE

Leading the Way through Technological Change

In an effort to catch potential errors in medication distribution, Jewish Hospital of Louisville, Kentucky (www.jhhs.org), became one of the first health care organizations in the United States to implement technology that relies on patient's wristbands with scannable bar codes and in-room touch-screen for comprehensive medication monitoring. To ease the organization through the transition to the computerized system, Jewish Hospital rolled out the new technology over an 18-month process, first implementing technology on surgical floors, then adding the service to long-term medical floors, and finally extending it to all clinic and out-patient facilities. In addition to medication monitoring, Jewish Hospital is considering enhancing the technology with additional capabilities over the next several years. Possible services to be rolled out in the future include intersite medical records transmission and electronic charting.

in making decisions that affect the planned change and the way it is implemented. Because shared power strategies entail a high level of involvement, they are often quite time consuming but result in long-lasting and internalized change.

A manager who shares power begins by recognizing that people have varied needs and complex motivations. He or she believes people behave as they do because of sociocultural norms and commitments to the expectations of others. Changes in organizations are understood to inevitably involve changes in attitudes, values, skills, and significant relationships, not just changes in knowledge, information, or intellectual rationales for action and practice. Thus, when seeking to change others, the manager is sensitive to the way group pressures can support or inhibit change. In working with people, managers make every attempt to gather opinions, identify feelings and expectations, and incorporate this information fully into the change process.

SELF-CHECK

- Identify and define **force-coercion strategy, rational persuasion strategy,** and **shared power strategy.**
- Compare the two force-coercion approaches: direct forcing and political maneuvering.
- Discuss characteristics of the three major change strategies.
- Describe appropriate workplace situations or environments for each of the three change strategies.

11.4 Resisting Change

Change typically brings with it resistance. When people resist change, they are defending something that is important and that appears to them as threatened by the attempted change.

Managers often view resistance as something that must be overcome in order for change to be successful. This is not always correct or helpful. **Resistance** is better viewed as feedback that indicates something can be done to achieve a better "fit" between the planned change, the situation, and the people involved.

Managers need to realize that several **group emotions** are triggered by change. These emotional responses can pervade an entire health care team and cause a group to resist—and even work against—the proposed change. As a health care leader, you must understand these emotions, their potential deleterious impact, and, most important, pragmatic approaches required to manage these emotions toward progressive change.

11.4.1 Understanding Why People Resist Change

Numerous reasons exist for why people in organizations resist planned change. Some of the more common include

- ▲ **disrupted habits:** Feeling upset when old ways of doing things can't be followed;
- ▲ **loss of confidence:** Feeling incapable of performing well under the new ways of doing things;
- ▲ **loss of control:** Feeling that things are being done *to* you rather than *by* or *with* you;
- ▲ **poor timing:** Feeling overwhelmed by the situation or that things are moving too fast;
- ▲ **work overload:** Not having the physical or psychic energy to commit to the change.

In addition to the preceding, *fear* is probably the most prevalent emotion cited by health care leaders as a major factor in the change process. Nearly everyone experiences uncertainty—fear of the unknown—when they don't understand what is happening or what is coming next.

Another prominent fear for steady players—who often represent the silent majority of a team—is fear of regression. Steady players often view any change with apprehension if the proposed change is not completely presented in a fashion that highlights its improvement value to the status quo. Managers can address fear of regression proactively by recognizing that most steady staff members eventually accept change, provided it is not simply change for the sake of change. As a leader, you have a responsibility to identify how the proposed change brings about new benefits for patients, your organization, your team, and individual team member. See section 11.2 for more ideas to address this type of fear.

Low-performing staff members often fear having to do more work. Change usually requires increased effort and higher contribution from all staff members. For low-performing staff, increased performance demands are ultimately threatening, because their current level of nonperformance and resistant behavior will be exacerbated by more pressure for optimum performance and an accelerated pace of action. Put bluntly, the need for change presents a great opportunity for low-performing staff to be exposed as incompetent, noncontributory, and detrimental to the provision of stellar health care.

If job descriptions and other substantiating criteria (see section 5.1) are in place for assessing performance, the change dynamic can provide an excellent opportunity to appraise the low-performing employee's contributions and provide the impetus for termination. This strategy is "rightsizing the right way," because successful health care organizations can only afford to employ individuals who are motivated, competent, and aware that the organization is more important in the work scheme than individual preferences, dissenting opinion, and other me-first mentalities.

11.4.2 Responding to Change Resistance

After a manager recognizes and understands resistance to change, he or she can deal with it in various ways:

▲ **Education and communication:** Manager uses discussions, presentations, and demonstrations to educate people beforehand about a change.

▲ **Participation and involvement:** Manager allows others to contribute ideas and help design and implement the change.

▲ **Facilitation and support:** Manager provides encouragement and training, actively listens to problems and complaints, and helps others to overcome performance pressures.

▲ **Facilitation and agreement:** Manager provides incentives that appeal to those who are actively resisting or ready to resist. With this approach, the manager typically makes trade-offs in exchange for assurances that change will not be blocked.

▲ **Manipulation and co-optation:** Manager tries to influence others covertly by providing information selectively and structuring events in favor of the desired change.

▲ **Explicit and implicit coercion:** Manager forces people to accept change by threatening resistors with a variety of undesirable consequences if they do not go along as planned.[6]

Obviously, the last two approaches carry great risk and potential for negative side effects.

FOR EXAMPLE

Small-Scale Changes on a Trial Basis

In 2005, Trillium Health Centre (www.trilliumhealthcentre.org) in Mississauga, Ontario, Canada, set an aggressive goal for itself—to reduce the number of cardiac arrests by 60% within its facilities. To meet this goal, Trillium created Rapid Response Teams and new protocols that require specially trained RNs and respiratory therapists to collaborate with ward nurses to quickly assess patients and implement life-saving procedures. What made the change at Trillium unique was that rather than implementing Rapid Response Teams throughout dozens of departments and facilities, the plan has been introduced on a small, year-long trial basis in only four departments (GI, Respiratory, Oncology and General Internal Medicine). The more manageable rollout of the plan is allowing Trillium to more carefully monitor and adjust the procedures.

SELF-CHECK

- Identify and define **resistance** and **group emotion.**
- Discuss common reasons for resisting change.
- List fears related to change resistance.
- Describe strategies for responding to change resistance.

11.5 Incorporating Organization Development Interventions

The foundations of organization development include respect for people and a commitment to their full participation in self-directed change processes. This is the very definition of employee involvement in action. OD rallies an organization's staff through teamwork and in support of constructive change.

This rallying process is evident in the various OD **interventions,** or activities that are initiated to directly facilitate the change processes. (See section 11.1.3 for more information about where interventions fit into the overall OD process.)

The following sections cover the most common types of interventions.

11.5.1 Organization-wide Interventions

OD practitioners operate on the premise that any change in one part of an organization also affects other parts. Additionally, an organization's culture is considered to have an important impact on member attitudes and morale. Furthermore, its structures and jobs can be designed to bring together people, technology, and systems in highly productive and satisfying working combinations.

Some common OD interventions that emphasize organizational effectiveness include

▲ **survey feedback:** Comprehensive and systematic data collection to identify attitudes and needs, analyze results, and plan for constructive action;

▲ **confrontation meeting:** Intensive, structured meetings to gather data on workplace problems and plan for constructive actions;

▲ **structural redesign:** Realigning the organization structure to meet the needs of environmental and contextual forces;

▲ **management by objectives (MBO):** Formalizing MBO throughout the organization to link individual, group, and organizational objectives. (See section 7.5 for more information on MBO.)

11.5.2 Team Interventions

Team plays a very important role in organization development. OD practitioners recognize two principles in this respect. First, teams are viewed as important vehicles for helping people satisfy important needs. Second, by improving collaboration within and among teams, organizational performance also improves.

Typically OD interventions designed to improve team effectiveness include

▲ **team building:** Structured experiences to help team members set goals, improve interpersonal relations, and become a better functioning team;

▲ **process consultation:** Third-party observation and advice on critical team processes (for example, communication, conflict, and decision making);

▲ **intergroup team building:** Structured experiences to help two or more teams set shared goals, improve relations, and become better coordinated.

Interdependence among all members of the group is essential to achieving change successfully. The following guidelines can help managers and their teams effectively implement change in a cohesive, integrated manner.

▲ **Identify problems promptly and pragmatically.** Doing so mandates a timely response to cited problems, a practical approach to gathering potential solutions from each staff member, and emphasis on defining new solutions, not reiterating old problems.

▲ **Elicit solutions from staff members.** Managers must do this constantly and consistently asking all group members, "How can we do X better?"

▲ **Use interactive feedback.** Present critical information to the group on a timely basis, acknowledge and use suggestive feedback, and reward any new innovations that contribute to the process with group recognition and other appropriate methods.

▲ **Resolve short-term problems and focus on the long term.** Put the responsibility for a solution on the individuals who identify the problem first, then charge the group with the responsibility of devising a solution that helps make the long-term objective of change a reality.

▲ **Reinforce the need for change.** Provide reinforcement throughout the change process by asking team members to help identify new benefits that the change may generate. These benefits can be any advantages the organization, department, or individual may realize that were not identified initially but are now readily apparent and tangible for the group to identify and discuss.

▲ **Cite examples of positive change.** Whenever possible, link past examples of positive group change and current challenges. You probably can easily identify a past action that was so daunting that by comparison a current change project is seemingly easy.

11.5.3 Individual Interventions

Organization development practitioners generally recognize that the need for individual growth and development is most likely to be satisfied in a supportive and challenging work environment. They also accept the premise that most people are capable of assuming responsibility for their own actions and of making positive contributions to organizational performance.

Based on these principles, some of the more popular OD interventions designed to help improve individual effectiveness include

▲ **sensitivity training:** Unstructured group sessions where participants learn interpersonal skills and increased sensitivity to other people;

▲ **management training:** Structured educational opportunities for developing important managerial skills and competencies;

▲ **role negotiation:** Structured interactions to clarify and negotiate role expectations among people who work together;

▲ **job redesign:** Realigning task components to better fit the needs and capabilities of the individual;

▲ **career planning:** Structured advice and discussion sessions to help individuals plan career paths and programs of personal development.

FOR EXAMPLE

IHI Interventions to Save 100,000 Lives

Founded in 1991, the Institute for Healthcare Improvement, or IHI (www.ihi.org), is a not-for-profit organization dedicated to improving the quality and value of health care throughout the United States. In response to discouraging patient mortality reports, IHI launched the 100,000 Lives Campaign in a collaborative effort to help hospitals substantially decrease in-house patient deaths. The campaign focuses on just six interventions, including techniques for preventing adverse drug events, central line infection, and ventilator-associated pneumonia. IHI supplies free online information, training materials, a discussion forum, and e-mail-based newsletters relating to the six interventions. Hospitals can choose to implement all or some of the six interventions. To learn more about the 100,000 Lives campaign and track the program's progress, visit www.ihi.org/IHI/Programs/Campaign.

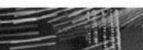

SELF-CHECK

- Identify and define **intervention.**
- Describe characteristics and appropriate uses of organization-wide interventions.
- Discuss strategies for using team interventions to foster interdependence.
- Compare individual intervention techniques.

11.6 Dealing with Stress

In a health care setting, the jobs that people perform—and the relationships and circumstances under which they have to do them—are often causes of significant stress. Formally defined, **stress** is a state of tension experienced by individuals facing extraordinary demands, constraints, or opportunities.[7] Any look toward a health care career is incomplete without considering stress as a challenge that you are sure to encounter along the way—and a challenge you must be prepared to help others learn to deal with.

11.6.1 Sources of Stress

The things that cause stress are called **stressors.** Whether stressors originate directly in the work setting or emerge in personal and nonwork situations, they all have the potential to influence work attitudes, behavior, and job performance.

Work factors have an obvious potential to create job stress. Some 46% of workers in one survey reported that their jobs were highly stressful; 34% said that their jobs were so stressful that they were thinking of quitting.

Today, most workers experience stress in long hours of work, excessive e-mails, unrealistic work deadlines, difficult bosses or co-workers, and unwelcome or unfamiliar work.[8] Stress is also associated with excessively high or low task demands, role conflicts or ambiguities, poor interpersonal relations, or career progress that is too slow or too fast. Stress tends to be high during periods of work overload, when office politics are common, and among people working for organizations undergoing staff cutback and downsizing. (This latter situation and lack of "corporate loyalty" to the employee can be especially stressful to employees who view themselves as "career" employees and who are close to retirement age.)

A variety of personal factors are also sources of potential stress for people at work. Such individual characteristics as needs, capabilities, and personality can influence how one perceives and responds to work situations. Researchers, for example, identify a **type A personality** that is high in achievement orientation,

---

FOR EXAMPLE

Personal Wellness

Personal wellness is a form of preventative stress management, in which employers help their employees recognize their responsibility to enhancing their physical, emotional, and relational health through educational resources and programming. As health care costs continue to rise, many employers are placing greater emphasis on personal wellness programs and a way to avoid health problems—or at least identify problems earlier, when they are more treatable. Personal wellness addresses dozens of health-related topics, including smoking, using alcohol, maintaining a nutritious diet, engaging in regular exercise, preventing the spread of sexually transmitted disease, and much more. The Wellness Council of America (www.welcoa.org) is a nonprofit, multidisciplinary organization that offers support, programming ideas, education materials, online tools, and other resources for individuals and organizations who want to make ongoing personal wellness a priority. The organization's free e-mail-based newsletter, *The Well Workplace,* highlights scientific studies and real-world techniques that you can use to make every day a healthy experience.

impatience, and perfectionism. Type A people are likely to create stress in circumstances that others find relatively stress-free. Type A people, in a sense, bring stress on themselves. Stressful behavior patterns of type A personalities include[9]

▲ always moving, walking, and eating rapidly;
▲ acting impatient, hurrying others, disliking waiting;
▲ doing, or trying to do, several things at once;
▲ feeling guilty when relaxing;
▲ trying to schedule more in less time;
▲ using nervous gestures such as a clenched fist;
▲ hurrying or interrupting the speech of others.

Finally, stress from nonwork factors can have spillover effects on an individual's work. Stressful life situations, including such things as family events (for example, the birth of a child), economics (a sudden loss of extra income), and personal affairs (a preoccupation with a bad relationship), are often sources of emotional strain. Depending on the individual and his or her ability to deal with them, preoccupation with such situations can affect one's work and add to the stress of work-life conflicts.

11.6.2 Consequences of Stress

Many people mistakenly assume that stress always has a negative influence on people's lives. Stress actually has two faces—one constructive and one destructive.[10]

▲ **Constructive stress** acts in a positive way for the individual and/or the organization. It occurs in moderation and proves energizing and performance enhancing.[11] The stress is sufficient to encourage increased effort, stimulate creativity, and enhance diligence in one's work, while not overwhelming the individual and causing negative outcomes. Type A individuals, for example, are likely to work long hours and to be less satisfied with poor performance. For them, challenging task demands imposed by a supervisor may elicit higher levels of task accomplishment. Even nonwork stressors such as new family responsibilities may cause them to work harder in anticipation of greater financial rewards.

▲ **Destructive stress**, or distress, is dysfunctional for the individual and/or the organization. It occurs as intense or long-term stress that, as Figure 11-5 shows, overloads and breaks down a person's physical and mental systems. Destructive stress can lead to **job burnout**—a form of physical and mental exhaustion that can be incapacitating both personally and with respect to one's work.

Figure 11-5

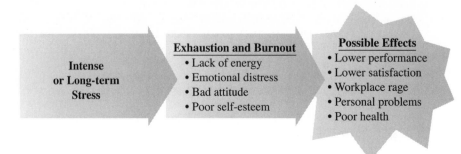

Potential negative consequences of destructive job stress.

Productivity can suffer as people react to very intense stress through turnover, absenteeism, errors, accidents, dissatisfaction, and reduced performance.

Today there is increased concern for another job consequence of excessive stress: **workplace rage,** or overtly aggressive behavior toward co-workers and the work setting in general. Lost tempers are a common example; the unfortunate extremes are tragedies involving physical harm to others.

Medical research is also concerned that too much stress can reduce resistance to disease and increase the likelihood of physical and mental illnesses, such as hypertension, ulcers, substance abuse, overeating, depression, muscle aches, and more.

Managers must be alert to signs of excessive stress in themselves and the people with whom they work. The multiple and varied symptoms of excessive stress include changes in work attitudes and performance as well as personal restlessness, irritability, and stomach upset. The best stress management alternative is to prevent it from ever reaching excessive levels in the first place. By recognizing stressors emerging from personal and nonwork factors, action can be taken to prevent stressors from adversely affecting the work experience. For example, family difficulties may be relieved by a change of work schedule.

SELF-CHECK

- Identify and define **stress, stressor, personal wellness program, type A personality, job burnout,** and **workplace rage.**
- List common factors that cause stress, including work factors and personal factors.
- Describe characteristics of a type A personality.
- Compare destructive stress and constructive stress.
- Discuss effects of stress on the workplaces and on workers.

SUMMARY

In many ways, change is the only constant in today's health care workplace. Managers, by responding positively to change, can become change leaders for their teams, staffs, and entire organizations. The process of planned change provides a structured way for organizations to evolve and improve. Managers can utilize several change strategies to implement and encourage positive changes. Interventions at the organization, team, or individual level can help respond to change resistance. Change frequently causes stress, but aware managers can monitor workplace stress and help employees to cope more effectively.

KEY TERMS

Bottom-up change	Initiatives for change come from people throughout an organization and are supported by the efforts of middle- and lower-level managers acting as change agents.
Career planning	Structured advice and discussion sessions to help individuals plan career paths and programs of personal development.
Change leader	A person or group who takes leadership responsibility for changing the existing pattern of behavior of another person or social system.
Changing stage	The phase of planned change in which something new takes place in a system, and change is actually implemented.
Confrontation meeting	Intensive, structured meetings to gather data on workplace problems and plan for constructive actions; an organization-wide OD intervention.
Constructive stress	Stress that acts in a positive way for the individual and/or the organization. It occurs in moderation and proves energizing and performance enhancing.
Destructive stress	Distress, or dysfunctional stress, for the individual and/or the organization. It occurs as intense or long-term stress that overloads and breaks down a person's physical and mental systems.
Direct forcing strategy	A force-coercion strategy in which a manager takes direct and unilateral action to "command" that change take place.
Force-coercion strategy	Change strategy that uses the power of legitimacy, rewards, and punishments as the primary inducements to change.

Group emotions	Emotional responses can pervade an entire team and cause a group to resist—and even work against—a proposed change.
Interventions	Within OD, activities that are initiated to directly facilitate the change processes.
Job burnout	A form of physical and mental exhaustion that can be incapacitating both personally and with respect to one's work.
Job redesign	Realigning task components to better fit the needs and capabilities of the individual.
Management training	Structured educational opportunities for developing important managerial skills and competencies.
Nonplayer	A team member who does not agree with a change and even works against it.
Organization development (OD)	A comprehensive approach to planned organizational change that involves applying behavioral science in a systematic and long-range effort to improve organizational effectiveness.
Outcome goals	In organization development, goals that focus on task accomplishments.
Performance gap	A discrepancy between the desired and actual state of affairs.
Personal wellness	A form of preventative stress management, in which employers help their employees recognize their responsibility to enhancing their physical, emotional, and relational health through educational resources and programming.
Planned change	Change that occurs as a result of the specific efforts of a change leader; usually in direct response to a perceived performance gap
Political maneuvering	A force-coercion strategy in which a manager works indirectly to gain special advantage over other people and thereby make them change. Political maneuvering involves bargaining, obtaining control of important resources, or granting small favors.
Process goals	In organization development, goals that focus on the way people work together.
Rational persuasion strategy	Informational change strategy that focuses on persuasion backed by special knowledge, data, and rational argument.

Refreezing stage	The phase of planned change in which a manager is concerned about stabilizing the change and creating the conditions for its long-term continuity.
Resistance	Feedback that indicates something can be done to achieve a better "fit" between the planned change, the situation, and the people involved.
Role negotiation	Structured interactions to clarify and negotiate role expectations among people who work together.
Sensitivity training	Unstructured group sessions where participants learn interpersonal skills and increased sensitivity to other people.
Shared power strategy	A change strategy that engages people in a collaborative process of identifying values, assumptions, and goals from which support for change will naturally emerge.
Stress	A state of tension experienced by individuals facing extraordinary demands, constraints, or opportunities.
Stressors	The things that cause stress.
Structural redesign	Realigning the organization structure to meet the needs of environmental and contextual forces; an organization-wide OD intervention.
Survey feedback	Comprehensive and systematic data collection to identify attitudes and needs, analyze results, and plan for constructive action; an organization-wide OD intervention.
Top-down change	Strategic and comprehensive changes are initiated by top management levels with the goal of comprehensive impact on the organization and its performance capabilities.
Type A personality	People who tend to be achievement orientated, impatient, and perfectionists. Type A people are likely to create stress in circumstances that others find relatively stress-free.
Unfreezing stage	The phase of planned change in which the need for change is recognized and a situation is prepared for change.
Workplace rage	Overtly aggressive behavior toward co-workers and the work setting in general, resulting for excessive stress.

ASSESS YOUR UNDERSTANDING

Go to www.wiley.com/college/Lombardi to evaluate your knowledge of the basics of leadership transfer.
Measure your learning by comparing pretest and post-test results.

Summary Questions

1. Planned changed is often in response to a performance gap, which is a discrepancy between the desired and actual state of affairs in the organization. True or false?

2. Within an organization, targets for change can include
   (a) tasks, technology, and culture.
   (b) upper, middle, and lower management.
   (c) the external and internal environments.
   (d) none of the above.

3. A traditional OD process consists of five steps: establishing a change relationship, diagnosing, intervening, evaluating, and achieving a terminal relationship. True or false?

4. The three phases of the planned change process are
   (a) identification, implementation, and evaluation.
   (b) brainstorming, testing, and feedback.
   (c) auditing, altering, and augmenting.
   (d) unfreezing, changing, and refreezing.

5. A proactive strategy for implementing planned change is
   (a) planning in detail.
   (b) dealing with nonplayers.
   (c) focusing on benefits.
   (d) all of the above.

6. When a nonplayer who is resistant to change says he should just go find another job, an appropriate managerial response would be, "Have patience with this current situation, and we can try to figure things out together." True or false?

7. When a manager uses special knowledge, data, and logical arguments to bring about change, she is engaging in
   (a) shared power change leadership.
   (b) post-evaluation change leadership.
   (c) rational persuasion change leadership.
   (d) force-coercion change leadership.

8. In today's health care workplace, force-coercion strategies of change leadership are generally inappropriate. Instead, managers should strive for solutions based on shared power. True or false?

9. Resistance is not necessarily negative energy that managers must work to overcome within the teams and department. Instead, resistance can be viewed as feedback that something can be done to achieve a better fit between the planned change and the situation. True or false?

10. The most common apprehension of steady-performing team members in regards to change is
    (a) fear of having to do more work.
    (b) fear of regression.
    (c) fear of the unknown.
    (d) fear of termination.

11. When a manager responds to employee resistance by providing encouragement and training, the manager is utilizing a participation and involvement strategy. True or false?

12. At the organizational level, an effective OD intervention might include
    (a) survey feedback.
    (b) team building.
    (c) career planning.
    (d) management training.

13. The goal of most team-level interventions is interdependence. True or false?

14. An individual intervention in which an employee learns interpersonal skills in an unstructured session is
    (a) role negotiation.
    (b) management by objectives (MBO).
    (c) confrontation meeting.
    (d) sensitivity training.

15. Stress is ultimately always detrimental to employee job performance. True or false?

16. Work factors that can cause stress include all the following except
    (a) long work hours.
    (b) role conflicts and ambiguities.
    (c) high achievement orientation.
    (d) difficult co-workers.

17. Individuals with type A personalities are more likely to create stressful circumstances for themselves. True or false?

Review Questions

1. In what three ways does a change leader contrast with status-quo manager?

2. When a new team leader and her teammates propose a new job-sharing strategy that increases job performance and saves the organization money, what type of change is occurring?

3. What needs to happen in the traditional organizational development (OD) process before a manager can begin suggesting new departmental procedures?

4. When a manager rewards staff for their performances and positive responses to change, she is engaging in which phase of the planned change process?

5. Planning in detail is a vital part of successful planned change. What are four critical questions that managers should ask themselves about their planned changes?

6. Force-coercion change strategies produce fast but more temporary results. What sorts of power are required for successful force-coercion change?

7. A manager who bargains with staff, obtains control of important resources, and grants small favors in an effort to lead change is engaging in what specific type of force-coercion strategy?

8. A shared power strategy of change leadership is based on empowerment and group participation. What are the pros and cons of this strategy?

9. Group emotions are often triggered by change. What is the most common emotion health care employees site when confronted with change?

10. A nurse manager tells her staff that any employee who refuses to work 8 hours of overtime in the next week will lose any scheduling privileges going forward. What response to change resistance is the manager using?

11. OD interventions often emphasize changes for overall organizational effectiveness. When data is systematically collected to identify attitudes and needs, what specific type of intervention is occurring?

12. When a manager seeks to elicit solutions for a problem from his staff members, the manager is utilizing which type of intervention?

13. OD practitioners recognize the need for individual growth and development. What are some common interventions at the individual level?

14. Stress can be created by a variety of factors. What are three major categories of stress-related factors?

15. Destructive stress can lead to extremely detrimental conditions for individuals and organizations. What are some possible negative consequences of destructive job stress?

Applying This Chapter

1. A busy suburban emergency room is planning to institute a new digital charting process for all patients. In the past, staff has been extremely reluctant to changes in the charting process and working with new technologies. Based on traditional OD processes, what are some things a manager can do to ensure the change to a digital charting process is successful?

2. What might be a proactive, positive response to a staff member who is resisting change and complains that "we've already changed several times in the last few years and nothing got better"?

3. Although force-coercion strategies for implementing change are quite traditional, they can be effective when utilized appropriate. Describe a situation in which a force-coercion strategy of change leadership is more appropriate rational persuasion or shared power strategies.

4. The communications team at a large research hospital has been charged with producing and distributing six additional newsletters each year to potential investors. The existing staff is resisting the new obligations, claiming that they already overworked and underappreciated. The team's manager has been given an additional $10,000 but no new staff to meet the new goal. How can the manager respond to her resistant team?

5. How might a health care manager respond with organization-wide, team, and individual interventions to the elimination of on-site radiology technician services from a small community hospital?

6. Maria, a lab technician recently returning from maternity leave, finds that her department was significantly altered during her absence. Several new pieces of equipment were added to the lab, and two of her favorite co-workers where reassigned to another facility within the organization. Maria was very interested in applying for a team leader position before taking leave, but now she just wants to do her job and leave a workplace she considers too stressful. How might Maria's stress relate to the three factors covered in section 11.6?

Identifying Bottom-up Change

When you're applying and interviewing for your first health care management position, you probably will not have work experiences to share with a hiring manager that involve your ability to introduce top-down changes. Instead, consider times that you were involved in suggesting, implementing, or producing bottom-up changes (see section 11.1.1). Bottom-up changes come from people (probably like yourself) who are actually doing the daily work and seeing the real-world challenges that the organization faces. Rather than complaining about the next challenging work or educational situation that arises, consider it an opportunity to create bottom-up change. You can make your situation better while gaining a useful experience to share in future job interviews.

Your Barriers to Change

On a blank sheet of paper, write down a description of a significant change that has happened in your career, your personal life, or your education. Why did the change happen? How did you feel about the change? Did you resist the change? Look at the typical reasons for resistance to change (listed in section 11.4.1)—disrupted habits, loss of confidence, loss of control, poor timing, and work overload. Which of these did you experience? Write down your responses to all these questions. Understand that while resisting change is normal and understandable, change is an indisputable fact of today's health care workplace. Fortunately, you probably resist change for similar reasons, regardless of the specific change. So after you identify how you tend to resist change, you can begin preparing yourself with rational, positive responses to your most typical change-resisting thoughts.

Thinking Strategically

Imagine a difficult situation involving others at work, school, or in your personal life. (Perhaps your department has been asked to cut $25,000 from its annual operating budget, you have group presentation on a complex health care topic due in 3 days, or you and your partner must relocate to a new apartment or home in the next 2 months.) What would be a possible response to the situation utilizing a force-coercion strategy? What would be a response based on rational persuasion? How about shared power? Although no single strategy is completely right or wrong, some strategies work better in some situations. Which strategy feels best to you personally? What sort of change leader might you prefer to be in your career?

Examples of Positive Change

Your interactions with bosses, co-workers, employees, professors, classmates, and even family and friends, will always involve some aspect of change. While change can be difficult, time-consuming, frustrating, and even scary, you can always choose to focus on examples of positive change. Take a moment and write a brief description (three or four sentences will do) about a time when you experienced a positive change in your education, work, or personal life. What made the change difficult? What made the change ultimately positive? Was there a particular lesson you learned in the change process? The next time you're confronted with change, think back on the example of positive change you identified. If appropriate, consider sharing your example with someone else.

Stress Diaries

Keeping a personal stress diary can help you better understand what stresses you and how you can react more effectively to everyday stress. Various forms of stress diaries are available online, and many are free. Whether you record your stressors in an electronic document or a blank notebook, the key is to write down your stress status on a regular basis (for example, every hour). Each entry in your stress diary should note date, time, description of your mood, how stressed you feel (on a scale of 0 to 10), any symptoms or emotions you're feeling, and what may be causing the stress. After 2 weeks, review all the entries and look for patterns: common stressors, typical responses, and times of day when you feel most stressed. Knowing the sorts of situations that cause you stress can help you prepare for and manage future stress better.

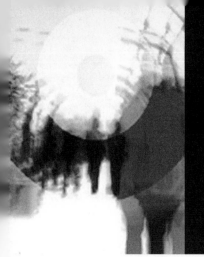

12

COMMUNICATING
Developing Outstanding Interpersonal Skills

Starting Point

Go to www.wiley.com/college/Lombardi to assess your knowledge of basic communication skills.
Determine where you need to concentrate your effort.

What You'll Learn in This Chapter

▲ Key elements of the communication process
▲ Typical sources of communication messaging
▲ Common communication barriers
▲ Perceptions that affect communication
▲ Strategies for improving communications
▲ Conflict management techniques
▲ Steps and pitfalls in the negotiation process

After Studying This Chapter, You'll Be Able To

▲ Compare effective communications and efficient communication
▲ Differentiate between incoming and outgoing communication
▲ Analyze the ways in which perceptions can alter a communication message
▲ Apply the strategies for improving communications
▲ Practice techniques for effective conflict management
▲ Compare negotiation methods and tools

Goals and Outcomes

▲ Master the terminology, tools, and techniques associated with the communication process
▲ Use effective communication techniques
▲ Respond to communication barriers
▲ Evaluate perceptions and their effects on communication
▲ Choose and use effective communication strategies
▲ Employ conflict management tools
▲ Apply common negotiating principles

INTRODUCTION

As a health care manager, the strength of your communication skills directly connects to your overall performance effectiveness. The communication process happens almost constantly during the workday because the sources of communication messages are numerous. A range of communication barriers and perceptions can negatively impact the communication process. Savvy managers can improve communications by focusing on mutual benefit, tailoring their messages, actively listening, and using effective communication techniques. Workplace conflict may be inevitable, but proactive managers can respond effectively to conflicts, often improving situations. In particularly, negotiation is complex set of tools that managers can utilize to minimize conflict and encourage positive workplace interaction and communication.

12.1 Understanding the Communication Process

The ability to communicate well, both orally and in writing, is a critical management skill. Through communication, people exchange and share information with one another, and influence one another's attitudes, behaviors, and understandings. Communication allows one to establish and maintain interpersonal relationships, listen to others, and gain information. No manager can handle conflict, negotiate successfully, and succeed at leadership without being a good communicator. It is no wonder that "communication skills" often top the list of attributes employers look for in job candidates.

12.1.1 Communication Essentials

Formally defined, **communication** is an interpersonal process of sending and receiving symbols with messages attached to them. The key elements in the communication process are shown in Figure 12-1. They include a **sender,** who is responsible for encoding an intended message into meaningful symbols, both verbal and nonverbal. The message is sent through a communication channel to a **receiver,** who then decodes or interprets its meaning. This interpretation may or may not match the sender's original intentions. **Feedback,** when present, reverses the process and conveys the receiver's response back to the sender.

Another way to view the communication process is as a series of questions. "Who?" (sender) "says what?" (message) "in what way?" (channel) "to whom?" (receiver) "with what result?" (interpreted meaning).

Effective communication occurs when the intended message of the sender and the interpreted meaning of the receiver are one and the same. Although this may seem like the goal in any communication attempt, it is not always achieved. **Efficient communication** occurs at minimum cost in terms of resources

Figure 12-1

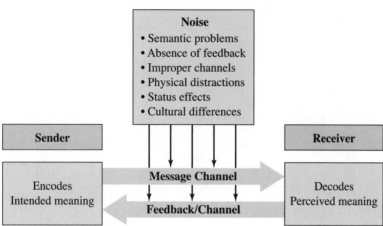

The process of interpersonal communication.

expended, such as the amount of time involved. Efficiency is one reason why so many people rely on voice mail and e-mail, rather than visiting others personally to communicate a message.

Efficient communication is not always effective. A low-cost approach such as an e-mail note to a distribution list may save time, but it does not always result in everyone getting the same meaning from the message. Without opportunities to ask questions and clarify the message, erroneous interpretations are possible.

By the same token, an effective communication may not always be efficient. If a manager visits each team member individually to explain a new change in office procedures, this process may guarantee that everyone truly understands the change. But it may also be very costly in the demands it makes on the manager's time. A team meeting is more efficient. In these and other ways, potential trade-offs between effectiveness and efficiency must be recognized in communication.

12.1.2 Identifying Communication Sources

Two types of communication are important to all members of health care teams, especially managers:

▲ **Incoming communication** includes directives, mandates, directions, guidance, support, feedback, questions, consultation, advice, demands, and expectations.

▲ **Outgoing communication** includes compliance, professional development, action, growth, support, team insight, leadership, contribution and expertise, and finally satisfaction and expectation fulfillment.

Figure 12-2

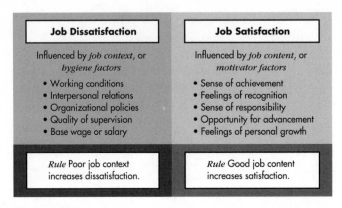

Incoming communication for health care managers.

For health care managers, six sources provide most incoming communication and are the target of outgoing communication: the organization, supervisors, family and friends, staff, peers, and patients. Figure 12-2 depicts incoming channels (from the six specific sources to the manager), and Figure 12-3 shows outgoing channels (from manager to the six sources).

Figure 12-3

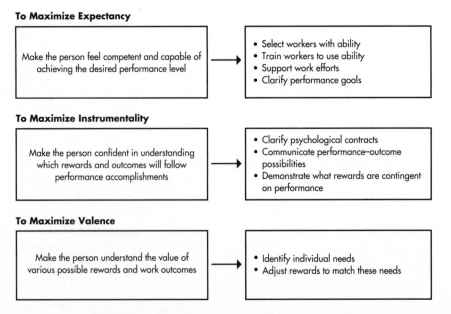

Outgoing communication for health care managers.

Additionally, communication can be classified by the source of the message. Some of the common communication sources include

▲ **the organization itself:** All health care organizations generate directives to managers regarding how to manage staff, the ways to conduct technical activities, and the quality of contributions expected from staff. These directives may be presented in written or oral form, and the information may be implicit or explicit. For example, an implicit directive may be that you maintain the highest moral and ethical standards in the delivery of your particular segment of health care service. However, if this directive is written into the organization's code of conduct, its mission statement, or a set of organizational standards, it is explicit. Additionally, newsletters, annual reports, newspaper articles, and other sources of information can clarify the values of a health care organization;

▲ **supervisors:** Your manager provides you with a certain amount of direction in how to conduct your job. This direction may include a history of departmental responsibilities, background into the department's prior performance, or some insight into individual members. Supervisor also should provide a set of detailed expectations they hold for your department.

▲ **family and friends:** The demands of a health care management job pretty much dictates a manager's working hours. For example, if an emergency requires your presence, most likely you will be there— even if it is your scheduled day off or hours past the end of your shift. Being a manager can put a strain on personal relationships, and family and friends may have difficulty adjusting to health care management work hours. Take a proactive, rather than reactive, approach to this potential problem. From the start, orient family and friends to the realities and expectations of your job. Remind them that a health care management job is not a 9-to-5 position; rather, job demands are the primary determinants of your working hours. Above all, keep communication constant and open between with your family and friends;

▲ **staff:** As a manager, you seek and receive feedback from your staff on a variety of issues. Feedback can include technical issues involving your department, individual concerns relative to the job, and suggestions on improving performance across the department. Conversely, as a manager, share information as appropriate with your staff and get their input and suggestions. This vital exchange can help you form a progressive frame of reference for dealing with management issues. For example, suppose your organization plans to implement a bonus-incentive compensation system. After attending several management meetings on this issue, you are curious about employee reaction to the new program. You may choose to discuss the issue in a department meeting, in one-on-one meetings with key employees, or informally within the context of ongoing discussions with staff. These communication efforts can give you a frame of reference that you can then use in your management discussions to help further refine the bonus-incentive compensation system within the organization;

▲ **peers and colleagues:** Peers and colleagues—that is, fellow managers—rely on you to provide technical expertise in key areas. In exchange, they provide their technical expertise and real-life management experiences to you, when appropriate;

▲ **patients:** The most important source of incoming information is the patient. In a sense, health care managers receive *all* communications from patients—or at least are party to all communications. Managers must take the lead in answering patients' requests, handling their complaints, and incorporating their input into the general management strategy of patient service. For example, the manager of a physical rehabilitation department of a small hospital may receive specific complaints or compliments about the way physical therapy was provided for a particular patient. However, the same patient may also comment on the hospital's billing system, its parking facilities, or how cooperative the security and reception personnel were in helping the patient find your department. All feedback—both positive and negative—should be incorporated into a manager's ongoing notes and relayed to appropriate individuals within the organization.

FOR EXAMPLE

Wireless Communication Systems

As wireless technology becomes cheaper and more reliable, hospitals are beginning to incorporate wireless computer networks and various hand-held devices into their communication plans and day-to-day work procedures. For example, the nursing call system at St. Agnes Hospital in Baltimore (www.stagnes.org) recently switched to an all-wireless network system from a leading communications and technology manufacturer. In the new system, each patient is given a wireless call unit that transmits bedside calls to wireless badges worn by nurses and other staff. Within the first 6 months of use, the new call system radically improved patient/nurse communication, reducing the time it took caregivers to respond to patient requests by more than 50%.

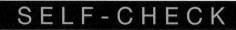

SELF-CHECK

- Identify and define **communication, communication channel,** and **feedback.**
- Describe the key aspects of the communication process, including sender, receiver, message, communication channel, and feedback.
- Compare characteristics of effective communication and efficient communication.
- Identify common incoming and outgoing sources of communication.

12.2 Recognizing Communication Barriers

Communication is a two-way process that requires effort and skill on the part of both the sender and the receiver. **Noise,** as Figure 12-1 shows, is anything that interferes with the effectiveness of the communication process. Common sources of noise include poor choice of channels, poor written or oral expression, failure to recognize nonverbal signals, physical distractions, and status effects.

12.2.1 Poor Choice of Channels

A **communication channel** is the medium through which a message is conveyed from sender to receiver.[1]

In general, **written channels** are acceptable for simple messages that are easy to convey and for those that require quick delivery to a wide audience. Written channels are also important, at least as follow-up communications, when formal policy or authoritative directives are being conveyed.

Oral channels work best for messages that are complex and difficult to convey, where immediate feedback to the sender is valuable. Oral channels are also more personal and can create a supportive, even inspirational, emotional climate.

12.2.2 Poor Written or Oral Expression

Communication is effective only to the extent that the sender expresses a message in a way that can be clearly understood by the receiver. The sender must choose her words well in order to express her intentions.

Consider the following confusing communication found among some top-level managers.

▲ A report reads: "Customer-patient elements are continuing to stress the fundamental necessity of a stabilization of the price structure at a lower

---

FOR EXAMPLE

Center for Creative Leadership

More than 30% of managers report some difficulties in dealing with communication and interpersonal relations. The Center for Creative Leadership (CCL; www.ccl.org), a not-for-profit training center in Greensboro, North Carolina, helps managers and other leaders address communication issues via role-playing exercises, self-evaluative tools, classes, online resources, and group exercises. Although participants in CCL programs come from a variety of disciplines, developing good communication skills is part of every CCL program. As CCL's Michael Wakefield notes, "Leaders who are trusted—even in times of great difficulty—are skilled communicators."

---

level than exists at the present time." (Translation: Patients keep saying that service prices need to go down and stay down.)

▲ A manager says: "Substantial economies were affected in this division by increasing the time interval between distribution of data-eliciting forms to outside entities." (Translation: The division was saving money by sending fewer questionnaires to suppliers.)

Both written and oral communication requires skill. It isn't easy, for example, to write a concise letter or to express your thoughts in an e-mail report. Your message can easily be misunderstood. It takes practice and hard work to express yourself well. The same holds true for oral communication that takes place via the spoken word in telephone calls, face-to-face meetings, formal briefings, video conferences, and the like.

12.2.3 Failure to Recognize Nonverbal Signals

Nonverbal communication takes place through such things as hand movements, facial expressions, body posture, eye contact, and the use of interpersonal space. Nonverbal communication can be a powerful means of transmitting messages. Eye contact or voice intonation can be used intentionally to accent special parts of an oral communication. Astute observers note how body language may express listeners' attitudes, even while they're maintaining silence.

When people do speak, a *mixed message* may occur when words communicate one message and actions, body language, appearance, or use of interpersonal space communicate something else. For example, watch how people behave in a meeting. A person who feels under attack may move back in a chair or lean away from the presumed antagonist, even while expressing verbal agreement. Such actions are done quite unconsciously, but they send messages to others who are alert enough to pick them up.

12.2.4 Physical Distractions

Any number of physical distractions can interfere with the effectiveness of communication. Some, such as telephone interruptions, drop-in visitors, and lack of privacy, can be avoided or minimized with proper managerial attention.

12.2.5 Status Effects

"Criticize my boss? I don't have the right to." "I'd get fired." "It's her company, not mine." These comments show how the hierarchy of authority creates another potential barrier to effective communications. Simply put, people often find it difficult to communicate with bosses and others of higher organizational status.

Filtering is the intentional distortion of information to make it appear favorable to the recipient. Filtering most often involves someone telling the boss what he or she wants to hear. Whether the reason behind this is a fear of retribution for bringing bad news, an unwillingness to identify personal mistakes, or just a general desire to please, the end result is the same. The person receiving filtered communications can end up making poor decisions because of a biased and inaccurate information base.

SELF-CHECK

- Identify and define **noise, communication channel, nonverbal communication,** and **filtering.**
- Discuss the impact of communication channel on a message.
- Explain the importance of good written and oral expression during the communication process.
- Describe how body language can lead to sending out a mixed message.
- Discuss how filtering and status effects can alter a message.

12.3 Understanding How Perceptions Affect Communication

Communication is also influenced by the way people receive and interpret information from the environment, a process called **perception.**[2] As Figure 12-4 shows, perception acts as a screen or filter through which information passes in interpersonal communication. The results of this screening process vary because individual perceptions are influenced by such things as values, cultural background, and other circumstances of the moment.

Figure 12-4

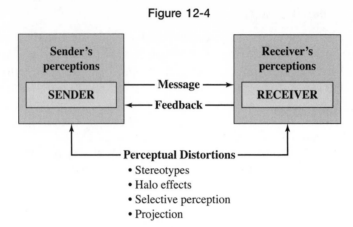

The process of interpersonal communication.

Because people can and do perceive the same things or situations very differently, perception can be an important influence on communication and interpersonal relations. In particular, a variety of tendencies toward perceptual distortions can impact communication. These tendencies include the use of stereotypes, halo effects, selectivity, and projections.

12.3.1 Stereotypes

A **stereotype** occurs when someone is identified with a group or category, and then oversimplified attributes associated with the group or category are attributed to the individual. Common stereotypes are those of young people, old people, teachers, students, union members, males, and females, among others. The phenomenon in each case is the same: A person is classified into a group on the basis of one piece of information, such as age or gender.

Characteristics commonly associated with the group are then assigned to the individual. What is generalized about the group (for example, "Young people dislike authority") may or may not be true about the individual. Stereotypes based on such factors as gender, age, and race can, and unfortunately still do, bias perceptions in some work settings. Consider this example of gender stereotypes:[3] "He's talking with co-workers." (Interpretation: He's discussing a new business strategy.). "She's talking with co-workers." (Interpretation: She's gossiping.)

12.3.2 Halo Effects

A **halo effect** occurs when one attribute is used to develop an overall impression of a person or situation. When meeting someone new, for example, the halo effect may cause one trait, such as a pleasant smile, to result in a positive first impression. By contrast, a particular hairstyle or manner of dressing may create a negative reaction. Halo effects, like stereotypes, cause individual differences to become obscured.

FOR EXAMPLE

Toward Greater Workplace Fairness

Unfortunately, the perceptions that section 12.3 covers continue to play a part in workplace discrimination. The not-for-profit news and advice resources Workplace Fairness.Org (www.workplacefairness.org) is a comprehensive online destination for help identifying and responding effectively to negative perceptions from managers, co-workers, and employees. The site outlines every U.S. employee's legal rights, recent news and research on discrimination, and recommended ways (both large and small) to take action against negative perceptions on the job.

Paying close attention to halo effects is especially significant in terms of communication about someone's work performance. One factor, such as a person's punctuality, may become the "halo" for a positive overall performance evaluation. Even though the general conclusion seems to make sense, it may or may not be true in a given circumstance.

12.3.3 Selectivity

Selective perception is the tendency to single out for attention those aspects of a situation or person that reinforce or appear consistent with one's existing beliefs, values, or needs.[4] What selectivity often produces in an organization is that people from different departments or functions—such as marketing and patient-care—tend to see things from their own points of view and fail to recognize or listen to other points of view. One way to reduce the impact of selectivity is to actively gather inputs from a variety of people and perspectives.

12.3.4 Projection

Projection is the assignment of personal attributes to other individuals. A classic projection error is to assume that other people share your needs, desires, and values.

Suppose, for example, that you enjoy considerable responsibility and challenge in your work. Suppose, too, that you are the newly appointed leader for a team whose work you consider dull and routine. You may move quickly to start a program of job enrichment to help members experience more responsibility and challenge. This action may or may not be a good decision. Instead of designing jobs to best fit others' needs, you have designed their jobs to fit yours. In fact, team members may be quite satisfied with jobs that, to you, seem routine.

Projection errors can be minimized by self-awareness and a willingness to communicate and empathize with others—that is, to try to see things through their eyes.

- Identify and define **perception, stereotype, halo effect, selective perception,** and **projection.**
- Discuss ways in which various perception impacts communication.
- Describe the potentially negative effects of stereotypes, halo effects, selectivity, and projection.

12.4 Improving Communication

A number of things can be done to overcome barriers, minimize perceptual distortions, and improve the process of communication. They include active listening, constructive feedback, open communication channels, the use of space and technology, and valuing diversity, among other techniques covered in the following section.

12.4.1 Underscoring Mutual Benefit

No matter what psychological or communication tactics you use to communicate messages as a health care manager, underscoring the mutual benefit of an action is a strong tactic for garnering the desired response. Generally five recipients receive the mutual benefit of a message:

▲ The message sender
▲ The message receiver
▲ The team-staff
▲ The organization
▲ The patient

Try to identify the individual and operational benefits of an action simply by asking, What are the benefits to each of these parties and to each facet of the business? Some possible answers (or payoffs) are

▲ greater effectiveness;
▲ increased efficiency;
▲ new programs or evidence of organization progress;
▲ short-term production gains;
▲ long-term positive gains;
▲ staff growth and development.

By articulating the potential payoffs, you lend maximum clarity to the communication process and stress the contribution needed from each individual in the department. If potential recipients fail to respond to the appeal for mutual benefits, you can logically assume that they are not interested in the positive success of the organization. Put simply, if people cannot respond to an appeal to help their colleagues and organization, they probably should not be there.

12.4.2 Evaluating Your Message

Communication involves not only what is said or written but how information is delivered. As one hospital administrator notes, "If you really want your staff to get your message, tell them three different ways." For example, a manager may communicate a change in policy via a group e-mail, the hospital newsletter, and an announcement at a quarterly meeting. (Ideally all three communications take place within a 2-week period or less.)

In addition to selecting the best delivery method, a message needs to be worded and presented in a clear, appropriate manner. As a manager, you can use the following to assess your communication style. Consider these 10 components as guidelines for analyzing all communication activity:

▲ **Core:** What is the root of the message? How direct is the message? Is it delivered clearly, understood easily, and capable of being acted on by the receiver?

▲ **Clarity:** Is the message clear in intent and purpose? What are its basic elements? What action must be undertaken to support this message?

▲ **Comprehensiveness:** What is the full scope of the message? Does it provide all information needed for the desired outcome?

▲ **Conciseness:** Did I get to the point? What is the main point of my message? Did I get to the point quickly? Did I get to the point too quickly, without providing enough foundation? Am I taking too long to get to the point?

▲ **Cleverness:** Am I using an appropriate "hook" to get attention? Am I being too gimmicky in delivering this message? Can I be more creative in delivering this message?

▲ **Character:** Does this message support the basic mission of the organization? Does this message seem consistent with other activities in my department? Does this message relate to something that ultimately better serves patients?

▲ **Credibility:** How believable is this message? Do I have enough credibility to garner support on the basis of this message? What points should I detail to get the receiver to buy in to this message?

▲ **Conviction:** Am I stressing the importance of this message enough? Am I displaying how much I believe in the action this message will generate?

FOR EXAMPLE

Execugrams

The use of periodic *execugrams,* which are correspondence from the CEO of an organization to all working staff members and volunteers, is an easily implemented management tool. At the Mercy Health System (www.mercyok.net) in Oklahoma City, execugram messages are coded in green and can contain information ranging from a favorable bond rating to news about the opening of a new clinic. The use of a color other than white for the execugram ensures that the document stands out from other notices, usually delivered on white paper stock.

▲ **Ability to compel:** What action am I asking for? Am I providing enough direction on how to support this message? Am I specifying the time, money, and other quantitative elements of this message strongly enough?

▲ **Consequence:** What is the desired outcome of this message? What positive consequences can be realized if this message is followed through? What are some secondary effects of this message? What impact does this message have on the receiver and other individuals in the department?

Prior to delivering any message, consider all 10 of the preceding C-guidelines. If you follow these guides in your management communications, the likelihood of misunderstanding and inaction will be diminished.

12.4.3 Making Successful Presentations

Presentations are a frequent responsibility for health care managers. Audiences for presentations can be your team, your peers, your supervisors, or perhaps a combination of the three groups.

Keep the following strategies in mind to make presentations as successful as possible:

▲ **Be prepared:** Know what you want to say; know how you want to say it; and rehearse saying it.

▲ **Set the right tone:** Give the audience your complete focus—make eye contact and be pleasant, confident, and engaging.

▲ **Organize your message into points:** State your purpose, make important points, follow with details, and then summarize.

▲ **Support your points:** Give specific reasons for your points and state them in understandable terms.

▲ **Accent the presentation:** Use good visual aids and provide supporting handouts when appropriate.

▲ **Add the right amount of polish:** Attend to the details, such as having the room, materials, and other arrangements ready to go.

▲ **Check your technology:** Check everything ahead of time. Make sure it works and know how to use it.

▲ **Don't bet on the Internet:** Beware of plans to make real-time Internet visits during a presentation. Save Web site and other content on a disk or your hard drive and then use a browser to open the file.

12.4.4 Active Listening

When people talk, they are trying to communicate something. That "something" may or may not be what they are saying. **Active listening** is the process of helping the source of a message say exactly what he or she really means.[5]

Active listening requires considerable effort, but the effects on the communication process can be beneficial. Keep in mind the following guidelines for active listening:

▲ **Stop talking:** You can't listen if you're talking.

▲ **Show that you want to listen:** Remove any potential distractions and try to physically put the other person at ease.

▲ **Listen for message content:** Try to hear exactly what content is being conveyed in the message.

▲ **Listen for feelings:** Try to identify how the source feels about the content in the message.

▲ **Respond to feelings:** Let the source know that her or his feelings are being recognized. Empathize with the other person, as appropriate.

▲ **Note all cues:** Be sensitive to nonverbal and verbal messages. Also, be mindful of mixed messages.

▲ **Take it easy:** Don't get mad; hold your temper. Go easy on arguments and critical responses.

▲ **Paraphrase and restate:** State back to the source what you think you are hearing.

Consider the following responses in terms of the active listening ideals previously listed:

Question: *"Don't you think employees should be promoted on the basis of seniority?"*

Passive listening response: *"No, I don't!"*

Active listening response: *"It seems to you that they should, I take it?"*

Question: *"What does the supervisor expect us to do about these out-of-date computers?"*

Passive listening response: *"Do the best you can, I guess."*

Active listening response: *"You're pretty disgusted with those machines, aren't you?"*

The preceding examples show how active listening can facilitate and encourage communication in difficult circumstances, rather than discourage it.

12.4.5 Providing Constructive Feedback

The process of telling other people how you feel about something they did or said, or about the situation in general, is called *feedback*.

The art of giving feedback is an indispensable skill, particularly for those who must regularly give performance feedback to others. When poorly done, feedback can be threatening and cause resentment. When well done, feedback—even performance criticism—is listened to, accepted, and used to good advantage by the receiver.[6]

The following are guidelines for giving effective, constructive feedback:[7]

▲ Give feedback directly and with real feeling, based on trust between you and the receiver.

▲ Make sure that feedback is specific rather than general. Use good, clear, and preferably recent examples to make your points.

▲ Give feedback at a time and in a location where the receiver seems most willing or able to accept it.

▲ Make sure the feedback is valid and limit it to things the receiver can be expected to do something about.

▲ Give feedback in small doses; never give more than the receiver can handle at any particular time.

12.4.6 Using Space Appropriately

An important but sometimes neglected aspect of communication is **proxemics**, or the use of interpersonal space.[8] The distance between people suggests varying intentions in terms of intimacy, openness, and status.

The physical layout of an office is an often-overlooked form of nonverbal communication. For example, an office with two or more chairs available for side-by-side seating, for example, convey a different message than having the manager's chair behind the desk and those for visitors directly in front.

Office and workspace layouts and architecture are becoming increasingly valued for their communicative qualities. Many work places (including some health care organizations) now include public spaces designed to encourage communication among people from different departments. In many work places, you must pass through a public space before reaching private offices. More meeting areas now have partial walls or glass walls to encourage greater openness and collaboration.

12.4.7 Using Technology Effectively

The new age of communication is one of e-mail, voice mail, online discussions, videoconferencing, virtual or computer-mediated meetings, and more. A related and important development is the growing use of in-house or corporate intranets to provide opportunities for increased communication and collaboration. Many progressive health care organizations use database programs to facilitate continuous electronic forums for communication, knowledge sharing, reference, and record keeping. The purpose of such programs is to encourage fast and regular communication and to provide a source of up-to-date information for problem-solving and work implementation.

Technology offers the power of the electronic grapevine, speeding messages and information from person to person within—as well as outside of—organizations. The results can be both functional—when the information is accurate, appropriate, and useful, as well as dysfunctional—when the information is false, private, distorted, or simply based on rumor.

Managers must be quick to correct misimpressions and inaccuracies. Managers need to model ways to utilize these modern grapevines as a means to quickly transfer factual and relevant information among organizational members.

12.4.8 Valuing Culture and Diversity

Health care workers don't have to travel abroad to come fact-to-face with diversity. Just going to work today can be a cross-cultural journey. The workplace abounds with subcultures based on gender, age, ethnicity, race, and other factors. As a result, the importance of cross-cultural communication skills applies at home just as well as it does in a foreign country.

Cultural skills are gained by reaching out, crossing cultural boundaries, and embracing and respecting differences. And they include an awareness of **ethnocentrism,** or the tendency to consider one's culture superior to others. Ethnocentrism can adversely affect communication in at least three major ways. Specially, ethnocentrism may

- ▲ cause someone to not listen well to what others have to say;
- ▲ cause someone to address or speak with others in ways that alienate them;
- ▲ lead to the use of inappropriate stereotypes when dealing with people from another culture.

SELF-CHECK

- Identify and define **active listening, feedback, proxemics, and ethnocentrism.**
- Discuss the impact of mutual benefit on five key recipients.
- List examples of a mutual benefit messages.
- Describe 10 characteristics of an effective message.
- Explain strategies for giving strong presentations.
- Compare characteristics of active listening and passive listening.
- Offer tips for giving constructive feedback, using space appropriately, and using technology effectively.
- Explain the importance of diversity in today's workplace.

12.5 Delving into Conflict Management

Among essential communication skills, the ability to deal with interpersonal conflicts is critical. **Conflict** is a disagreement between people on substantive or emotional issues.[9] Managers and leaders spend a lot of time dealing with conflicts of various forms.

Substantive conflicts involve disagreements over such things as goals, the allocation of resources, the distribution of rewards, policies and procedures, and job assignments. **Emotional conflicts** result from feelings of anger, distrust, dislike, fear, and resentment, as well as from personality clashes.

12.5.1 Responding to Conflict

In terms of interpersonal styles, people respond to conflict in different ways.[10] **Cooperativeness** is the desire to satisfy another party's needs and concerns; **assertiveness** is the desire to satisfy one's own needs and concerns.

Figure 12-5 shows five interpersonal styles of conflict management that result from various combinations of cooperativeness and assertiveness. Briefly stated, the following conflict management styles (and behaviors) can result:

▲ **Avoidance:** Being uncooperative and unassertive. Behaviors include downplaying disagreement, withdrawing from the situation, or staying neutral at all costs.

▲ **Accommodation, or smoothing:** Being cooperative but unassertive. Behaviors include letting the wishes of others rule, smoothing over, or overlooking differences to maintain harmony.

Figure 12-5

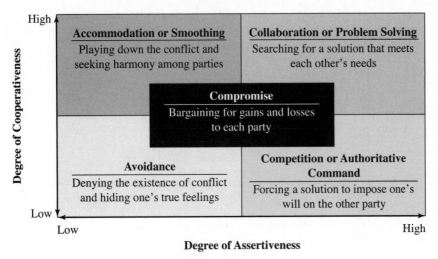

Alternative conflict management styles.

▲ **Competition, or authoritative command:** Being uncooperative but assertive. Behaviors include working against the wishes of the other party, engaging in win-lose competition, or forcing through the exercise of authority.

▲ **Compromise:** Being moderately cooperative and assertive. Behaviors include bargaining for acceptable solutions in which each party wins a bit and loses a bit.

▲ **Collaboration, or problem-solving:** Being both cooperative and assertive. Behaviors include trying to satisfy everyone's concerns fully by working through differences; finding and solving problems so that everyone gains.[11]

The various conflict management styles can result in quite different outcomes.[12] Conflict management by avoidance or accommodation often creates a lose-lose conflict. No one achieves her or his true desires, and the underlying reasons for conflict often remain unaffected. Although a lose-lose conflict may appear settled or may even disappear for a while, it tends to recur in the future.

Competition and compromise tend to create win-lose conflict. Here, each party strives to gain at the other's expense. In extreme cases, one party achieves its desires to the complete exclusion of the other party's desires. Because win-lose methods fail to address the root causes of conflict, future conflicts of the same or a similar nature are likely to occur.

Collaboration uses problem-solving to reconcile underlying differences and is often the most effective conflict management style. It creates win-win conflict

Figure 12-6

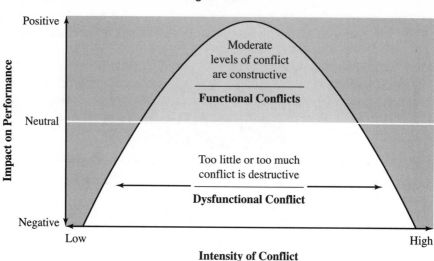

Positive and negative relationship between conflict and performance.

whereby issues are resolved to the mutual benefit of all conflicting parties. This is typically achieved by openly confronting the issues and through the willingness of those involved to recognize that something is wrong and needs attention. Win-win methods are preferred approaches to conflict management.

12.5.2 Separating Functional and Dysfunctional Conflicts

Conflict in organizations can have both positive and negative aspects. Figure 12-6 shows that conflict of moderate intensity can actually be good for performance. This **functional conflict** stimulates people toward greater work efforts, cooperation, and creativity.

At very low or very high intensities, **dysfunctional conflict** occurs. Too much conflict is distracting and interferes with other more task-relevant activities; too little conflict may promote complacency and the loss of a creative, high-performance edge. For example, the negative side of conflict can occur when two team members are unable to work together because of interpersonal hostilities (an emotional conflict) or when members of a committee can't agree on common goals (a substantive conflict).

12.5.3 Resolving Conflict

Conflicts can either be **resolved,** in the sense that their causes are corrected, or they can be **suppressed,** in that the causes remain but the conflict is controlled for a period of time. Suppressed conflicts run the risk of recurring at a later time.

True conflict resolution, by contrast, eliminates the underlying causes of conflict and reduces the potential for similar conflicts in the future. The following are ways that work situations can be restructured to resolve conflicts:

▲ **An appeal to superordinate goals** can focus the attention of conflicting parties on one mutually desirable objective. This approach offers a common frame of reference against which to analyze and reconcile disagreements.

▲ **Expanding the resources available to everyone** can resolve conflicts whose causes lie in competition for scarce resources.

▲ **By altering one or more human variables**—that is, by replacing or transferring one or more of the conflicting parties—conflicts caused by poor interpersonal relationships can be eliminated.

▲ **By altering the physical environment**—rearranging facilities, workspace, or workflows you can decrease opportunities for conflict.

▲ **Using integrating devices**—such as liaison personnel, special task forces, and cross-functional teams, and even the matrix form of organization (see section 3.1.4)—can change communication patterns and assist in conflict resolution.

▲ **Changing the reward system** may reduce the competition among individuals and groups for rewards. Creating systems that reward cooperation can encourage teamwork and keep conflict within constructive limits.

FOR EXAMPLE

Conflict Coaching at John Hopkins

As one of the most dynamic research hospitals in the United States, John Hopkins Hospital (www.hopkinsmedicine.org) also takes a dynamic approach to encouraging and facilitating employee conflict resolutions. What John Hopkins calls "conflict coaching" is the first of three officially recognized techniques within the organization. (Visit www.hopkinsmedicine.org/jhhr/PoliciesProcedures/HR604 for details on the organization's comprehensive conflict resolution program.) Conflict coaching, which is free and available to all employees, is confidential, voluntary, and one-on-one. A trained coach talks the employee through a past or present dispute, helping the employee identify options. After the employee selects a path of action, the coach can help the employee prepare for a "conflict conversation," mapping out an agenda for a meeting and preparing responses to likely questions. If the employee is unable to resolve the conflict via conflict coaching, the employee can then move on to mediation, a process that John Hopkins can fully facilitate as well.

▲ **Creating new policies and procedures** that direct behavior in ways that minimize the likelihood of negative conflict situations can help.

▲ **Training** can help prepare people to communicate and work more effectively in situations that are conflict-prone.

SELF-CHECK

- Identify and define **conflict, cooperativeness,** and **assertiveness.**
- Compare substantive conflict and emotional conflict.
- Describe the five interpersonal styles of conflict management: avoidance, accommodation, competition, compromise, and collaboration.
- List characteristics of functional conflict and dysfunctional conflict, and resolved conflict and suppressed conflict.
- Discuss techniques for resolving conflict.

12.6 Negotiating

As a manager, how would you behave, and what would you do if

▲ you have been offered a promotion and would really like to take it, but the pay raise offered is less than you hoped?

▲ you have enough money to order one new computer for your department, but you have requests for two new machines?

These are but two examples of the many situations in today's health care workplace that involve **negotiation,** the process of making joint decisions when the parties involved have different preferences. People negotiate over such diverse matters as salary, merit raises and performance evaluations, job assignments, work schedules, work locations, special privileges, and many other considerations. All such situations are susceptible to conflict and require exceptional communication skills.

Most new health care managers are not born negotiators, skilled negotiators, or educated negotiators. Few health care curriculums offer courses of practicum experiences on negotiating.

And yet, in the course of a given day, health care managers may negotiate a fee-for-services contract, establish new performance standards for a nonperforming employee, or set a new schedule for an operating room. All these interactions, like many of the interpersonal interactions managed by an effective physician leader, call for negotiation skill, strategy, and savvy.

FOR EXAMPLE

Negotiation Teams

Many workers within health care organizations today are forming *negotiation teams* to address major changes, such as new facility construction, contract negotiation, or operations expansion. Negotiating teams (typically three to eight members total) form for a limited time and have a specific goal. Successful teams often include a balance of listeners, talkers, presenters, and perceivers because the type of communicator brings something different and important to the negotiation process. For example, at Devon Health Services, Inc. (www.devonhealth.com), a "Claims Negotiation team" composed of nonmedical health care professionals was established to negotiate discounts on medical claim. The group has helped patients receive discounts of 25% and more on medical claims by negotiating special reimbursement solutions with doctors and hospitals.

This section, although hardly exhaustive, offers an overview of the negotiation process, as well as some basic strategies that health care managers can implement into their daily managerial duties.

12.6.1 Choosing a Negotiation Approach

In general, two types of goals exist in the world of negotiation:

▲ **Substance goals** are concerned with outcomes. They are tied to the "content" issues of the negotiation.

▲ **Relationship goals** are concerned with processes. They are tied to the way people work together while negotiating and how they (and any constituencies they represent) will be able to work together again in the future.

Negotiation can be considered successful when issues of substance are resolved and working relationships among the negotiating parties are maintained or even improved.[13]

The way each party approaches a negotiation can have a major impact on its outcomes.[14]

▲ In **distributive negotiation,** each party makes claims for certain preferred results. This is a competitive win-lose approach in which one party can gain only if the other loses. Relationships are often sacrificed as the negotiating parties focus only on their respective self-interests.

▲ In **principled negotiation,** a win-win orientation operates.[15] The interests of all parties are considered, and the goal is to base the final outcome on the merits of individual claims. Everyone looks for ways for all claims to be satisfied if possible, with no one "losing" in the process.

Many health care managers approach negotiation as a series of *appeals* that they make to the other party. Although appeals can be an effective way of gaining your opponent's attention, appeals alone are not typically enough to reach a win-win agreement.

Essentially, negotiating appeals fall into the following basic types:

▲ **Appeal to ego:** A negotiator uses an array of compliments, ego-stroking, and other self-esteem gratification techniques to reach a favorable settlement. Using expressions like, "A smart individual like you," "Someone who is a real go-getter," or "An intelligent manager like yourself," as preambles to statements helps to build an appeal-to-ego strategy. This strategy may be effective in the short term, but over the long term it can be seen as manipulative, less than genuine, and basically phony.

▲ **Appeal to authority:** In this case, an individual uses an authority such as a state regulation board, the board of directors, or other proverbial "powers that be" as the driving factor in why a negotiation settlement should be reached quickly and favorably. This tactic is not only somewhat disingenuous, as it connotes a power play by the negotiator who uses it, but is also an abdication of authority relative to the basic responsibility of the individuals present at the negotiation table.

▲ **Appeal to the norm:** This appeal is in evidence when one negotiator cites the need for commonality or normalcy as a driving force for reaching a settlement. Statements such as, "Most physicians would take this deal" or "Every hospital in the state does it" are examples of appeal-to-norm strategies. This technique may be effective in some cases, where standards and practices are the prominent feature of the need to reach a negotiated settlement, but in all cases it is a less-than-effective strategy.

▲ **Appeal to emotion:** Anger, pride, friendship, gravity (such as "If we don't do this, the hospital will close!"), and other emotional drivers are used to trigger a negotiated settlement in an appeal-to-emotion ploy. Appealing to emotion is a perilous tactic for a health care leader to use. Fundamentally, most people who have had any sort of tenure in health care have witnessed a wide array of emotionalism displayed by patients and employees on any given day. Therefore, they are not likely to be motivated by someone crying, yelling, threatening, conjoining, or displaying any other type of emotional behavior that is not specifically related to the negotiation objective at hand.

▲ **Appeal to a vision:** Here, a negotiator presents a picture of what the final negotiating outcome may be. Appealing to a vision is perhaps the only effective strategy among the appeal-process negotiation techniques. In painting a picture of a harmonious workplace, effective emergency room, progressive medical service organization, or any other favorable vision of health care excellence, a negotiator can create a vision that is equally alluring to their opponent as to themselves. The vision can be not only the objective for the negotiation but also the driving motivation for reaching a settlement. However, the vision must be one that is equally shared and desired by both negotiation parties; otherwise the tactic is doomed to fail.

▲ **Appeal to mission:** A negotiator constantly cites the mission of the health care organization as the driving force for reaching a negotiated settlement. This can be an effective appeal only if coupled with the vision appeal and other artful negotiation.

▲ **Appeal to personal relationships:** Friendship, collegiality, past history, and other personal notes are used as catalysts for obtaining a progressive settlement. Though a certain amount of strength of interpersonal relationship can be drawn on in any negotiation, the effective negotiator does not rely strictly on personal friendship as the centerpiece for negotiation. Simply put, if an individual uses personal friendship as a mainstay of negotiation, her opponent can simply say something along the lines of "Friendship is one thing, business is another—let's get down to the brass tacks of reaching a good agreement."

Many elements of the psychological win-win approach can be incorporated into a more effective strategy of the **mutual-benefit logical approach** to negotiation. The mutual-benefit logical approach is based on several basic beliefs:

▲ **Preparation is key:** If you are prepared and your opponent is not, or is not as well prepared as you are, the odds increase in your favor that you can prevail in the negotiation. Preparation takes several forms in logical negotiation: knowing your opponent, preparing your bargaining position, preparing counterarguments, and planning overall negotiation strategies are all examples of well-prepared negotiation techniques.

▲ **Knowledge of your opponent is crucial:** By understanding your opponent's position, analyzing potential methods and approaches of your opponent, and counteracting your opponent's forays in the negotiation process, the likelihood of a negotiation victory is enhanced. Again, preparation is key, and the requirement that the negotiator does the homework is paramount to success.

▲ **Establish a negotiation range:** Prepared negotiators understand the differences between wants and needs and negotiate by focusing on needs. Often, two negotiating parties reach an immediate impasse because both sides endeavor to move the other party toward the "want" position. By focusing on needs, there exists the opportunity for a well-negotiated settlement that can be favorable to both parties.

12.6.2 Knowing an Opponent's Position

At the outset of the negotiation process, a savvy negotiator tries to ascertain his or her opponent's position. This can be achieved by asking your opponent to prioritize the list of most important agenda items for the negotiation. You can then ascertain the primary and secondary agenda items for your opponent.

Furthermore, try to determine the strategic position of your opponent on mutually beneficial needs range. By asking a sequence of questions, you can elicit more specific information about your opponent's desired outcomes for the negotiation. The following questions force your opponent to be more specific about his or her position:

▲ What do you need to have happen here at the negotiation table?

▲ Specifically what do you need from our discussions?

▲ Why is this particular initiative important to you?

▲ Which one of these items is the most important to you?

▲ What are you looking for from this negotiation?

▲ Would you please list for me—so we all understand—what your priorities are, listed in numerical order?

▲ What do you need to get done here at the negotiating table, or what do we need to get done?

▲ What do you want to get done, or what do we want to get done here at the table? (Note: By using this and the preceding question in concert, you may be able to get a sense of an opponent's "dream objective".)

▲ How can we make this happen?

▲ Can you directly, honestly, and specifically tell us what your ultimate objectives are for this negotiation?

In seizing the initiative in trying to unveil your opponent's position, you are better prepared to list priorities for the negotiation and identify not only the primary and secondary needs of the opponent, but your potential trade-off positions for the negotiation.

Once again, by simply being prepared and taking a proactive stance in the negotiation process, you gain an upper hand that helps facilitate a more favorable result to the negotiation process.

12.6.3 Avoiding Negotiating Pitfalls

The negotiation process is admittedly complex. Negotiators must guard against several common mistakes. Many obstacles can stand in the way of success in reaching an agreement.

Pitfalls such as the following can too easily create win-lose situations, which can ultimately result in poor final results:[16]

▲ **The myth of the fixed pie:** When you fall prey to this pitfall in negotiation, you assume that in order for you to gain, the other person must give up something. Negotiating this way fails to recognize the possibility that sometimes the pie can be expanded or utilized to everyone's advantage.

▲ **Nonrational escalation of conflict:** In this pitfall, the negotiator becomes committed to previously stated demands and allows concerns for ego and face-saving to increase the perceived importance of satisfying these demands.

▲ **Overconfidence and ignoring the other's needs:** The error here is becoming overconfident that your position is the only correct one and failing to see the needs of the other party and the merits in its position.

▲ **Too much telling, too little hearing:** When committing a telling problem, you don't really make yourself or your side understood. When committing a hearing problem, you don't listen sufficiently to understand what the other is saying.

12.6.4 Reaching Agreement

At a certain point—a point that is difficult to define because each negotiation is different—you should move to close the deal.

Generally, you will want to close the deal when you have ascertained that your opponent has reached a position of agreement with you within the mutually beneficial need range that is amenable to both parties. At that point, you can choose among the following options:

▲ Verify the position of both parties
▲ Take the deal
▲ Reject the deal
▲ Consider the long-range ramifications of accepting or rejecting the deal
▲ Consider alternative deals with other parties
▲ Reevaluate the benefits provided by the impending deal
▲ Perhaps most important, listen to and trust your gut-level comfort level with the deal
▲ Summarize and reiterate the tenets of the deal so that both parties understand

If the answers to all the items on this checklist are relatively positive, you should embrace the deal that has been generated through the negotiation strategy.

Unfortunately, it may not always be possible to achieve integrative agreements. When negotiations reach the point of impasse, dispute resolution through mediation or arbitration can be useful.

▲ **Mediation** involves a neutral third party who tries to improve communications between negotiating parties and keep them focused on relevant issues. This mediator does not issue a ruling or make a decision, but can take an active role in discussions. Mediation often includes making suggestions in an attempt to move the parties toward agreement.

▲ **Arbitration** is a stronger form of dispute resolution. Arbitration involves a neutral third party, the arbitrator, who acts as a judge and issues a binding decision. The arbitration process usually includes a formal hearing in which the arbitrator listens to both sides and reviews all facets of the case before making a ruling.

As in all leadership endeavors, no right or wrong answers exist in the negotiation process. However, by following the introductory guidelines in this chapter—and more important, trusting your intrinsic intelligence and negotiation savvy—the art of mutually beneficial negotiation is well within your grasp as a health care manager.

SELF-CHECK

- Identify and define **negotiation, mutual-benefit logical approach, mediation,** and **arbitration.**
- Compare substantive goals and relationship goals within the negotiation process.
- Define distributive negotiation and principled negotiation approaches.
- Discuss the seven basic negotiating appeals.
- Describe three key strategies for successful negotiation.
- List questions that can help determine your opponent's position.
- Contrast arbitration and mediation.

SUMMARY

Health care managers receive and send out communication in a variety of forms, all day, every day. At its most basic, communication involves a sender, a receiver, and a message. The sender, or source, of a message can include the organization, supervisors, staff, and others. Barriers (such as nonverbal signals or a poor choice of channel) and perceptions (such as stereotypes or projections) cause communication messages to be blocked or distorted. Improving communication skills does take effort, but the results can increase the likelihood of a message being effectively, efficiently, and correctly received. Conflict naturally occurs in today's dynamic health care workplace; proactive managers utilize conflict management techniques—especially negotiation—to help their departments continue to operate smoothly.

KEY TERMS

Accommodation	In conflict management, being cooperative but unassertive; also known as *smoothing*.
Active listening	The process of helping the source of a message say exactly what he or she really means.
Arbitration	A stronger form of dispute resolution than mediation, arbitration involves a neutral third party who acts as a judge and issues a binding decision.
Assertiveness	The desire to satisfy one's own needs and concerns.
Avoidance	In conflict management, being uncooperative and unassertive.
Collaboration	In conflict management, being both cooperative and assertive; problem-solving.
Communication	An interpersonal process of sending and receiving symbols with messages attached to them.
Communication channel	The medium through which a message is conveyed from sender to receiver.
Competition	In conflict management, being uncooperative but assertive; also known as *authoritative command*.
Compromise	In conflict management, being moderately cooperative and assertive.
Conflict	A disagreement between people on substantive or emotional issues.
Cooperativeness	The desire to satisfy another party's needs and concerns.
Distributive negotiation	Each party makes claims for certain preferred results; decisions are often win-lose.
Dysfunctional conflict	Conflict at very low or high intensities that distracts and interferes with other more task-relevant activities.

Effective communication	The intended message of the sender and the interpreted meaning of the receiver are one and the same.
Efficient communication	Communication that occurs at minimum cost in terms of resources expended and the amount of time involved.
Emotional conflicts	Disagreements over feelings of anger, distrust, dislike, fear, and resentment, as well as from personality clashes.
Ethnocentrism	The tendency to consider one's culture superior to others.
Feedback	The reverse of the communication process; the receiver responds back to the send.
Filtering	The intentional distortion of information to make it appear favorable to the recipient.
Functional conflict	Conflict of moderate intensity that can actually be good for performance, stimulating greater work efforts, cooperation, and creativity.
Halo effect	Communication problem that occurs when one attribute is used to develop an overall impression of a person or situation.
Mediation	A neutral third party tries to improve communications between negotiating parties and keep them focused on relevant issues. The mediator does not issue a ruling or make a decision, but can take an active role in discussions.
Mutual-benefit logical approach	A negotiation strategy that focus on win-win psychology.
Negotiation	The process of making joint decisions when the parties involved have different preferences.
Noise	Anything that interferes with the effectiveness of the communication process.
Nonverbal communication	Communication takes place through such things as hand movements, facial expressions, body posture, eye contact, and the use of interpersonal space.
Perception	The way people receive and interpret information from the environment.
Principled negotiation	The interests of all parties are considered, and the goal is to base the final outcome on the merits of individual claims; a win-win orientation operates.

Projection	The assignment of personal attributes to other individuals.
Proxemics	The use of interpersonal space in communication.
Receiver	In the communication process, the personal who decodes or interprets the meaning of a message.
Relationship goal	In negotiation, a goal that is concerned with processes and is tied to the way people work together while negotiating and how they can work together again in the future.
Resolved conflict	The causes of a conflict are corrected.
Selective perception	The tendency to single out for attention those aspects of a situation or person that reinforce or appear consistent with one's existing beliefs, values, or needs.
Sender	In the communication process, the person who is responsible for encoding an intended message into meaningful symbols, both verbal and nonverbal.
Stereotype	Communication problem that occurs when someone is identified with a group or category, and then oversimplified attributes associated with the group or category are attributed to the individual.
Substance goal	In negotiation, a goal that is concerned with outcomes and is tied to content issues of the negotiation.
Substantive conflicts	Disagreements over such things as goals, the allocation of resources, the distribution of rewards, policies and procedures, and job assignments.
Suppressed conflict	The causes of a conflict remain, but the conflict is controlled for a period of time.

ASSESS YOUR UNDERSTANDING

Go to www.wiley.com/college/Lombardi to evaluate your knowledge of basic communication skills.
Measure your learning by comparing pretest and post-test results.

Summary Questions

1. Communication is an interpersonal process of sending and receiving symbols with messages attached to them. True or false?
2. Managerial directives and organizational mandates are examples of
   (a) outgoing communication.
   (b) efficient communication.
   (c) incoming communication.
   (d) inefficient communication.
3. Communication sources for health care managers can include
   (a) supervisors, staff, and peers.
   (b) newspapers, memos, and e-mails.
   (c) human resources, public relations, and information technology.
   (d) consultants, technicians, and subject specialists.
4. Conducting an employee review primarily via e-mail is an example of which type of communication barrier?
   (a) Status effect
   (b) Poor written communication
   (c) Failure to recognize nonverbal signs
   (d) Poor choice of channels
5. Nonverbal communication includes all the following except
   (a) eye contact.
   (b) dress.
   (c) hand movements.
   (d) use of interpersonal space.
6. When an employee tells his or her boss only information the boss wants to hear, the communication barrier that occurs is known as *fabrication*. True or false?
7. Which of the following statements about stereotypes is true?
   (a) Stereotypes classify a person into a group based on one piece of information.
   (b) Stereotypes about gender are the most common workplace stereotype.
   (c) Stereotypes are an exaggeration of a commonly held belief.
   (d) None of these

8. An example of projection in the workplace is
   (a) blaming a low-performing staff member for not meeting a departmental goal.
   (b) assigning unpopular tasks to a staff member who is difficult to get along with.
   (c) preferring to hire male nurses for third-shift positions.
   (d) signing up a staffer for a management course that was helpful to your own career.

9. A well-crafted piece of communication has credibility and sense of consequence. True or false?

10. Active listening requires you block out all visual information and focus on the message someone else is saying. True or false?

11. In order for constructive feedback to be effective, you should
    (a) present the feedback in a public forum.
    (b) make sure the feedback is specific rather than general.
    (c) give four pieces of positive feedback for every negative piece.
    (d) ask the feedback recipient to repeat the feedback to you.

12. Substantive conflicts involve personality clashes and resentment, while emotional conflicts involve disagreements over goals, resources, rewards and assignments. True or false?

13. What conflict management strategy is coming into play when a receptionist refuses to get involved in a disagreement between the billing manager and the nursing staff manager?
    (a) Compromise
    (b) Accommodation
    (c) Competition
    (d) Avoidance

14. Collaboration and problem-solving strategies for conflict management tend to create win-lose situations. True or false?

15. Which of the following statements is true about principled negotiation?
    (a) Each party makes claims for a preferred result.
    (b) The interests of each party are considered.
    (c) A competitive, win-lose approach produces better results.
    (d) Negotiating teams prepare their cases in advance.

16. When a manager tells his emergency-room staff to reach a compromise quickly because the needs of the ER patients are a life-or-death matter, the manager is using an appeal to
    (a) honor.
    (b) mission.

(c) emotion.

(d) the norm.

17. In the negotiating pitfall known as the *myth of the fixed pie,* you believe that in order for anyone to gain, someone else must give up something. True or false?

18. Mediation involves a neutral third party who

(a) listens to the situation and hands down a decision.

(b) interprets legal codes and assigns responsibilities.

(c) reviews decisions in previous cases.

(d) tries to improve communication between parties.

Review Questions

1. The shift manager posts a memo in the break room that tells all staff to submit their time sheets a day earlier than originally scheduled. Who or what are the sender, message, channel, and receiver in this communication scenario?

2. A new manager reviews her department's written handbook to determine the course of action to deal with a problem employee. What communication source is the manager relying on?

3. For health care managers, what is the more important source of incoming communication?

4. In the communication process, anything that interferes with the effectiveness of a message is noise. What are the most common forms of noise?

5. Physical distractions are one form of noise that managers can typically deal with quite effectively. What are some common physical distractions related to a manager's office space?

6. Over one weekend last year, a laboratory tech at a large urban hospital put in nearly 25 hours of overtime to keep the facility operating while several employees were ill or on vacation. The laboratory manager frequently recalls the tech's service and praises her nearly a year after the event. What sort of perception issue is happening here?

7. Perceptions act as a screen through which information must pass during interpersonal communication. What influences a person's perceptions?

8. Selectivity is the tendency to single out attention on those aspects of a situation or person that supports your beliefs, values, or needs. What is one way to minimize the impact of selectivity?

9. Highlighting a message of mutual benefit can dramatically improve your effectiveness as a communicator. What are the five typical recipients of a mutual benefit message?

10. The layout of a workspace impacts a staff's ability to communicate. What are same layout ideas that encourage greater communication?

11. Ethnocentrism, or the tendency to consider your culture superior to others, can negatively affect communication in the workplace. What are two ways that ethnocentrism has a negative impact?

12. When you disagree with team members, you tend to debate issues until you near the breaking point. You frequently use your authority to force the resolution you want. What sort of conflict management strategy do you tend to use?

13. An individual with a high degree of assertiveness and a high degree of cooperativeness will more gravitate toward what type of conflict management?

14. During a health care benefits negotiation, your opponent tells you that "the board of directors is giving employees everything they possibly can" and that you must remember that the most important thing about your job is "providing outstanding services to hospital patients." What sort of appeal is your opponent using?

15. During the process of negotiating for a pay raise, you try to focus on the interests of yourself and your department, creating a win-win situation. What approach to negotiation are you taking?

16. During negotiation, Ray tends to fixate on the one or two "injustices" that he feels were done against him, rather than trying to come up with solutions for the future. Which of the negotiating pitfalls is Ray experiencing?

Applying This Chapter

1. Effective communication isn't always efficient, and efficient communication isn't always effective. Can you provide an example of both situations?

2. Your staff has complained lately that your communication isn't always clear. You send out daily status e-mails and frequently tell staff that your "door is always open," and yet your messages don't seem to be getting through. What are some communication barriers you should evaluate?

3. After successfully working in a fast-paced emergency room for 10 years, Janice was promoted to nursing staff manager for the entire hospital. Although Janice tries to assign tasks fairly and consistently among the hospital's five nursing staffs, she tends to project her ER experiences on all employees, telling them to focus on efficiency and quick decision making. What could Janice do to minimize her projection tendencies and potentially improve staff effectiveness?

4. Due to recent changes in state law, the staff of the medical records department you manage must complete an additional piece of paperwork

for every patient treated and assign all accounts an additional billing code. What are some mutual benefits you might be able to highlight for your staff to ensure compliance?

5. The five-member customer service team that Bettina leads has two star representatives and three average workers. The two stars frequently try to outshine each other, bragging about their successes or diminishing the success of the other. The rest of the team sometimes takes sides with one or the other of the stars, but for the most part they're annoyed by the stars' egos and in-fighting. What is something Bettina can do to respond the ongoing conflict in her department?

6. As the nursing staff manager at a university hospital, the salary negotiation team you've been serving on for 8 months is deadlocked with the hospital's upper management. Your staff has been working without a contract for 6 months and is threatening a strike. What options do you have to reach resolution?

Considering Multiple Information Sources

Consider the most common information sources for health care managers (section 1.1.2). While each of these sources can provide you important, useful information, which sources do you anticipate will provide you with the most valuable information while working in a health care environment? Rank the information sources based on your own perspective, and then ask a full-time health care work or manager to rank the same list of information resources. In what ways did your rankings differ?

Boost Your Writing Skills

Written communication skills are still key to managerial success. While managers today typically write fewer official memos than managers 10 years go, today's managers write often dozens of e-mails each day. Each of these messages needs to effectively and efficiently communicate your meaning. Good grammar is essential to crafting a good e-mail. Assess your grammar with more than 100 free, interactive quizzes available at http://grammar.ccc.commnet.edu/grammar/quiz_list. htm. The main site (http://grammar.ccc.commnet. edu/grammar) is also a good resource if you have a question while writing a message.

360-Degree Roundup

Three-hundred-sixty-degree feedback, an approach advocated by author and health care management consultant Donald N. Lombardi, helps managers become more aware of the feelings and perceptions of staff, peers, and supervisors. The technique involves gathering feedback from a manager's subordinates, as well as from peers and bosses. A self-assessment is also part of the process. The goal of 360-degree feedback is to gain awareness and information that can be used for constructive improvement. Conduct your own version of a 360-degree roundup, collecting feedback on a specific aspect of a job you have (your communication style, or the overall quality of your charting or a specific type of report, perhaps). Seek out feedback from someone at your level, as well as from someone

below and above you. If you don't have a job where you can conduct a roundup, use the information-gathering approach suggested here and have people at various levels evaluate your resume, a research paper, or school project.

Your Nonverbal Communication Style

Nonverbal communication—body language, facial expressions, and body positioning—can say as much as the actual words you use. Identify your nonverbal communication traits by reading about 200 words of text in front of a mirror several times. (The text you use can be just about anything: the first few paragraphs of a paper you've written, a page or two from a favorite book, an interesting newspaper article.) First, read the piece as naturally as possible, attempting to make eye contact with yourself in the mirror. What facial expressions did you use? Did you sit or stand as you read the piece? Did you use hand gestures or other physical actions? What felt natural and comfortable? What felt forced and uncomfortable? Now, read the piece several more times. Slouch in a chair and cross your arms. Stand perfectly straight with your arms behind your back and avoid any hand gestures. Read the piece with a big smile on your face. Again, which of these readings felt natural and comfortable? Which felt forced and uncomfortable? Finally, read the piece as naturally as possible, incorporating what you've previously observed.

Your Response to Conflict

Review the five types of responses to conflict based on personality type as outlined in 12.5.1. Each of these responses may be appropriate options for any given situation. Consider a conflict you recently experienced in your job, education, or personal life. How could you respond to the same situation using avoidance, accomodation, competition, compromise, or collaboration? Which response feels most appropriate for the situation? Do you feel that response fits best with your personality?

Know Your Negotiation Strengths

Successful negotiation is much more than being able to argue more aggressively than your opponent and get your way. Before you begin your next negotiation (perhaps for something as important as a pay raise, as critical as an extension on a homework deadline, or as mundane as which movie you and your friends will see), identify the strongest interpersonal skill or skills you bring to the negotiating table. Some effective negotiation strengths include effective communication, accurate presentation of complex facts, keen observation of the other side, or compassionate listening and understanding. After you identify your strength (or strengths), plan your negotiation around your skill. For example, if you identify that accurate presentation of complex facts is your greatest strength, plan ways to quickly summarize information, guide your opponent through complex data, and highlight accuracies (and inaccuracies) in the information you're both reviewing. By capitalizing your strengths, you are more likely to reach a resolution that truly satisfies your personality.

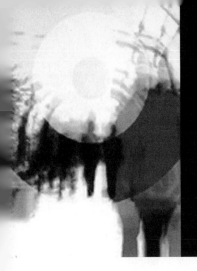

ENDNOTES

Chapter 1

1. See Dave Ulrich, "Intellectual Capital = Competence Commitment," *Sloan Management Review* (Winter 1998), pp. 15–26.

2. For a perspective on the first-level manager's job, see Leonard A. Schlesinger and Janice A. Klein, "The First-Line Supervisor: Past, Present and Future," pp. 370–82, in Jay W. Lorsch (editor), *Handbook of Organizational Behavior* (Englewood Cliffs, N.J.: Prentice-Hall, 1987).

3. R. Roosevelt Thomas Jr., "From Affirmative Action to Affirming Diversity," *Harvard Business Review* (March–April 1990): pp. 107–117; see also Mary Gentile (editor), *Differences That Work: Organizational Excellence through Diversity* (Boston: Harvard Business School Press, 1996).

4. Taylor Cox Jr., "The Multicultural Organization," Academy of Management Executives vol. 5 (1991), pp. 34–47, and *Cultural Diversity in Organizations: Theory, Research and Practice* (San Francisco: Berrett-Koehler, 1993).

5. Quotation from *Business Week,* August 8, 1990, p. 50.

8. Mintzberg, op. cit., p. 46. For a related discussion see also Henry Mintzberg, "Covert Leadership: Notes on Managing Professionals," *Harvard Business Review* (November–December, 1998), pp. 140–147.

6. Hal Lancaster, "Middle Managers Are Back—But Now They're 'High-Impact' Players," *Wall Street Journal,* April 14, 1998, p. B1.

7. Based on Jay A. Conger, *Winning 'em Over: A New Model for Managing in the Age of Persuasion* (New York: Simon & Schuster, 1998), pp. 180–181; Stewart D. Friedman, Perry Christensen and Jessica DeGroot, "Work and Life: The End of the Zero-Sum Game, *Harvard Business Review* (November–December, 1998), pp. 119–129; and, Argyris, C., "Empowerment: The emperor's new clothes," *Harvard Business Review* (May–June, 1998), pp. 98–105.

9. For a classic study see Thomas A. Mahoney, Thomas H. Jerdee, and Stephen J. Carroll, "The Job(s) of Management," *Industrial Relations, vol. 4* (February 1965), pp. 97–110.

Chapter 2

1. Reported in Barbara Ley Toffler, "Tough Choices: Managers Talk Ethics," *New Management, vol. 4* (1987): 34–39. See also Barbara Ley Toffler, *Tough Choices: Managers Talk Ethics* (New York: Wiley, 1986).

2. Linda K. Trevino and Katherine A. Nelson, *Managing &* (New York: John Wiley & Sons, 1995), pp. 47–60.

3. See Trevino and Nelson, op. cit., 1995.

4. Interactional justice is described by Robert J. Bies, "The Predicament of Injustice: The Management of Moral Outrage," in L.L. Cummings & B.M. Staw (eds.), *Research in Organizational Behavior, vol. 9* (Greenwich, CT: JAI Press, 1987), pp. 289–319. The example is from Carol T. Kulik and Robert L. Holbrook, "Demographics in Service Encounters: Effects of Racial and Gender Congruence on Perceived Fairness," *Social Justice Research,* vol. 13 (2000), pp. 375–402.

5. Saul W. Gellerman, "Why 'Good' Managers Make Bad Ethical Choices," *Harvard Business Review,* vol. 64 (July–August, 1986): 85–90.

6. The discussion and subsequent case are developed from Steven N. Brenner and Earl A. Mollander, "Is the Ethics of Business Changing?" *Harvard Business Review, vol. 55* (January–February 1977): 57.

7. Archie B. Carroll, "A Three-Dimensional Model of Corporate Performance," *Academy of Management Review,* vol. 4 (1979): 497–505.

Chapter 3

1. The classic work is Alfred D. Chandler, *Strategy and Structure* (Cambridge, MA: MIT Press, 1962).

2. See Alfred D. Chandler Jr., "Origins of the Organization Chart," *Harvard Business Review,* March–April 1988, pp. 156–157.

3. See David Krackhardt and Jeffrey R. Hanson, "Informal Networks: The Company Behind the Chart," *Harvard Business Review,* July–August 1993, pp. 104–111.

4. Kenneth Noble, "A Clash of Styles: Japanese Companies in the U.S," *New York Times,* January 25, 1988, p. 7.

5. Henry Mintzberg, "The Structuring of Organizations," in *The Strategy Process: Concepts, Contexts, and Cases,* James Brian Quinn, Henry Mintzberg, and Robert M. James, eds (Englewood Cliffs, NH: Prentice-Hall, 1988), pp. 276–304.

6. Susan Albers Mohrman, Susan G. Cohen, and Allan M. Mohrman Jr., *Designing Team-Based Organizations* (San Francisco: Jossey-Bass, 1996).

7. See, for example, Johnathon Rosenoer, Douglas Armstrong, J. Russell Gates, *The Clickable Corporation* (New York: The Free Press, 1999).

8. See George P. Huber, "A Theory of Effects of Advanced Information Technologies on Organizational Design, Intelligence, and Decision Making," *Academy of Management Review,* vol. 15 (1990): 67–71.

9. See Jay R. Galbraith, *Organizational Design* (Reading, MA: Addison Wesley, 1977).

10. Max Weber, *The Theory of Social and Economic Organization,* A. M. Henderson trans. and H. T. Parsons (New York: The Free Press, 1947).

11. For classic treatments of bureaucracy, see Alvin Gouldner, *Patterns of Industrial Bureaucracy* (New York: The Free Press, 1954); Robert K. Merton, *Social Theory and Social Structure* (New York: The Free Press, 1957).

12. Tom Burns and George M. Stalker, *The Management of Innovation* (London: Tavistock, 1961, republished by Oxford University Press, London, 1994).

13. See Rosabeth Moss Kanter, *The Changing Masters* (New York: Simon & Schuster, 1983).

14. Alfred D. Chandler Jr., *Strategy and Structure: Chapter in the History of American Industrial Enterprise* (Cambridge, MA: MIT Press, 1962).

15. Paul R. Lawrence and Jay W. Lorsch, *Organizations and Environment* (Boston: The Division of Research, Graduate School of Business Administration, Harvard University, 1967).

16. See Jay R. Galbraith, *Organizational Design* (Reading, MA: Addison-Wesley, 1977); and, Susan Albers Mohrman, "Integrating Roles and Structure in the Lateral Organization," chapter 5 in Galbraith, Lawler and Associates, op. cit., 1993.

17. Michael Hammer, *Beyond Reengineering* (New York: Harper Business, 1997).

18. Michael Hammer and James Champy, *Reengineering the Corporation: A Manifesto for Business Revolution* (New York: Harper Business, 1993).

19. Michael Hammer, *Beyond Reengineering* (New York: Harper Business, 1993), pp. 28–30.

20. Jon R. Katzenbach and Douglas K. Smith, *The Wisdom of Teams: Creating the High Performance Organization* (Boston: Harvard Business School Press, 1993).

21. See Marvin E. Shaw, *Group Dynamics: The Psychology of Small Group Behavior, 2d ed.* (New York: McGraw-Hill, 1976); Harold J. Leavitt, "Suppose We Took Groups More Seriously," in *Man and Work in Society* Eugene L. Cass and Frederick G. Zimmer, eds. (New York: Van Nostrand Reinhold, 1975), pp. 67–77.

22. See W. Jack Duncan, "Why Some People Loaf in Groups While Others Loaf Alone," *Academy of Management Review,* vol. 8 (1004): 79–80.

23. For insights on how to run an effective meeting see Mary A. De Vries, *How to Run a Meeting* (New York: Penguin, 1994).

24. For a good discussion of quality circles, see Edward E. Lawler III and Susan A. Mohrman, "Quality Circles after the Fad," *Harvard Business Review,* vol. 63 (January–February 1985): 65–71; Gerald E. Ledford Jr., Edward E. Lawler III, and Susan A. Mohrman, "The Quality Circle and Its Variations," chapter 10 in John R. Campbell, Richard J. Campbell and *Productivity in Organizations* (San Francisco: Jossey-Bass, 1988); and Lawler, Mohrman, and Ledford, 1992, *Employee Involvement.*

25. Wanda J. Orlikowski and J. Debra Hofman, "An Improvisational Model for Change Management: The Case of Groupware Technologies," *Sloan Management Review,* fall 1993, pp. 27–36.

26. R. Brent Gallupe and William H. Cooper, "Brainstorming Electronically," *Sloan Management Review,* winter 1997, pp. 11–21.

27. See, for example, Paul S. Goodman, Rukmini Devadas, and Terri L. Griffith Hughson, "Groups and Productivity: Analyzing the Effectiveness of Self-Managing Teams," chapter 11 in John R. Campbell, Richard J. Campbell, *Productivity in Organizations* (San Francisco: Jossey-Bass, 1988); Jack Orsbrun, Linda Moran, Ed Musslewhite, and John H. Zenger, with Craig Perrin, *Self-Directed Work Teams: The New American Challenge* (Homewood, IL: Business One Irwin, 1990); Dale E. Yeatts and Cloyd Hyten, *High Performing Self-Managed Work Teams* (Thousand Oaks, CA: Sage, 1997).

Chapter 4

1. For a review of research on group effectiveness, see J. Richard Hackman, "The Design of Work Teams," in Handbook of Organizational Behavior Jay W. Lorsch, ed. (Englewood Cliffs, NJ: Prentice-Hall, 1987), pp. 315–342.

2. See Patricia Doyle Corner and Angelo J. Kinicki, "A Proposed Mediator between Top Team Demography and Financial Performance," *Academy of Management Proceedings* '97, pp. 7–11.

4. Bruce W. Tuckman, "Development Sequence in Small Groups" *Psychology Bulletin,* vol. 63 (1965): 38499: Bruce W. Tuckman and Mary Ann C. Jensen, "Stages of Small-Group Development Revisited," *Group & Organization Studies,* vol. 2 (1977): 419–427. For a slightly different model, see also J. Steven Heinen and Eugene Jacobson, " A Model of Task Group Development in Complex Organizations and a Strategy of Implementation," *Academy of Management Review,* vol. 1 (1976):98–111.

5. For a good discussion, see Robert F. Allen and Saul Pilnick, "Confronting the Shadow Organization: How to Detect and Defeat Negative Norms," Organizational Dynamics, Spring 1973, pp. 13–17.

6. See Edgar H Schein, Process Consultation, Volumes I & II, Second Edition (Englewood Cliffs, NJ.: Prentice-Hall, 1998.

7. A classic work in this area is the 1948 article in the *Journal of Social Issues,* vol. 2:42–47, by K. Benne and P. Sheets. See also op. cit, 1988.

8. Research on communication networks is found in Alex Bavelas," Communication Patterns in Task-Oriented Groups," *Journal of the Accuostical Society of America,* vol. 22 (1950): 725–730: see also Marvin E. Shaw, Group Dynamics: *The Psychology of Small Group Behavior* (New York: McGraw-Hill, 1976).

9. See William D. Dyer, *Team-Building* (Reading, MA: Addison-Wesley, 1977).

10. Schein, op. cit., 1988.

11. See Kathleen M. Eisenhardt, Jean L. Kahwajy, and L.J. Bourgeois III, " How Management Teams Can Have a Good Fight," *Harvard Business Review,* July-August 1997, pp. 77–85.

12. Victor H. Vroom and Arthur G. Jago, *The New Leadership: Managing Particiaption in Organizations* (Engelwood Cliffs, NJ: Prentice-Hall, 1988).

13. Norman F. Maier, "Assets and Liabilities in Group Problem Solving" *Psychological Review,* vol. 74 (1967):239–249.

14. See Irving L. Janis, "Groupthink," Psychology Today, November 191, pp. 43–46: *Victims of Groupthink,* 2d ed. (Boston: Hougton Mifflin, 1982).

15. Both the symptoms and guidelines are from Ibid.

16. Katzenbach and Smith, 1993.

Chapter 5

1. Quote from William Bridges, "The End of the Job," *Fortune,* September 19, 1994, p. 68.

2. For a discussion of affirmative action see R. Roosevelt Thomas, Jr. "from 'Affirmative Action' to 'Affirming Diversity,' " *Harvard Business Review* (November–December 1990), pp. 107–117; and Thomas, *Beyond Race and Gender,* op.cit., 1998).

3. See discussion by David A. DeCenzo and Stephen P. Robbins, *Human Resource Management, 6th ed.* (New York: Wiley, 1999), pp. 66–68 and 81–83.

4. See example and discussion of BFOQs in David A. DeCenzo and Stephen P. Robbins, *Human Resource Management, 6th ed.* (New York: Wiley, 1999), pp.77–79.

5. See discussion by David A. DeCenzo and Stephen P. Robbins, *Human Resource Management,* 6th ed. (New York: Wiley, 1999), pp. 79–90.

6. See "Reinventing Labor: An Interview with Union President Lynn Williams," *Harvard Business Review,* July–August 1993, pp. 115–125.

7. See Boris Yavitz, "Human Resources in Strategic Planning," in *Executive Talent: Developing and Keeping the Best People,* Eli Ginzberg (ed.)(New York: Wiley, 1988), p. 34.

8. See John P. Wanous, *Organizational Entry: Recruitment, Selection, and Socialization of Newcomers* (Reading, MA: Addison-Wesley, 1980), pp. 34–44.

9. "Would You Hire This Person Again?" *Business Week,* Enterprise issue, June 9, 1997, pp. ENT32.

10. For a scholarly review, see John Van Maanen and Edgar H. Schein, "Toward a Theory of Socialization," in *Research in Organizational Behavior, vol. 1,* Barry M. Staw, ed. (Greenwich, CT: JAI Press, 1979), pp. 209–64; for a practitioner's view, see Richard Pascale, "Fitting New Employees into the Company Culture," *Fortune,* May 28, 1984, pp. 28–42.

11. This involves the social information processing concept as discussed in Gerald R. Salancik and Jeffrey Pfeffer, "A Social Information Processing Approach to Job Attitudes and Task Design," *Administrative Science Quarterly, vol. 23* (June 1978): 224–253.

12. Larry L. Cummings and Donald P. Schwab, *Performance in Organizations: Determinants and Appraisal* (Glenview, IL: Scott, Foresman, 1973).

13. See Betty Friedan, *Beyond Gender: The New Politics of Work and the Family* (Washington, DC: Woodrow Wilson Center Press, 1997) and James A. Levine, *Working Fathers: New Strategies for Balancing Work and Family* (Reading, MA: Addison-Wesley, 1997).

14. Information from David Coburn, "Balancing Home, Work Still Big Concern," *Columbus Dispatch,* February 16, 1998, pp. 8, 9.

Chapter 7

1. See, for example, Robert C. Camp, Business Process Benchmarking (Milwaukee: ASQ Quality Press, 1994); Michael J. Spendolini, The Benchmarking Book (New York: AMACOM, 1992); and Christopher E. Bogan and Michael J. English, Benchmarking for Best Practices; Winning Through Innovative Adaptation (New York: McGraw-Hill, 1994).

2. Harold Koontz and Cyril O'Donnell, Essentials of Management (New York: McGraw-Hill, 1974), pp. 362–365.

3. See William Newman, Constructive Control: Design and Use of Control Systems (Englewood Cliffs, NJ: Prentice-Hall, 1975).

4. Douglas McGregor, The Human Side of Enterprise (New York: McGraw-Hill, 1960).

5. The "hot stove rules" are developed from R. Bruch McAfee and William Poffenberger, Productivity Strategies: Enhancing Employee Job Performance (Englewood Cliffs, NJ: Prentice-Hall, 1982), pp. 54–55. They are originally attributed to Douglas McGregor, "Hot Stove Rules of Discipline," in Personnel: The Human Problems of Management, G. Strauss and L. Sayles, eds. (Englewood Cliffs, NJ: Prentice-Hall, 1967).

6. See Dale D. McConkey, How to Manage by Results, 3d ed. (New York: AMACOM, 1976); Stephen J. Carroll Jr. and Henry J. Tosi Jr., Management by Objectives: Applications and Research (New York: Macmillan, 1973); and Anthony P. Raia, Managing by Objectives (Glenview, IL: Scott, Foresman, 1974).

7. For a discussion of research, see Carroll and Tosi, Management by Objectives; Raia, Managing by Objectives; 1974; Steven Kerr, "Overcoming the Dysfunctions of MBO," Management by Objectives 5, no. 1 (1976).

8. See Douglas McGregor, The Human Side of Enterprise (New York: McGraw-Hill, 1960). The work on goal setting and motivation is summarized in Edwin A. Locke and Gary P. Latham, Goal Setting: A Motivational Technique That Works! (Englewood Cliffs, NJ: Prentice-Hall, 1984).

Chapter 8

1. Gary Hamel and C. K. Prahalad, "Strategic Intent," Harvard Business Review, May–June, 1989, pp. 63–76.

2. See Michael E. Porter, Competitive Strategy: Techniques for Analyzing Industries and Competitors (New York: The Free Press, 1980), and Competitive Advantage: Creating and Sustaining Superior Performance (New York: The Free Press, 1986); and Richard A. D'Aveni, Hyper-Competition: Managing the Dynamics of Strategic Maneuvering (New York: The Free Press, 1994).

3. Peter F. Drucker, "Five Questions," Executive Excellence, November 6, 1994, pp. 6–7.

4. Peter F. Drucker, Management: Tasks, Responsibilities, Practices (New York: Harper & Row, 1973), p. 122.

5. Henry Mintzberg, "Planning on the Left Side and Managing on the Right," Harvard Business Review, vol. 54 (July–August 1976): 46–55; Henry Mintzberg and James A. Waters, "Of Strategies, Deliberate and Emergent," Strategic Management Journal, vol. 6 (1985): 257–72; Henry Mintzberg, "Crafting Strategy," Harvard Business Review, vol. 65 (July–August 1987): 66–75.

6. See Richard A. D'Aveni, Hyper-Competition: Managing the Dynamics of Strategic Maneuvering (New York: The Free Press, 1994), pp.13–16, 21–24.

7. Richard G. Hammermesh, "Making Planning Strategic," Harvard Business Review, vol. 64 (July–August 1986): 115–120.

8. See Gerald B. Allan, "A Note on the Boston Consulting Group Concept of Competitive Analysis and Corporate Strategy," Harvard Business School, Intercollegiate Case Clearing House, ICCH9-175-175 (Boston: Harvard Business School, June 1976).

9. Matt Murray, "As Huge Companies Keep Growing, CEOs Struggle to Keep Pace," Wall Street Journal (February 8, 2001), pp. A1, A6.

Chapter 9

1. Max DePree, "An Old Pro's Wisdom: It Begins with a Belief in People," New York Times, September 10, 1989, p. F2; Max DePree, Leadership Is an Art (New York: Doubleday, 1989); David Woodruff, "Herman Miller: How Green Is My Factory," Business Week, September 16, 1991, pp. 54–56; Max DePree, Leadership Jazz (New York: Doubleday, 1992).

2. Tom Peters, "Rule #3: Leadership Is Confusing as Hell," Fast Company (March 2001), pp. 124–140.

3. Abraham Zaleznick, "Leaders and Managers: Are They Different?" Harvard Business Review, May–June, 1977, pp. 67–78.

4. See Kouzes and Posner, "The Leadership Challenge," The Leadership Challenge: How to Get Extraordinary Things Done in Organizations. See also James C. Collins and Jerry I. Porras, "Building Your Company's Vision," Harvard Business Review, September–October 1996, pp. 65–77.

5. Rosabeth Moss Kanter, "Power Failure in Management Circuits," Harvard Business Review, vol. 47 (July–August 1979): 65–75.

6. For a good managerial discussion of power, see David C. McClelland and David H. Burnham, "Power Is the Great Motivator," Harvard Business Review, vol. 54 (March–April 1976): 100–110.

7. See John R. P. French Jr. and Bertram Raven, "The Bases of Social Power," in Group Dynamics: Research and Theory Darwin Cartwright, ed. (Evanston, IL: Row, Peterson, 1962), pp. 607–613. For managerial applications of this basic framework, see Gary Yukl and Tom Taber, "The Effective Use of Managerial Power," Personnel, vol. 60 (1983): 37–49; Robert C. Benfari, Harry E. Wilkinson, and Charles D. Orth, "The Effective Use of Power," Business Horizons, vol. 29 (1986): pp. 12–16.

8. Gary A. Yukl, Leadership in Organizations, 4th ed. (Englewood Cliffs, NJ: Prentice-Hall, 1998), includes "information" as a separate, but related, power source.

9. Jay A. Conger, "Leadership: The Art of Empowering Others," Academy of Management Executive, vol. 3 (1989): 17–24.

10. Conger, op. cit.

11. The early work on leader traits is well represented in Ralph M. Stogdill, "Personal Factors Associated with Leadership: A Survey of the Literature," Journal of Psychology, vol. 25 (1948): 35–71. See also Edwin E. Ghiselli, Explorations in Management Talent (Santa Monica, CA: Goodyear, 1971), and Shirley A. Kirkpatrick and Edwin A. Locke, "Leadership: Do Traits Really Matter?" Academy of Management Executive (1991): 48–60.

12. See also John W. Gardner's article, "The Context and Attributes of Leadership," New Management, vol. 5 (1988): 18–22; John P. Kotter, The Leadership Factor (New York: The Free Press, 1988); and Bernard M. Bass, Stogdill's Handbook of Leadership (New York: The Free Press, 1990).

13. See Bass, Stogdill's Handbook of Leadership.

14. Robert R. Blake and Jane Srygley Mouton, The New Managerial Grid III (Houston: Gulf Publishing, 1985).

15. For a good discussion of this theory, see Fred E. Fiedler, Martin M. Chemers, and Linda Mahar, The Leadership Match Concept (New York: Wiley, 1978); Fiedler's current contingency research with the cognitive resource theory is summarized in Fred E. Fiedler and Joseph E. Garcia, New Approaches to Effective Leadership (New York: Wiley, 1987).

16. Paul Hersey and Kenneth H. Blanchard, Management and Organizational Behavior (Englewood Cliffs, NJ: Prentice-Hall, 1988). For an interview with Paul Hersey on the origins of the model, see John R. Schermerhorn Jr., "Situational Leadership: Conversations with Paul Hersey," Mid-American Journal of Business, fall 1997, pp. 5–12.

17. See, for example, Robert J. House, "A Path-Goal Theory of Leader Effectiveness," Administrative Sciences Quarterly, vol. 16 (1971): 321–38; Robert J. House and Terrence R. Mitchell, "Path-Goal Theory of Leadership," Journal of Contemporary Business, autumn 1974, pp. 81–97; the path-goal theory is reviewed by Bernard M. Bass in Stogdill's Handbook of Leadership, and Yukl in Leadership in Organizations. A supportive review of research is offered in Julie Indvik, "Path-Goal Theory of Leadership; A Meta-Analysis," in Academy of Management Best Paper Proceedings 1986, John A. Pearce II and Richard B. Robinson Jr., eds. pp. 189–92.

18. See Steven Kerr and John Jermier, "Substitutes for Leadership: Their Meaning and Measurement," Organizational Behavior and Human Performance, vol. 22 (1978): 375–403; Jon P. Howell and Peter W. Dorfman, "Leadership and Substitutes for Leadership among Professional and Nonprofessional Workers," Journal of Applied Behavioral Science, vol. 22 (1986): 29–46.

19. Victor H. Vroom and Arthur G. Jago, The New Leadership: Managing Participation in Organizations (Englewood Cliffs, NJ: Prentice-Hall, 1988). This is based on earlier work by Victor H. Vroom, "A New Look in Managerial Decision-Making," Organizational Dynamics (spring 1973), pp. 66–80; and Victor H. Vroom and Phillip Yetton, Leadership and Decision-Making (Pittsburgh: University of Pittsburgh Press, 1973).

20. For a good discussion see Edgar H. Schein, Process Consultation Revisited: Building the Helping Relationship (Reading, MA: Addison-Wesley, 1999).

21. See the discussion by Victor H. Vroom, "Leadership and the Decision Making Process," Organizational Dynamics, vol. 28 (2000), pp. 82–84.

22. The distinction was originally made by James McGregor Burns, Leadership (New York: Harper & Row, 1978) and was further developed by Bernard Bass, Leadership and Performance Beyond Expectations (New York: The Free Press, 1985) and Bernard M. Bass, "Leadership: Good, Better, Best," Organizational Dynamics, vol. 13 (winter 1985): 26–40.

23. This list is based on Kouzes and Posner, op. cit.; Gardner, op. cit.

24. See Daniel Goleman, Emotional Intelligence (New York: Bantam Books, 1995) and Working with Emotional Intelligence (New York: Bantam Books, 1998).

25. Daniel Goleman, "What Makes a Leader?" Harvard Business Review (November–December, 1998), pp. 93–102.

26. A. H. Eagly, S. J. Daran, and M. G. Makhijani, "Gender and the Effectiveness of Leaders: A Meta-Analysis," Psychological Bulletin, vol. 117 (1995), pp. 125–45.

27. Research on gender issues in leadership is reported in Sally Helgesin, The Female Advantage: Women's Ways of Leadership (New York: Doubleday, 1990); Judith B. Rosener, "Ways Women Lead," Harvard Business Review, (November–December 1990), pp. 119–125; and Alice H. Eagly, Stephen J. Karau, and Blair T. Johnson, "Gender and Leadership Style Among School Principals: A Meta Analysis" Administrative Science Quarterly, vol. 27 (1992). pp. 76–102. See also the discussion of women leaders in Chapter 11, Jean Lipman-Blumen, Connective Leadership: Managing in a Changing World (New York: Oxford University Press, 1996).

28. Vroom, op.cit. (2000).

29. Rosener, op.cit. (1990).

30. For debate on whether some transformational leadership qualities tend to be associated more with female than male leaders, see "Debate: Ways Women and Men Lead," Harvard Business Review, (January–February 1991), pp. 150–60.

31. Gardner, "The Context and Attributes of Leadership," op. cit., 1988.

32. See Steven R. Covey, Principle-Centered Leadership (New York: Free Press, 1992); and, Lee G. Bolman and Terrence E. Deal, Leading With Soul (San Francisco: Jossey-Bass, 1995).

Chapter 10

1. See Abraham H. Maslow, *Eupsychian Management* (Homewood, IL: Richard D. Irwin, 1965); Abraham H. Maslow, *Motivation and Personality,* 2d ed. (New York: Harper & Row, 1970). For a research perspective, see Mahmoud A. Wahba and Lawrence G. Bridwell, "Maslow Reconsidered: A Review of Research on the Need Hierarchy," *Organizational Behavior and Human Performance,* vol. 16 (1976): 212–240.

2. The complete two-factor theory is in Frederick Herzberg, Bernard Mausner, and Barbara Block Snyderman, *The Motivation to Work, 2d ed.* (New York: Wiley, 1967); Frederick Herzberg, "One More Time: How Do You Motivate Employees?" *Harvard Business Review,* vol. 47 (January–February 1968): 53–62, and reprinted as an HBR classic in vol. 65, September–October 1987, pp. 109–120.

3. Critical reviews are provided by Robert J. House and Lawrence A. Wigdor, "Herzberg's Dual-Factor Theory of Job Satisfaction and Motivation: A Review of the Evidence and a Criticism," *Personnel Psychology,* vol. 20 (winter 1967): 369–389; Steven Kerr, Anne Harlan, and Ralph Stogdill, "Preference for Motivator and Hygiene Factors in a Hypothetical Interview Situation," *Personnel Psychology,* vol. 27 (winter 1974): 109–124.

4. For a collection of McClelland's work, see David C. McClelland, The Achieving Society (New York: Van Nostrand, 1961); "Business Drive and National Achievement," *Harvard Business Review,* vol. 40 (July–August 1962): 99–112; David C. McClelland and avid H. Burnham, "Power Is the Great Motivator," *Harvard Business Review,* vol. 54 (March–April 1976): 100–110; David C. McClelland, Human Motivation (Glenview, IL: Scott, Foresman, 1985); David C. McClelland and Richard E. Boyatsis, "The Leadership Motive Pattern and Long-Term Success in Management," *Journal of Applied Psychology,* vol. 67 (1982): 737–743.

5. See, for example, J. Stacy Adams, "Toward an Understanding of Inequity," *Journal of Abnormal and Social Psychology,* vol. 67 (1963): 422–436; J. Stacy Adams, "Inequity in Social Exchange," in *Advances in Experimental Social Psychology,* vol. 2, L. Berkowitz, ed. (New York: Academic Press, 1965), pp. 267–300.

6. Victor H. Vroom, *Work and Motivation* (New York: Wiley, 1964, republished by Jossey-Bass, 1994).

7. The work on goal-setting theory is well summarized in Edwin A. Locke and Gary P. Latham, *Goal Setting: A Motivational Technique That Works!* (Englewood Cliffs, NJ: Prentice-Hall, 1984). See also Edwin A. Locke, Kenneth N. Shaw, Liso A. Saari, and Gary P. Latham, "Goal Setting and Task Performance, 1969–1980," *Psychological Bulletin,* vol. 90 (1981): 125–152; Mark E. Tubbs, "Goal Setting; A Meta-Analytic Examination of the Empirical Evidence," *Journal of Applied Psychology,* vol. 71 (1986): 474–483.

8. E. L. Thorndike, *Animal Intelligence* (New York: Macmillan, 1911), p. 244.

9. For an overview, see Paul E. Spector, *Job Satisfaction* (Thousand Oaks, CA: Sage, 1997).

10. Herzberg, op.cit., 1987, pp. 109–20.

11. For a complete description of the job characteristics model, see J. Richard Hackman and Greg R. Oldham, *Work Redesign* (Reading, MA: Addison-Wesley, 1980); additional descriptions of directions in job

design research and practice are available in Ramon J. Aldag and Arthur P. Brief, *Task Design and Employee Motivation* (Glenview, IL: Scott, Foresman, 1979); and Ricky W. Griffin, *Task Design: An Integrative Approach* (Glenview, IL: Scott, Foresman, 1982).

12. See Michelle Conlin, "9 to 5 Isn't Working Anymore," *Business Week* (September 20, 1999), p. 94.

13. A good overview is Allen R. Cohen and Herman Gadon, *Alternative Work Schedules: Integrating Individual and Organizational Needs* (Reading, MA: Addison-Wesley, 1978).

14. Daniel Eisenberg, "Rise of the Permatemp," Business Week (July 12, 1999), p. 48.

15. "A Leg Up for the Lowly Temp," *Business Week* (June 21, 1999), pp. 102–103.

Chapter 11

1. See Edward E. Lawler III, "Strategic Choices for Changing Organizations," chapter 12 in Allan M. Mohrman Jr., Susan Albers Mohrman, Gerald E. Ledford Jr., Thomas G. Cummings, Edward E. Lawler III, and associates, Large Scale Organizational Change (San Francisco: Jossey-Bass, 1989).

2. The classic description of organizations on these terms is by Harold J. Leavitt, "Applied Organizational Change in Industry: Structural, Technological and Humanistic Approaches," in *Handbook of Organizations* James G. March, ed. (Chicago: Rand McNally, 1965), pp. 1144–1170. Another timely approach is described by Ralph H. Kilmann in *Beyond the Quick Fix* (San Francisco: Jossey-Bass, 1984).

3. Kurt Lewin, "Group Decision and Social Change," in *Readings in Social Psychology*, G. E. Swanson, T. M. Newcomb and E. L. Hartley, eds. (New York: Holt Rinehart, 1952), pp. 459–473.

4. The change strategy examples in this section are developed from an exercise reported in J. William Pfeiffer and John E. Jones, *A Handbook of Structured Experiences for Human Relations Training*, vol. 2 (La Jolla, CA: University Associates, 1973).

5. John P. Kotter and Leonard A. Schlesinger, "Choosing Strategies for Change," *Harvard Business Review*, vol. 57 (March-April 1979): 109–112.

6. Overviews of organization development are provided by Wendell L. French and Cecil H. Bell Jr., *Organization Development*, 6th ed. (Englewood Cliffs, MJ: Prentice-Hall, 1999).

7. See Arthur P. Brief, Randall S. Schuler, and Mary Van Sell, *Managing Job Stress* (Boston: Little, Brown, 1981), pp. 7, 8.

8. Sue Shellenbarger, "Do We Work More or Not? Either Way, We Feel Frazzled," *Wall Street Journal*, (July 30, 1997), p. B1; "Desk Rage," *Business Week* (November 27, 2000), p. 12.

9. The classic work is Meyer Friedman and Ray Roseman, *Type A Behavior and Your Heart* (New York: Knopf, 1974).

10. See Hans Selye, *Stress in Health and Disease* (Boston: Butterworth, 1976).

11. See Steve M. Jex, *Stress and Job Performance* (San Francisco: Jossey-Bass, 1998).

12. Robert Kreitner, "Personal Wellness: It's Just Good Business," *Business Horizons*, (May-June 1982), pp. 28–35.

Chapter 12

1. See Robert H. Lengel and Richard L. Daft, "The Selection of Communication Media as an Executive Skill," *Academy of Management Executive*, vol. 2 (August 1988): 225–232.

2. See H. R. Schiffman, *Sensation and Perception: An Integrated Approach*, 3d ed. (New York: John Wiley, 1990).

3. These examples are from Natasha Josefowitz, *Paths to Power* (Reading, MA: Addison-Wesley, 1980), p. 60.

4. The classic work is Dewitt C. Dearborn and Herbert A. Simon, "Selective Perception: A Note on the Departmental Identification of Executives," *Sociometry*, vol. 21 (1958): 140-144. See also, J. P. Walsh, "Selectivity and Selective Perception: Belief Structures and Information Processing," *Academy of Management Journal* vol. 24 (1988): 453–470.

5. This discussion is based on Carl R. Rogers and Richard E. Farson, "Active Listening" (Chicago: Industrial Relations Center of the University of Chicago), n.d.

6. A useful source of guidelines is John J. Gabarro and Linda A. Hill, "Managing Performance," Note 9-96-022, Harvard Business School Publishing, Boston, MA.

7. Developed from John Anderson, "Giving and Receiving Feedback," in Paul R. Lawrence, Louis B. Barnes, and Jay W. Lorsch, *Organizational Behavior and Administration*, 3d ed. (Homewood, IL: Richard D. Irwin, 1976), p. 109.

8. A classic work on proxemics is Edward T. Hall's book *The Hidden Dimension* (Garden City, NY: Doubleday, 1986).

9. Richard E. Walton, *Interpersonal Peacemaking: Confrontations and Third-Party Consultation* (Reading, MA: Addison-Wesley, 1969, p. 2.

10. See Kenneth W. Thomas, "conflict and conflict Management," in *Handbook of Industrial and Organizational Behavior*, M. D. Dunnett, ed. (Chicago: Rand McNally, 1976), pp. 889–935.

11. See Robert R. Blake and Jane Strygley Mouton, "The Fifth Achievement," *Journal of Applied Behavioral Science*, vol. 6 (1970), pp. 413-427; Alan C. Filley, *Interpersonal Conflict Resolution* (Glenview, IL: Scott Foresman, 1975).

12. This discussion is based on Filley, op. cit.; and, Vincent L. Ferraro and Sheila A. Adams, "Interdepartmental Conflict: Practical Ways to Prevent and Reduce It," *Personnel*, vol. 61 (1984), pp. 12–23.

13. Roger Fisher and William Ury, *Getting to Yes: Negotiating Agreement without Giving In* (New York: Penguin, 1983) and William L. Ury, Jeanne M. Brett, and Stephen B. Goldberg, *Getting Disputes Resolved* (San Francisco: Jossey-Bass, 1997).

14. Fisher and Ury, *Getting to Yes*; see also James A. Wall Jr., *Negotiation: Theory and Practice* (Glenview, IL: Scott Foresman, 1985).

15. Ibid.

16. Developed from Max H. Bazerman, *Judgment in Managerial Decision Making*, 3d ed. (new York: Wiley, 1994), chap. 7; and Fisher and Ury, *Getting to Yes*, pp. 10–14.

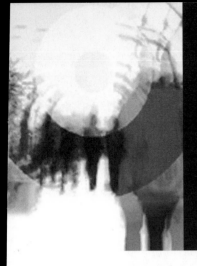

GLOSSARY

Accommodation   In conflict management, being cooperative but unassertive; also known as *smoothing*.

Accountability   The requirement of one person to answer to higher authority and show results achieved for assigned duties.

Action analysis   The process of a manager examining the viability of a plan and predicting whether a decision is sound and the courses of action effective.

Action orientation   A state of mind in which you and your organization act and react confidently and quickly to new situations.

Active listening   The process of helping the source of a message say exactly what he or she really means.

Adaptive organizations   Organizations with a minimum of bureaucratic features and with cultures that encourage worker empowerment and participation.

Affective skills   Abilities managers use to manage their own emotions and their interaction with others in the workplace.

Affirmative action   Preference in hiring and promotion to women and minorities, including veterans, the aged, and the disabled.

Agendas   Action plans set by managers that include specific long- and short-term goals.

Arbitration   A stronger form of dispute resolution than mediation, arbitration involves a neutral third party who acts as a judge and issues a binding decision.

Assertiveness   The desire to satisfy one's own needs and concerns.

Asset management   The ability to use resources efficiently and operate at minimum cost.

Authority decision   Decision made by the leader and then communicated to the group.

Avoidance   In conflict management, being uncooperative and unassertive.

Base compensation   An employee's salary or hourly wage.

Benchmarking   Using external comparisons to evaluate an organization's current performance and identify possible future actions.

Bona fide occupational qualification   Criteria for employment that can be clearly justified as being related to a person's capacity to perform a job.

Bottom-up change   Initiatives for change come from people throughout an organization and are supported by the efforts of middle- and lower-level managers acting as change agents.

Boundaryless organization   An increasingly common structure in the business world, which combines teams and network structures for temporary purposes.

Budget   Financial plans that commit resources to activities, projects, or programs.

Bureaucracy   A form of organization based on logic, order, and the legitimate use of formal authority.

Business strategy   Top- and mid-level management set the direction for a single business unit.

Career planning   Structured advice and discussion sessions to help individuals plan career paths and programs of personal development.

Career planning   The process of systematically matching career goals and individual capabilities with opportunities for their fulfillment.

Centralization   Traditional, top-down decision.

Chain of command   Line of authority that vertically links all positions with successively higher levels of management.

Change leader   A person or group who takes leadership responsibility for changing the existing pattern of behavior of another person or social system.

Change Readiness Index (CRI)   Scorecard system asks team members to rate their health care organization and specific teams or groups in the categories such as patient service, organizational reaction and readiness to change.

Changing stage   The phase of planned change in which something new takes place in a system, and change is actually implemented.

Codes of ethics   Official written guidelines on how to behave in situations where ethical dilemmas are likely to occur.

Coercive power   The ability to influence through punishment, a type of position power.

Cohesiveness   The degree to which members are motivated to remain part of a team.

Collaboration   In conflict management, being both cooperative and assertive; problem-solving.

Collective bargaining   The process of negotiating, administering, and interpreting labor contracts.

Committee   Organizational group that usually operates with a continuing purpose while its membership may change over time.

Communication   An interpersonal process of sending and receiving symbols with messages attached to them.

Communication channel   The medium through which a message is conveyed from sender to receiver.

Comparable worth   The notion that persons performing jobs of similar importance should be paid at comparable levels.

Competition   In conflict management, being uncooperative but assertive; also known as *authoritative command*.

Competitive advantage   An attribute or combination of attributes that allows an organization to outperform its rivals.

Compressed workweek   Any work schedule that allows a full-time job to be completed in less than the standard 5 days of 8-hour shifts.

Compromise   In conflict management, being moderately cooperative and assertive.

Concentration   Growth strategy that uses existing strengths in new and productive ways.

Conceptual skill   The ability to think analytically and solve complex problems.

Concurrent controls   Controls that focus on what actually happens during the work process, also called *steering controls*.

Conflict   A disagreement between people on substantive or emotional issues.

Confrontation meeting   Intensive, structured meetings to gather data on workplace problems and plan for constructive actions; an organization-wide OD intervention.

Control   Meeting the desired outcomes as efficiently as possible.

Control equation   Need for Action = Desired Performance − Actual Performance.

Constructive stress   Stress that acts in a positive way for the individual and/or the organization. It occurs in moderation and proves energizing and performance enhancing.

Consultative decision   Decision made by the leader after asking group members for information, advice, or opinions.

Contingency leadership theory   Leadership theory in which a leader's success depends on a match between leadership style and situational demands.

Contingency planning   The process of identifying alternative courses of action that you can implement if and when an original plan proves inadequate because of changing circumstances.

Continuous business development (CBD)   A building-block approach to all departmental activities in management efforts. Every effort undertaken by the department should be done to make the department a stronger, more progressive entity than it was prior to the effort.

Continuous quality improvement (CQI)   Ongoing quality enhancement as the incentive that fuels everyday activities associated with optimum health care delivery.

Continuous reinforcement schedule   Rewarding behavior each time a desired behavior occurs.

Continuum of care   The complete spectrum of available health care services.

Controlling   The managerial process of measuring work performance, comparing results to objectives, and taking corrective action as needed.

Control process   A four-step method for measuring performance.

Cooperativeness   The desire to satisfy another party's needs and concerns.

Core characteristics model   Richard Hackman's motivation theory with five core job characteristics, skill variety, task identity, task, significance, autonomy, and feedback from the job itself.

Core competencies   Special strengths that an organization has or does exceptionally well in comparison with competitors.

Core values   Principles that affect and guide the action of an organization.

Corporate strategy   Top management directs an organization as a whole toward sustainable competitive advantage.

Cost-benefit analysis   Comparing alternative costs (time, money, resources, human capital, etc.) to the expected benefits.

Crisis   An unexpected and demanding problem that can result in disaster.

Cross-functional teams   Within a matrix structure, workers belong to at least two formal groups at the same time—a functional group and a product, program, or project team.

Customer-patient   Individual who utilizes the goods and services produced by health care organizations.

Decentralization   Dispersed decision making.

Deficit principle   In Maslow's needs theories, only an unsatisfied need—one for which a deficit exists—can be a motivator of behavior.

Delegation   The process of distributing and entrusting work to other people.

Destructive stress   Distress, or dysfunctional stress, for the individual and/or the organization. It occurs as intense or long-term stress that overloads and breaks down a person's physical and mental systems.

Differentiation   The degree of difference that exists between the internal components of the organization.

Direct forcing strategy   A force-coercion strategy in which a manager takes direct and unilateral action to "command" that change take place.

Disciplinary probation   The final step before termination, generally a 3-month process in which poor performers are given the opportunity to turn performance around to an acceptable level.

Discipline   The act of influencing behavior through reprimand.

Distributed leadership   A team in which all members share responsibility for both task and maintenance activities.

Distributive negotiation   Each party makes claims for certain preferred results; decisions are often win-lose.

Diversification   Growth strategy that focuses on acquiring or investing in new businesses and services.

Divisional structures   Organization strategy in which you group together people who provide the same services, work within the same processes, serve similar audiences, or are located in the same area or geographical region.

Documentation   The process of objectively recording performance and performance levels.

Dysfunctional conflict   Conflict at very low or high intensities that distracts and interferes with other more task-relevant activities.

Economic order quantity (EOQ)   A quantitative method of inventory control that involves ordering a fixed number of items every time an inventory level falls to a predetermined point.

Effective communication   The intended message of the sender and the interpreted meaning of the receiver are one and the same.

Effective skills   Managerial abilities that support the effort to complete work on time and within budget.

Efficient communication   Communication that occurs at minimum cost in terms of resources expended and the amount of time involved.

Emergent strategy   Strategy that develops progressively over time as managers learn from and respond to work situations.

Emotional conflicts   Disagreements over feelings of anger, distrust, dislike, fear, and resentment, as well as from personality clashes.

Emotional intelligence   The ability to understand emotions in one's self and others and then use this understanding to guide behavior.

Employee involvement team   Group of workers who meet on a regular basis outside of their formal assignments, with the goal of applying their expertise and attention to continuous improvement.

Employment discrimination   Situation in which someone is denied a job or a job assignment for reasons that are not job relevant.

Empowerment   The process through which managers enable and help others to gain power and achieve influence within the organization.

Engineering comparison   Comparison that uses standards set scientifically through such methods as time and motion studies.

Environment analysis   Analysis that takes into account the theoretical and physical environment in which you operate and in which the action plan will be undertaken.

Equal employment opportunity (EEO)   The right to employment without regard to race, color, national origin, religion, gender, age, or physical and mental ability.

Equity theory   Motivation theory in which people who believe that they have been inequitably treated in comparison to others will try to eliminate the discomfort and restore a sense of equity to the situation.

Ethical behavior   What is accepted to be "good" and "right" as opposed to "bad" or "wrong" in the context of the governing code.

Ethical dilemma   A situation that requires you to make a choice or take action that, although offering the potential for personal or organizational benefit, may be considered unethical.

Ethics   Collection of moral principles within a group or organization that set standards of good or bad, or right or wrong, for one's conduct.

Ethics training   Structured programs to help participants understand the ethical aspects of decision making.

Ethnocentrism   The tendency to consider one's culture superior to others.

Expectancy   In expectancy theory, a person's belief that working hard will result in a desired level of task performance being achieved.

Expectancy theory   Victor Vroom's motivation theory based on an individual's willingness to work hard at tasks important to the organization.

Expert power   The ability to influence through special expertise; a type of personal power.

External control   Attempting to control the behavior of others through personal supervision or formal administrative systems.

Extinction   In operant conditioning, anything that decreases the frequency of or eliminates an undesirable behavior by making the removal of a pleasant consequence contingent on its occurrence.

Feedback   The reverse of the communication process; the receiver responds back to the sender.

Feedback controls   Controls that take place after work is completed, also called *postaction controls*.

Feedforward controls   Controls that are accomplished before a work activity begins, also called *preliminary controls*.

Filtering   The intentional distortion of information to make it appear favorable to the recipient.

Fixed budget   A financial plan that allocates a set amount of resources that can be used, but not exceeded, for a specified purpose.

Flexibility   The willingness or ability to change and adapt to shifting circumstances.

Flexible budget   A financial plan that allocates resources based on the need level of various departments or activities.

Flexible working hours   Any work schedule that gives employees some choice in the pattern of their daily work hours, also called *flexitime* or *flextime*.

Focus   Knowing what an organization does best, knowing the needs of customers and patients, and knowing how to serve customers and patients well.

Force-coercion strategy   Change strategy that uses the power of legitimacy, rewards, and punishments as the primary inducements to change.

Forecasting   The process of making assumptions about what will happen in the future.

Formal references   Information sources such as journals, management texts, or an organization's manual of standard operating procedures.

Formal structure   The intended or official structure of an organization.

Forming stage   The first stage of team development; involves the initial entry of individual members into a team.

Fringe benefits   The additional nonwage or nonsalary forms of compensation workers receive, including disability protection, health and life insurance, and retirement plans.

Functional chimneys   Negative effect of formal structures, in which members of a specific functional group develop self-centered and narrow viewpoints, become uncooperative with other groups, and lose the ability to focus on the larger picture.

Functional conflict   Conflict of moderate intensity that can actually be good for performance, stimulating greater work efforts, cooperation, and creativity.

Functional strategy   Middle and low-level management guide the use of resources to implement a specific business strategy.

Functional structure   Organization strategy in which people with similar skills and performing similar tasks are grouped together.

Function analysis   Analysis in which you evaluate every role affected by implementing and executing a strategic action plan.

General environment   The background and external conditions for an organization.

Glass-ceiling effect   The existence of an invisible screen that prevents disfavored people or minorities from rising above a certain level of organizational responsibility.

Goal-setting theory   Edwin Locke's theory that clear, desirable performance targets (goals) can motivate.

Group decision   All members to participate in making a decision and working together to achieve a consensus regarding the preferred course of action.

Group emotions   Emotional responses can pervade an entire team and cause a group to resist—and even work against—a proposed change.

Group process   The way the members of a team actually work together.

Groupthink   The tendency for highly cohesive groups to lose their critical evaluative capabilities.

Growth strategy   Strategy that pursues larger size and expanded operations.

Halo effect   Communication problem that occurs when one attribute is used to develop an overall impression of a person or situation.

Hard data   Any information that may have been generated by a test, questionnaire, form, or survey.

Health care network   Different medical services joining together to provide comprehensive health care, often sharing the services of one business office and laboratory.

Heterogeneous team   A team comprised of a more diversity array of members.

Hierarchy of objectives   Plans in which the goals for each area of the organization are linked together, scheduled chronologically, or ranked in terms of importance.

Historical analysis   Analysis that takes into account past precedents established in the organization.

Historical comparison   Comparison that uses past performance as a standard for evaluating current performance.

Homogeneous team   A team comprised of same or similar kinds of members.

Horizontal structures   New organizational models that emphasize integration and cross-functional teamwork, often while gaining the advantages of networking through information technology.

Human resource management (HRM)   Attracting, developing, and maintaining a talented and energetic workforce to support organizational mission, objectives, and strategies.

Human skill   The ability to work well with other people.

Hygiene factors   In two-factor theory, things relating more to the work setting.

Improvement objectives   MBO goals that document intentions for improving performance in a specific way and with respect to a specific factor.

Independent contracting   Specific health care-related tasks or projects are assigned to outsiders rather than full-time workers.

Individualism view   Based on the belief that your primary commitment is to the advancement of your long-term self-interests.

Informal structure   The unofficial but often critical working relationships among organizational members, regardless of formal titles and relationships.

Input standards   Control measurements that focus on the amount of work expended in task performance.

Instrumentality   In expectancy theory, a person's belief that successful performance will be followed by rewards and other potential outcomes.

Integration   The level of coordination achieved among an organization's internal components.

Integrity   Honesty, credibility, and consistency in putting one's values into action.

Intellectual capital   An organization's employees, including their talents, knowledge, and experience.

Interactive leadership   A leader focuses on building consensus and good interpersonal relations through communication and involvement.

Intermediate-range plan   A plans that covers 1 to 2 years.

Intermittent reinforcement schedule   Rewarding behavior only periodically.

Internal control   Allowing motivated individuals and groups to exercise self-discipline in fulfilling job expectations.

Interpersonal skills   Ability to learn more about others' personalities and professional preferences, relative to job performance.

Interventions   Within OD, activities that are initiated to directly facilitate the change processes.

Intradepartmental conflict   A conflict that takes place within a single department or work group.

Job analysis   The orderly study of just what is done, when, where, how, why, and by whom in existing or potential new jobs.

Job burnout   A form of physical and mental exhaustion that can be incapacitating both personally and with respect to one's work.

Job descriptions   Written statements of job duties and responsibilities.

Job design   The process of creating or defining jobs by assigning specific work tasks to individuals and groups.

Job enlargement   The process of increasing task variety by combining two or more tasks that were previously assigned to separate workers.

Job enrichment   The process of building more opportunities for satisfaction into a job by expanding not just job scope but also job depth.

Job performance   The quantity and quality of tasks accomplished by an individual or group at work.

Job redesign   Realigning task components to better fit the needs and capabilities of the individual.

Job rotation   The process of increasing task variety by periodically shifting workers between jobs involving different task assignments.

Job sharing   One full-time job is split between two or more people.

Job simplification   The process of streamlining work procedures so that people work in well-defined and highly specialized tasks.

Job specifications   Qualifications (educational level, prior experience, or skills) that should be met by any person hired for a given job.

Justice view   Based on the belief that all ethical decisions should treat people impartially and fairly, according to guiding rules and standards

Just-in-time scheduling (JIT)   A Japanese model for industrial productivity, JIT systems try to reduce costs and improve workflow by scheduling items to arrive just in time to be used.

Labor unions   Organizations to which workers belong that deal with employers on the workers' behalves.

Law of contingent reinforcement   In operant conditioning, for a reward to have maximum reinforcing value, it must be delivered only if the desirable behavior is exhibited.

Law of effect   In behavior reinforcement theory, behavior that results in a pleasant outcome is likely to be repeated; behavior that results in an unpleasant outcome is not likely to be repeated.

Law of immediate reinforcement   In operant conditioning, the more immediate the delivery of a reward after the occurrence of a desirable behavior, the greater the reinforcing value of the reward.

Leader-participation model   Leadership model in which a leader chooses the method of decision making that best fits the nature of the problem being faced.

Leadership   The process of inspiring others to work hard to accomplish important tasks.

Leadership style   The recurring pattern of behaviors exhibited by a leader.

Leadership through empowerment   Helping others use their knowledge and judgment to make a real difference in daily workplace affairs.

Leading   The managerial process of arousing people's enthusiasm to work hard to fulfill plans and accomplish objectives.

Legitimate power   The ability to influence through formal authority; a type of position power.

Leverage   The ability to earn more in returns than the cost of debt.

Liquidity   The ability to generate cash to pay bills.

Long-range plan   A plan that looks 3 or more years into the future.

Maintenance activities   Work activities that support the emotional life of the team as an ongoing social system.

Management   The process of organizing, planning, and controlling the use of resources, and leading to accomplish performance goals.

Management by exception   The practice of giving priority attention to situations that show the greatest need for action.

Management by objectives (MBO)   A structured process of regular communication in which a supervisor and subordinate jointly set performance objectives for the subordinate and review results accomplished.

Management training   Structured educational opportunities for developing important managerial skills and competencies.

Manager   Anyone in an organization who supports and is responsible for the work performance of one or more other persons.

Matrix structure   Organization strategy that combines elements of both the functional and divisional structures.

Mediation   A neutral third party who tries to improve communications between negotiating parties and keep them focused on relevant issues. The mediator does not issue a ruling or make a decision but can take an active role in discussions.

Mission statement   Precisely worded declaration that identifies where an organization intends to operate, who it serves, and what products or services it provides.

Moral leadership   Leadership that by actions and personal example sets high ethical standards for others to follow.

Moral-rights view   Respects and protects the fundamental rights of people. Decisions are made in response to an ideal or moral, not based on personal or individual circumstances.

Motivation   Forces within individuals that account for the level, direction, and persistence of effort they expend at work.

Mutual-benefit logical approach   A negotiation strategy that focus on win-win psychology.

Need for achievement   In acquired needs theory, the desire to do something better or more efficiently, to solve problems, or to master complex tasks.

Need for affiliation   In acquired needs theory, the desire to establish and maintain friendly and warm relations with other people.

Need for power   In acquired needs theory, the desire to control other people, to influence their behavior, or to be responsible for them.

Needs   Unfulfilled physiological or psychological desires of an individual.

Negative reinforcement   In operant conditioning, anything that increases the frequency of or strengthens desirable behavior by making the avoidance of an unpleasant consequence contingent upon its occurrence.

Negotiation   The process of making joint decisions when the parties involved have different preferences.

Networking   The process of building and maintaining positive relationships with people, typically outside of your current organization or business.

Noise   Anything that interferes with the effectiveness of the communication process.

Nonplayer   A team member who does not agree with a change and even works against it.

Nonverbal communication   Communication takes place through such things as hand movements, facial expressions, body posture, eye contact, and the use of interpersonal space.

Norm   A behavior expected of team members.

Norming stage   The third stage of team development; members begin to become coordinated as a working unit and tend to operate with shared rules of conduct.

Objectives   Short-term targets that direct activities toward key and specific results.

Operant conditioning   B. F. Skinner's concept of learning by reinforcement.

Operational plan   A plan that defines what needs to be done in specific areas to implement a strategic plan.

Operations management   The portion of management duties that emphasizes utilizing people, resources, and technology to the best advantage.

Opportunities   External factors of a SWOT analysis that include possible new markets, a strong economy, weaknesses in competitors, and emerging technologies.

Opportunity situation   Actual performance is above the standard.

Organization   A collection of people working together to achieve a common purpose.

Organizational design   The process of aligning organizational structures and cultures to best serve the organization's mission, strategy, and objectives.

Organization chart   Diagram that identifies key positions, job titles, lines of authority, and communication within an organization.

Organization development (OD)   A comprehensive approach to planned organizational change that involves applying behavioral science in a systematic and long-range effort to improve organizational effectiveness.

Organization structure   The system of tasks, workflow, reporting relationships, and communication channels that link the diverse parts of an organization.

Organizing   The managerial process of assigning tasks, allocating resources, and arranging and coordinating the activities of individuals and groups to implement plans.

Orientation   A set of activities designed to familiarize new employees with their jobs, co-workers, and key aspects of the organization as a whole.

Organization chart   Diagram that identifies key positions, job titles, lines of authority, and communication within an organization.

Organization structure   The system of tasks, workflow, reporting relationships, and communication channels that link the diverse parts of an organization.

Outcome goals   In organization development, goals that focus on task accomplishments.

Output standards   Control measurement results that focus on performance quantity, quality, cost, or time.

Outsourcing alliance   Contracting to purchase important services from another organization.

Participative planning   Involves the people who are affected by a plan or who are required to help implement the plan to aid in the planning process.

Path-goal theory   Leadership theory that suggests an effective leader is one who clarifies paths through which followers can achieve both task-related and personal goals.

Patient   Individual who utilizes the goods and services produced by health care organizations.

Perceived negative inequity   In equity theory, people who perceive negative inequity tend to reduce their work efforts to compensate for missing rewards.

Perception   The way people receive and interpret information from the environment.

Performance appraisal   Taking qualitative, subjective perceptions of performance and ascribing a quantitative, objective rating.

Performance gap A discrepancy between the desired and actual state of affairs.

Performance norm Any behavior expectation that defines the level of work that team members are expected to contribute.

Performing stage The fourth stage of team development; the team operates with a clear and stable structure, and members are motivated by team goals.

Permatemps Long-term temporary workers who supplement the full-time workforce.

Personal development objectives MBO goals that pertain to personal growth activities, often those resulting in expanded job knowledge or skills.

Personal power Power derived from a leader's unique personal qualities.

Personal values Morals, or the underlying beliefs and attitudes that help determine individual behavior.

Personal wellness A form of preventative stress management, in which employers help their employees recognize their responsibility to enhancing their physical, emotional, and relational health through educational resources and programming.

Planned change Change that occurs as a result of the specific efforts of a change leader; usually in direct response to a perceived performance gap.

Planning The managerial process of setting performance objectives and determining what actions should be taken to accomplish them.

Planning process Deciding exactly what you, your team, or your department wants to accomplish and how to best go about meeting your goals.

Policy Formal statements that communicate broad guidelines for making decisions and taking action in specific circumstances.

Political maneuvering A force-coercion strategy in which a manager works indirectly to gain special advantage over other people and thereby make them change. Political maneuvering involves bargaining, obtaining control of important resources, or granting small favors.

Portfolio-planning approach A basic method of formulating strategy and making decisions, in which managers allocate scarce organizational resources among competing opportunities.

Position power Power from a manager's official status in the organization's hierarchy of authority.

Positive reinforcement In operant conditioning, anything that strengthens or increases the frequency of desirable behavior by making a pleasant consequence contingent on its occurrence.

Power   The ability to get someone else to do something you want done; the ability to make things happen for the good of the group or organization as a whole.

Principled negotiation   The interests of all parties are considered, and the goal is to base the final outcome on the merits of individual claims; a win-win orientation operates.

Problem situation   Actual performance is below the standard.

Procedure   Statement that describes exact rules for dealing with specific situations.

Process goals   In organization development, goals that focus on the way people work together.

Process reengineering   The systematic and complete analysis of work processes and the design of new and better ones with the goal of focusing attention on the future, on patients, and on improving ways of doing things.

Process theory   Motivational theory focuses on how people actually make choices to work hard or not, based on their individual preferences, the available rewards, and possible work outcomes.

Process value analysis   Managers identify and carefully evaluate each step in a workflow. Each step must be important, useful, and add value to the overall purpose of the organization; if not, the step is eliminated.

Product outputs   The finished good or service that a team produces.

Productivity   Performance effectiveness and efficiency within the organization.

Profitability   The ability to earn revenues greater than costs.

Progression principle   In Maslow's hierarchy of needs, a need at one level does not become activated until the next lower-level need is already satisfied.

Progressive discipline   A disciple system in which reprimands are tied to the severity and frequency of misbehavior.

Projection   The assignment of personal attributes to other individuals.

Projects   Specific goals that can be accomplished by teams working under tight deadlines.

Project schedules   Time-focused places that identify the activities required to accomplish a specific major project.

Promotion   Movement of an employee to a higher-level position.

Proxemics   The use of interpersonal space in communication.

Punishment   In operant conditioning, anything that decreases the frequency of or eliminates an undesirable behavior by making an unpleasant consequence contingent on its occurrence.

Purpose   Why an organization exists; organizations exist to produce goods and/or services that satisfy the needs of customers.

Qualitative outcome   A nonmeasurable result, usually involving personalities and perceptions rather than specific figures.

Quality circle   A popular form of employee involvement team in which a group of workers meets regularly to discuss and plan specific ways to improve work quality.

Quality control   Checking processes, materials, products, and services to ensure that they meet high standards.

Quality of work life (QWL)   An indicator of the overall quality of human experiences in the workplace.

Quantitative outcome   A measurable result.

Rational persuasion strategy   Informational change strategy that focuses on persuasion backed by special knowledge, data, and rational argument.

Realistic job previews   Opportunities during the selection process that provide candidates with all pertinent information about the job and organization without distortion before the job is accepted.

Receiver   In the communication process, the person who decodes or interprets the meaning of a message.

Recruitment   A set of activities designed to attract a qualified pool of job applicants to an organization.

Reference checks   Inquiries to previous employers, academic advisors, co-workers, and/or acquaintances regarding the qualifications, experience, and past work records of a job applicant.

Referent power   The ability to influence the behaviors of other people because they admire you and want to identify positively with you; a type of personal power.

Refreezing stage   The phase of planned change in which a manager is concerned about stabilizing the change and creating the conditions for its long-term continuity.

Reinforcement theory   Motivational theory that explains human behavior as a result of one's external environment.

Relationship goal   In negotiation, a goal that is concerned with processes and is tied to the way people work together while negotiating and how they can work together again in the future.

Relative comparison Comparison that uses the performance achievements of other people, work units, or organizations as evaluation benchmarks.

Resistance Feedback that indicates something can be done to achieve a better "fit" between the planned change, the situation, and the people involved.

Resolved conflict The causes of a conflict are corrected.

Resource inputs The people and ideas that teams use to create outputs.

Restructuring The process of changing an organization's structure in an attempt to improve performance.

Retrenchment strategy Strategy that reduces the scale of operations in order to gain efficiency and improve performance.

Reward power The ability to influence through rewards; a type of position power.

Role definition Helps individuals identify with their work role and with the overall mission of their work group.

Role negotiation Structured interactions to clarify and negotiate role expectations among people who work together.

Satisfier factors In two-factor theory, things relating to the nature of a job itself.

Scenario planning Identifying alternative future states of affairs that may occur and then dealing hypothetically with each situation and formulating possible plans.

Selection The process of choosing from a pool of applicants the person or persons who offer the greatest performance potential.

Selective perception The tendency to single out for attention those aspects of a situation or person that reinforce or appear consistent with one's existing beliefs, values, or needs.

Self-managing work team Workers whose jobs have been redesigned to create a high degree of task interdependence and who have been given authority to make many decisions about how they go about doing the required work.

Sender In the communication process, the person who is responsible for encoding an intended message into meaningful symbols, both verbal and nonverbal.

Sensitivity training Unstructured group sessions where participants learn interpersonal skills and increased sensitivity to other people.

Sexual harassment Situation in which a person experiences conduct or language of sexual nature that affects his or her employment situation.

Shaping   The process of creating a new behavior by the positive reinforcement of successive approximations to it.

Shared power strategy   A change strategy that engages people in a collaborative process of identifying values, assumptions, and goals from which support for change will naturally emerge.

Short-range plan   Plan that covers 1 year or less.

Situational leadership model   Successful leaders adjust their styles depending on the readiness of followers to perform in a given situation.

Six Sigma   A collection of rigorous, systematic control tools that uses information and statistical analysis to measure and improve an organization's performance, practices, and systems.

Skill   An ability to translate knowledge into action that results in desired performance.

Social audit   A systematic assessment of an organization's commitments and accomplishments in the areas of social responsibility.

Socialization   The process of influencing the expectations, behavior, and attitudes of a new employee in a way considered desirable by the organization.

Social responsibility   Having concern for issues beyond business-related issues, including ecology and environmental quality, patient care and protection, and community involvement.

Span of control   The number of people reporting directly to a manager within an organizational structure.

Specific environment   The actual organizations, groups, and persons with whom an organization must interact in order to survive and prosper.

Stability strategy   Strategy that maintains a present course of action without major operating changes.

Stakeholders   The people, groups, and institutions who are affected in one way or another by the organization's performance.

Stereotype   Communication problem that occurs when someone is identified with a group or category, and then oversimplified attributes associated with the group or category are attributed to the individual.

Storming stage   The second stage of team development; tension often emerges between members over tasks and interpersonal concerns.

Strategic alliance   Two or more organizations join together in partnership to pursue an area of mutual interest.

Strategic human resource planning   A process of analyzing staffing needs and planning how to satisfy these needs in a way that best serves organizational mission, objectives, and strategies.

Strategic intent   The focusing of all organizational energies on a unifying and compelling target.

Strategic management   The process of formulating and implementing strategies that create competitive advantage and advance an organization's mission and objectives.

Strategic plan   Action plans, usually from uppermost management or executive management, that focus an entire organization's energies on a clear target or goal.

Strategy   A comprehensive action plan that identifies long-term direction and guides resource utilization to accomplish an organization's mission and objectives with sustainable competitive advantage.

Strategy formulation   Assessing existing strategies, organization, and environment to develop new strategies and strategic plans capable of delivering future competitive advantage.

Strategy implementation   Acting upon strategies successfully to achieve the desired results.

Strengths   Internal factors of a SWOT analysis.

Stress   A state of tension experienced by individuals facing extraordinary demands, constraints, or opportunities.

Stressors   The things that cause stress.

Structural redesign   Realigning the organization structure to meet the needs of environmental and contextual forces; an organization-wide OD intervention.

Structured problem   Familiar situations.

Substance goal   In negotiation, a goal that is concerned with outcomes and is tied to content issues of the negotiation.

Substantive conflicts   Disagreements over such things as goals, the allocation of resources, the distribution of rewards, policies and procedures, and job assignments.

Substitutes for leadership   Aspects of a work setting and the people involved that can reduce the need for a leader's personal involvement.

Subsystems   Small departments, work units, or teams headed by managers that perform specialized tasks within organizations.

Suppressed conflict   The causes of a conflict remain, but the conflict is controlled for a period of time.

Survey feedback   Comprehensive and systematic data collection to identify attitudes and needs, analyze results, and plan for constructive action; an organization-wide OD intervention.

Sustainable competitive advantage   An attribute that is difficult for competitors to imitate.

SWOT analysis   A common planning tool used to analyze strengths and weaknesses inside an organization, and opportunities and threats outside the organization.

Synergy   The creation of a whole that is greater than the sum of its parts; one of the benefits of teamwork.

Task activities   Work activities that contribute directly to the team's performance purpose.

Task force   Organizational group that is more temporary with official tasks that are very specific and time defined. Once its stated purpose has been accomplished, a task force typically disbands.

Task performance   The act of getting a job done.

Team   A small group of people with complementary skills who work together to achieve a shared purpose and hold themselves mutually accountable for its accomplishment; Group of workers organized to accomplish tasks; the building blocks of today's new and more horizontal organizational forms.

Team building   A sequence of planned activities used to gather and analyze information on how a team functions.

Team diversity   The different values, personalities, experiences, demographics, and cultures among the members of a team.

Teamwork   The process of people working together to accomplish goals.

Technical skill   The ability to use a special proficiency or expertise to perform particular tasks.

Telecommuting   A work arrangement that allows at least a portion of scheduled work hours to be completed outside of the office, facilitated by various forms of electronic communication and computer-mediated linkages to clients, patients, and a central office; sometimes called *flexiplace* or *cyber-commuting*.

Termination   The involuntary and permanent dismissal of an employee.

Threats   External factors of a SWOT analysis that include the emergence of new competitors, scarce resources, changing customer demands, and new government regulations, among other possibilities.

Top-down change   Strategic and comprehensive changes are initiated by top management levels with the goal of comprehensive impact on the organization and its performance capabilities.

Training   A set of activities that provides the opportunity to acquire and improve job-related skills.

Transactional leadership A leader adjusts tasks, rewards, and structures to help followers meet their needs while working to accomplish organizational objectives.

Transfer Movement of an employee to a different job at a similar level of responsibility.

Transformational leadership A leader uses charisma and related qualities to raise aspirations and shift people and organizational systems into new high-performance patterns.

Two-factor theory Frederick Herzberg's motivation theory that focuses on the nature of the job itself and the work setting.

Type A personality People who tend to be achievement orientated, impatient, and perfectionists. Type A people are likely to create stress in circumstances that others find relatively stress-free.

Unfreezing stage The phase of planned change in which the need for change is recognized and a situation is prepared for change.

Unity-of-command principle Each person in an organization should report to one and only one supervisor.

Unstructured problem Unexpected and ambiguous situations that lack critical information.

Upside-down pyramid Organizational mind-set that refocuses attention on the marketplace and patient needs by putting patients on top, served by workers in the middle, who are in turn supported by managers at the bottom.

Utilitarian view Also known as **results-oriented point of view,** this ethical standpoint tries to assess the moral implications of a decision in terms of its consequences.

Valence In expectancy theory, the value a person assigns to the possible rewards and other work-related outcomes.

Value-added worker Someone who does things that create eventual value for best serving customers.

Value-driven leadership Leaders incorporate certain values and ethical principles into the work environment.

Vertical structures Traditional top-down organizational models.

Virtual teams Teams that work together and solve problems through largely computer-mediated rather than face-to-face interactions.

Vision An overarching goal that the manager/leader has for his or her department or team.

Weaknesses Internal factors of a SWOT analysis.

Workforce diversity   Demographic differences among employees, principally differences in age, gender, race, ethnicity, able-bodiedness, religious affiliation, and sexual orientation.

Workplace rage   Overtly aggressive behavior toward co-workers and the work setting in general, resulting from excessive stress.

Work process   A related group of tasks that together create a result of value for the customer or patient.

Zero-based budget   A budget in which all projects or activities must compete anew for available funds in each budget cycle.

INDEX